# ATHLETIC & ORTHOPEDIC INJURY ASSESSMENT

## CASE RESPONSES AND INTERPRETATIONS

*David C. Berry,* Ph.D., ATC, EMT-B
SAGINAW VALLEY STATE UNIVERSITY

*Michael G. Miller,* Ed.D., ATC, CSCS
WESTERN MICHIGAN UNIVERSITY

*Leisha M. Berry,* MSPT, ATC

Routledge
Taylor & Francis Group
LONDON AND NEW YORK

First published 2011 by Holcomb Hathaway, Publishers, Inc.

Published 2017 by Routledge
2 Park Square, Milton Park, Abingdon, Oxon OX14 4RN
711 Third Avenue, New York, NY 10017, USA

*Routledge is an imprint of the Taylor & Francis Group, an informa business*



ISBN 978-1-934432-11-2 (pbk) 978-0-4157898-51- (hbk)

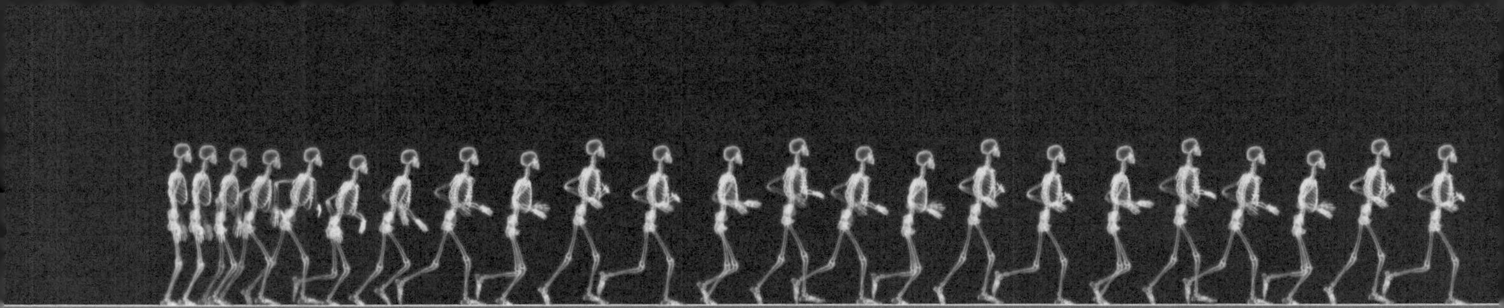

# Contents

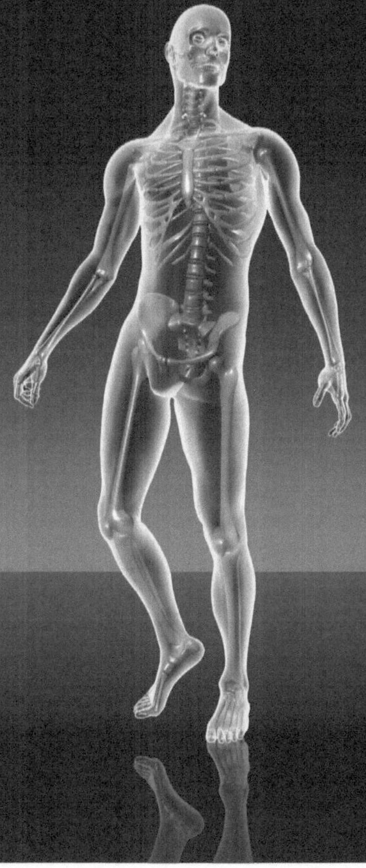

CHAPTER 1

# Introduction

Welcome to *Athletic & Orthopedic Injury Assessment: Case Responses and Interpretations*, a companion book to *Athletic & Orthopedic Injury Assessment: A Case Study Approach*. The case study text is designed to allow preprofessionals and students to step into the role of an evaluating clinician as they acquire, interpret, and attempt to make rational clinical decisions using classroom theory (i.e., knowledge and comprehension) and clinical reality (application). Each case includes a set of questions to aid in this process. In *Case Responses and Interpretations,* you will find possible responses and guidance for all questions that accompany the case studies. While the cases themselves are not reprinted in this book, the questions are provided. You'll find that the answers include identification of differential and clinical diagnoses; explanations of diagnostic tests; relevant anatomical information; splinting, spine boarding, and other techniques/procedures; and much more. We hope you find this book helpful, whether you are an instructor leading class discussions and analyzing student work, a preprofessional preparing for the case scenarios on the BOC national certification exam, or a student seeking to compare these suggested answers with your own analyses.

## USING THIS BOOK

In this book we use the same question-numbering format as in the case study book; for example, question 3.1/1 is the same in both books, indicating that it is Chapter 3, case 1, question 1. However, most of the figures in this answer manual are different from those in the case book, as they are specific to the answers. Thus, we have added the letter "A" (for Answer) to figures in this companion book, as in Figure A1.1.1 and so on.

We drew on research and our experience as practitioners to provide these answers. Where possible, we provide evidence-based treatment options, and reference lists at the end of each chapter support our responses. However, just as in the real world, many of these questions may have multiple answers, and you may find that your recommendations and interpretations vary from those provided here. In some cases we have indicated which questions might be answered in a variety of ways. We suggest that these questions will work well in group discussions. The key is for readers to be able to use their experience and knowledge to explain their answers and provide support for their suggested plans of action. In the classroom, instructors and students may find that sharing these differences of opinion will generate interesting and informative discussions.

In creating *Case Responses and Interpretations,* we have worked to provide accurate, up-to-date information based on the best practices currently available. If you would like to find out more about a particular answer, we recommend starting with the references cited in the answers. These references are a valuable tool for exploring and expanding upon answers, and they give an idea of the variety of resources available. New findings and revisions of standards do occur, so you may encounter additional or revised information that is not included in the answers we have provided. Please contact our publisher, Holcomb Hathaway, at info@hh-pub.com if you would like to offer suggestions regarding updated information.

## POSSIBLE ADDITIONAL QUESTIONS

The questions that follow each case are specifically designed to encourage readers to comprehend, apply, analyze, synthesize, and then evaluate. However, many additional questions can be explored to expand a reader's learning experiences. The following list provides examples of such questions, and you are welcome and encouraged to create your own supplementary questions. You may want to consider questions related to your areas of interest, your geographic region, or recent news or developments involving injury assessment.

- Identify the layperson's term for the clinical diagnosis.
- Identify the medical term for the clinical diagnosis.
- Identify the mechanism of injury related to the clinical diagnosis.
- Identify other potential mechanisms of injury for the clinical diagnosis that may not be athletically related.
- Identify and discuss the possible etiologies of the clinical diagnosis.
- What other clinical problems, if any, may the clinical diagnosis cause?
- Identify and discuss the differences between the differential diagnoses. What would lead you to believe one or more of the differential diagnoses is not possible given the information provided in the case?
- Discuss the possible differences in the etiology of the clinical diagnosis between an athletic population and the general population.
- Based upon the information presented in the case, determine what type of physician should the patient be referred to and explain why.
- Identify three to five additional history questions that could be asked by the clinician in order to properly evaluate this condition. Why are these questions important? What do they have to offer relative to the physical examination and/or patient outcomes?
- What anatomical structures, if any, were omitted as part of the physical examination that could have helped establish the clinical diagnosis?
- What ligamentous (provocative) or special tests were omitted that could/should have helped establish the clinical diagnosis? Describe how these test(s) are performed. What is the reliability and validity of these tests?
- Describe in detail how to perform procedures such as AROM, AAROM, RROM, relevant ligamentous and special tests, or tests to check neurological and circulatory status.
- What key finding(s) in the history and physical examination possibly led the clinician to refer the patient to a physician or the clinical diagnosis?
- What are some of the most common diagnostic tests used when diagnosing this clinical diagnosis?

- Using an algorithm, briefly outline the evaluation procedures you would perform during an on-field, sideline, or off-field assessment of the clinical diagnosis.
- Using an algorithm, briefly outline the treatment procedures you would perform in appropriately managing the clinical diagnosis.
- Identify and discuss the clinical criteria used in deciding the best course of action for the clinical diagnosis.
- What is the best approach to manage the clinical diagnosis?
- What are some ways that the clinical diagnosis can or could have been prevented?

Instructors may also wish to alter the cases, introducing additional ethical and legal issues, or adding "What if's?" to the cases.

## BEYOND THE CASE STUDIES

The case studies in *Athletic & Orthopedic Injury Assessment: A Case Study Approach*, together with *Athletic & Orthopedic Injury Assessment: Case Responses and Interpretations*, are intended to provide the opportunity for learning and practicing, so we encourage you to go beyond the cases, questions, and answers as they are presented. The ability to competently diagnose and treat injuries is critical in building a successful career as a clinician. Additional practice and discussion can further prepare readers for the situations and challenges they will face as they move from case studies to real-life cases. Please note that as an additional resource we have included in the appendix the Content Outline, Domain Descriptions and Task Statements, of the BOC Role Delineation/Practice Analysis (RD/PA), which identifies the essential knowledge and skills for the athletic training profession and serves as a blueprint for exam development.

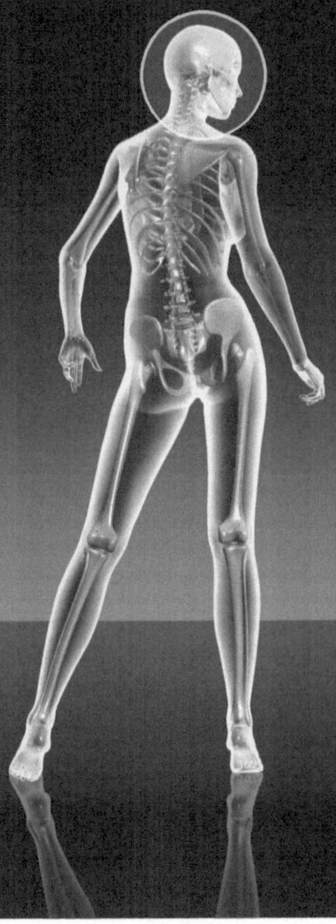

# CHAPTER 2
# Head and Face

## QUICK REFERENCE

# ANSWERS TO CASE QUESTIONS

## CASE 2.1 Orbital Blowout Fracture

2.1 / **1.** *Based on the information presented in the case, determine (a) the differential diagnoses and (b) the clinical diagnosis.*

a. Differential diagnoses: corneal abrasion/laceration, hyphema, retinal detachment, and ruptured globe[39,44]

b. Clinical diagnosis: orbital blowout fracture

2.1 / **2.** *Based on the clinical diagnosis, identify the harmful effects of being struck in the eye with a blunt force object larger than the diameter of the orbit.*

When a blunt force object larger than the orbital opening strikes the eye it compresses the floor of the orbit or the medial wall and increases the intra-orbital pressure. This increase in pressure causes the orbital bones to break at their weakest points, usually the posteriomedial portion of the orbital floor and medial orbital wall.[44,72,80] The breakage of these bones acts as a pressure valve release, preventing ruptures of the globe. When a blunt force object smaller than the orbit strikes the eye, however, unreleased compression can increase intra-ocular pressure to the point that the sclera tears and the globe ruptures.[65,72]

2.1 / **3.** *If Tom had also presented with changes in visual acuity and/or vision loss, what would be the clinical implication, and how could a clinician assess these changes?*

Changes in visual acuity and/or loss of vision may indicate trauma to the optic nerve (CN II)[65] and should be assessed by using a Snellen chart and examining the patient's peripheral vision. When completing an on-field evaluation, the Snellen chart may be replaced by assessing the athlete's ability to read the scoreboard. In place of a scoreboard or a Snellen chart, Mary may also consider having the athlete identify how many fingers she is holding up.

In cases of monocular diplopia (double vision looking through one eye) after sustaining trauma to the eye, issues such as hyphema, detached retina, or globe trauma should be suspected. Binocular diplopia (double vision looking through two eyes) may be caused by soft-tissue entrapment (zymgomatic fracture), hemorrhage, or edema.

2.1 / **4.** *During Mary's observation of the eye, suppose she notices subconjunctival hemorrhaging and a shallow anterior chamber in combination with the above signs. What steps should Mary take to manage this situation?*

A teardrop-shaped or irregular pupil, subconjunctival hemorrhaging, full-thickness laceration to the cornea, or deep or shallow anterior chamber are signs of a ruptured globe. In this situation, a protective eye shield in a loose-packed position should be used to cover the eye, and the athlete should be referred to an ophthalmologist for immediate care.[65]

2.1 / **5.** *Based on the information presented in the case, what if anything would you have done or added to help guide the physical examination?*

The answers to this question will vary from student to student; however, any trauma to the head requires a concussion assessment.[22] Perform a complete observation of the eye from all directions (superior, inferior, lateral, and medial). In this case, determining whether there is a zygomatic bone fracture would be warranted, as the zygomatic bone comprises infraorbital margin and floor of the orbit. Furthermore, cranial nerve testing of the optic (CN II), oculomotor (CN III), trochlear (CN IV), and abducens (CN VI) may be warranted.

2.1 / **6.** *After completing the physical examination, Mary documented her findings and sent a copy of the report to the administration office. Please document your findings as if you were the treating clinician. If the case did not provide information you believe is pertinent to the clinical diagnosis, please feel free to add this information to your documentation.*

Answers will vary. Students should consider writing a SOAP note (see textbook Appendix B) using the ABCD format when writing the short- and long-term goals.

## CASE 2.2 Corneal Abrasion/Laceration

2.2 / **1.** *Based on the information presented in the case, determine (a) the differential diagnoses and (b) the clinical diagnosis.*

a. Differential diagnoses: conjunctivitis, corneal laceration, corneal ulceration, iritis, foreign body, and blunt trauma[10,27,35]

b. Clinical diagnosis: corneal abrasion

2.2 / **2.** *Based on the information presented in the case, what type of physician should Tamara refer Sherrie to and why?*

The physician of choice would be an ophthalmologist if available. Ophthalmologists are physicians specializing in eye and vision care. They are trained to dispense medication and provide a full spectrum of eye care, including complex and delicate eye surgery. Some ophthalmologists specialize in a certain area of eye care, such as glaucoma, refractive surgery, or retinal surgery. If an ophthalmologist is not available, a referral to the team physician or emergency room is a viable option.

2.2 / **3.** *Tamara asked Sherrie several history questions to guide the physical examination. Based on the clinical diagnosis above, identify three to five specific history questions you as the evaluating clinician may have asked.*

The answers to this question will vary among students; however, according to the clinical diagnosis, there are several history questions a clinician could ask to assist in determining the clinical diagnosis.[27,87] These questions include but are not limited to:

a. Did you suffer any type of acute trauma to the eye (e.g., fingers, fingernails, self-inflicted rubbing)?

b. Do you have a sensation of a foreign body in your eye?

c. Do you remember getting any dirt in your eye and then rubbing your eye?

d. Do you wear contacts?

e. How long have you been wearing this pair of contacts?

f. When was the last time you cleaned your contacts?

g. Did you remove your contacts last night?

2.2 / **4.** *There is one mechanism of injury common to the case's clinical diagnosis that typically occurs outside of participating in athletics. Identify this MOI, and discuss how it causes the clinical diagnosis.*

Contact lenses put the wearer at greater risk of developing corneal abrasions because of the action of placing contacts into the eye. Inserting and removing contacts predisposes the wearer to corneal abrasions from fingernails.[27,87] Contacts that are dirty or damaged also increase the risk of damage to the corneas (scratch) as they move around. Contacts improperly placed in the eye also increase the risk of trauma.

2.2 / **5.** *(a) Overall, do you believe Tamara adequately evaluated Sherrie's condition, given the information provided in the case? (b) What, if any, tests or procedures were omitted that could have helped in establishing the clinical diagnosis? (c) Describe how these test(s) are performed.*

a. The answers for this question will vary among students.

b. Based on the information presented Tamara could have used a fluorescein strip and a cobalt blue light. A corneal abrasion is an epithelial defect that stains when a fluorescein dye is used. In conjunction with a cobalt light in a darkened room, the defect turns greenish-yellow.[27,93]

c. Begin the test by soaking a fluorescein strip in sterile saline. Ask the athlete to look up and gently touch the inside of the lower eyelid with the moistened strip, taking care not to touch the cornea (Figure A2.1.1). Touching the cornea may cause the athlete significant discomfort. Ask the athlete to blink her eye several times, and wash the eye thoroughly with eye wash or saline to irrigate the eye. Darken the room, shine a cobalt blue light into the affected eye, and observe for a defect.

FIGURE A.2.1.1 Using a fluorescein strip and cobalt blue light.

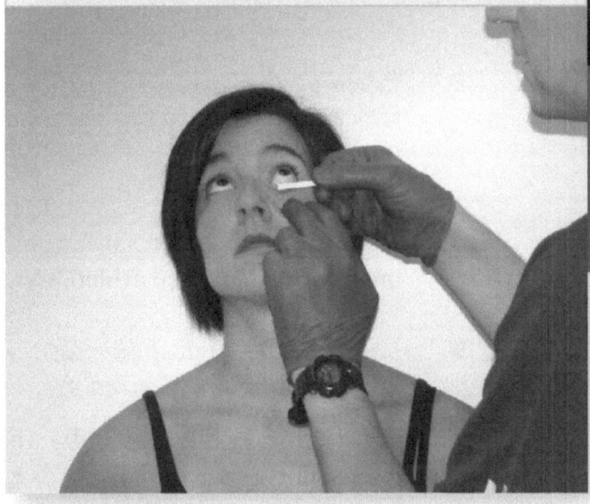

Tamara could have also inverted the upper eyelid to identify any foreign objects. If no fluorescein strips are available, Tamara could have used a penlight angled from the lateral and medial borders at the cornea while in a dark room. Tamara could have also suggested the use of sunglasses to assist with the photosensitivity.

## CASE 2.3 Conjunctivitis/Hordeolum

2.3 / **1.** *Based on the information presented in the case, determine (a) the differential diagnoses and (b) the clinical diagnosis.*

a. Differential diagnoses: chlamydia, conjunctivitis-viral, contact lens complications, corneal foreign body, corneal abrasion, scleritis, herpes, and Horner Syndrome[10,49]

b. Clinical diagnosis: conjunctivitis with a possible hordeolum

2.3 / **2.** *Based on the case, it is possible that Shelia should have spent more time evaluating Peter's eye. What type of functional and special tests, if any, would you have performed and why?*

Functional testing may include testing for motility of the eye and the ability to open and close the eyelids. Special testing to ensure proper functioning of the cranial nerves may include assessing the athlete's visual acuity and pupillary reflex and reaction.

2.3 / **3.** *Based on the clinical diagnosis, explain whether you would expect Peter to have difficulty opening the affected eye.*

Yes, Peter may have difficulty opening the eye, because the reported discharge emanating from the eye causes the eyelids to adhere together, particularly at night.

2.3 / **4.** *The yellow discharge noted during the inspection indicates what possible types of infection?*

Hyperacute and acute infective conjunctivitis can present with thick yellowish discharge. Two common bacterial infections are the *Staphylococcus aureus* and *Neisseria gonorrhoeae* bacterium.[28] Conjunctivitis may also be caused by the *Haemophilus, Streptococcus pneumoniae, Moraxella catarrhalis, H. influenza,* or *Pseudomonas aeruginosa* bacterium[28,29] or by the herpes virus.

2.3 / **5.** *What is/are the most common methods of contracting the above clinical diagnosis?*

The most common methods of contracting conjunctivitis is contact with a contaminated finger,[28] which can occur when dealing with contact lens,[9] sharing make-up, or sharing contaminated clothing and towels. To prevent the spread of this and many other bacterial and viral diseases, it is recommended that athletes not share towels or clothing during practice.

2.3 / **6.** *What behavior of Shelia's makes this case very disturbing?*

The most disturbing behavior in this case was Shelia's lack of protection against pathogenic agents. Conjunctivitis is a moderately contagious condition that demands the use of personal protective equipment and adequate hand washing. Compounding this situation Shelia disregarded OSHA standards, which state: "Eating, drinking, smoking, applying cosmetics or lip balm, and handling contact lenses are prohibited in work areas where there is a reasonable likelihood of occupational exposure"[58] in conjunction with the lack of work practice control (e.g., washing your hands after treating an athlete/patient).

## CASE 2.4 Ruptured Globe/Hyphema

2.4 / **1.** *Based on the information presented in the case, determine the likely clinical diagnoses and identify the difference between them.*

The most likely clinical diagnoses in this case would be a ruptured globe and hyphema. A hyphema is a common ocular injury resulting in a shearing of the iris's blood vessel, allowing for accumulation of blood cells in the aqueous humor.[78] A globe rupture is a much more serious injury that occurs when the integrity of the outer membranes of the eye is disrupted by blunt or penetrating trauma.[27,78] Ruptured globes present with the most severe pain and decreased vision, severe subconjunctival hemorrhaging, and a deep or shallow anterior chamber as compared with the contralateral eye.[27]

2.4 / **2.** *Based on the information presented in the case, discuss the manner in which Bud assessed Larry's visual acuity and why he chose to assess it this way.*

Because Bud was performing a pseudo on-field evaluation it is unlikely he had access to a Snellen chart. Therefore, Bud determined Larry's visual acuity by asking him to count the number of fingers Bud was holding up at a given distance.

2.4 / **3.** *If this athlete were evaluated in the athletic training room, discuss how Bud should then assess visual acuity and how the results should be interpreted?*

If the assessment occurred in the athletic training room, the use of a Snellen chart would be recommended to assess visual acuity during an off-field evaluation. A 20/20 vision score is often described as having "normal" eyesight. A score of 20/50 would describe a person who sees detail from 20 feet away with the same acuity as a person with normal eyesight would see it from 50 feet away. Essentially, the larger the denominator, the poorer an individual's vision.

2.4 / **4.** *Overall, do you believe that Bud adequately assessed Larry's condition? What if anything would you have done differently as the evaluating clinician?*

Rodriguez, Lavina, and Agarwal[72] recommend assessing for anisocoria and relative pupillary defects when assessing eye trauma by using reflex and reaction testing. Given the mechanism of injury, a concussion assessment is also probably warranted. The concussion assessment should evaluate the cranial nerves, focusing on the optic (II), oculomotor (III), trochlear (IV), and abducens (VI). It is also suggested that in situations where a globe rupture is suspected the clinician should limit the amount of manipulation in favor of immediate referral.[72]

2.4 / **5.** *If Larry's eyelid was too swollen to open, what strategies could you use to evaluate the eye, if any?*

Harrahill suggests that in situations where the eye is too swollen to open, the evaluator should attempt to shine a penlight over the eye to assess if the patient can, at a minimum, determine the presence of light and the direction it is coming from. This assesses the gross function of the retina. Inability of the examiner to gently open the eye requires immediate referral to an ophthalmologist or team physician.[25]

2.4 / **6.** *Do you believe Bud managed the current situation appropriately? What if anything would you have done differently?*

Calling Larry's parents and notifying EMS are appropriate steps; however, asking Larry to remain supine is an inappropriate action in the presence of a hyphema. If the patient must be laid down, he should do so with his head upright at a 30 degree flexion angle.[25] A rigid shield should be used to further protect the eye and prevent any undue pressure on the globe.[27] Excessive pressure applied to the globe may lead to leaking of the intraocular fluid.[25] Be sure to avoid the use of eyedrops, and do not allow the patient to eat or drink (as happened when the coach offered Larry water), in the event that surgery is necessary.[25,72]

## CASE 2.5 Detached Retina

2.5 / **1.** *Based on the information presented in the case, determine (a) the clinical diagnosis, and (b) the hallmark symptom reported in this case.*

a. Clinical diagnosis: retinal tear/retinal detachment

b. Floating spots and the mechanism of injury[27]

2.5 / **2.** *Describe the etiology of the clinical diagnosis.*

There are three basic mechanisms leading to a retinal detachment. In this case a tear or hole in the retina most likely allowed fluid from the vitreous cavity to seep between the retina and vitreous cavity, causing a separation and interruption of the nerve impulses being relayed to the optic nerve and the choroids of the retina.[17]

2.5 / **3.** *What type of physician should the athletic trainer refer this athlete to and why?*

All patients with acute onset of flashes or floaters should be referred to an ophthalmologist because proper care can prevent a retinal tear from becoming a retinal detachment.[17] If not treated appropriately, a retinal detachment may cause damage to the macula (structures of the macula are specialized for high-acuity vision), resulting in permanent vision loss.[17,27]

2.5 / **4.** *The mechanism of injury in this case was a direct blow causing a jarring force in the head. Identify another potential MOI for this condition that is not related to an athletic injury.*

A variety of risk factors predispose individuals to retinal detachments, including aging, cataract surgery, congenital eye diseases, and family history of detachment(s).[17] Because of these predisposing factors, forceful sneezing can also cause a retinal detachment.

2.5 / **5.** *As the evaluating clinician, imagine a patient presenting with the same MOI but with immediate changes in visual field and sudden onset of one large floater. What pre-hospital care would be necessary?*

The initial pre-hospital care may include the use of an eye shield to prevent the extrusion of intra-ocular material and avoid unwanted pressure on the eye's globe.[42]

## CASE 2.6 Auricular Hematoma

2.6 / **1.** *Based on the information presented in the case, determine the clinical diagnosis and its etiology.*

Clinical diagnosis: auricular hematoma. An auricular hematoma results from a shearing force or excessive friction to the auricle, which leads to a separation of the outer tissue (perichondrium, the dense, irregular connective tissue membrane around cartilage) from the cartilaginous plate[40] and a rupture of blood vessels within the perichondrium.[43] Over time, the accumulation of fluid between these two layers causes the cartilage to die from poor nutrition and poor oxygenation because the blood flow to the auricle is now diminished.[40,43] The cartilage is replaced by fibrocartilaginous scar tissue resulting in a "cauliflower ear."[19] This condition is most often seen in boxers and wrestlers.

2.6 / **2.** *During Dr. Cost's inspection of the ears, she noted swelling of the external ear structures. In addition to examining the external ear, Dr. Cost also evaluated the middle and inner ear. Explain the most appropriate procedure for evaluating the middle and inner ear.*

The use of an otoscope will allow for proper examination of the ear, particularly the external auditory canal and tympanic membrane, for the presence of blood, canal laceration, or tympanic membrane rupture.

2.6 / **3.** *Dr. Cost asked several history questions to guide the physical examination. Identify three to five history questions Dr. Cost or a clinician may have asked in order to properly evaluate this case.*

The answers will vary among students; however, based on the clinical diagnosis, a clinician could ask about:

a. The onset of pain and pain characteristics
b. Mechanism of injury
c. Previous history and/or treatment
d. Use of protective headgear, which is required by the NCAA for collegiate wrestlers[56]

2.6 / **4.** *How do you think Dr. Cost is going to manage this case?*

There are various treatments that can be used by a physician to relieve the hematoma; however, there is no clear consensus regarding which treatment produces the best cosmetic result with the least permanent deformity.[34] The treatment most advocated involves draining the hematoma in order to prevent any further tissue damage. Aspiration/incision and drainage appears to be one of the most common techniques used by physicians to remove fluid collections and clots.[21–23,26] Immediately after drainage of the fluid, an external compression dressing should be used to avoid re-accumulation of fluid.

2.6 / **5.** *What supplies will an athletic trainer need to lay out to assist the physician based on the question above?*

Probable supplies include: (a) aseptic wash, (b) lidocaine (which should normally be provided by and managed by the team physician and kept stored in a locked cabinet), (c) needles and syringe, (d) sterile surgical equipment, and (e) dressing and bandage material (e.g., gauze).

2.6 / **6.** *What steps, if any, will the team's athletic trainer need take to prevent this from occurring in the future.*

The athletic trainer and/or the team physician will need to schedule an appointment with the wrestling coaches to discuss the use of the recommended protective headgear. It should be stressed both to coaches and players that wearing the appropriately sized headgear required by the National Collegiate Athletic Association[56] decreases the shear forces applied to the ear's cartilage, and decreases the likelihood of tissue damage. Furthermore, although a cauliflower ear may be considered a "sign" of being a wrestler, continued participation without headgear can lead to permanent disfigurement of the ear. Consider providing some relevant literature dealing with the long-term complications of auricular hematomas. If this fails to resolve the issue, the athletic director may need to intervene in the situation.

## CASE 2.7 Impacted Cerumen

2.7 / **1.** *Based on the information presented in the case, determine the clinical diagnosis and its pathophysiology.*

The clinical diagnosis is impacted ear wax or cerumen. Cerumen production occurs as a result of the accumulation of lipids and peptides from sebaceous and cerumenous glands, respectively, in the auditory canal, mixed with other components such as dead skin (keratin), sweat, and oil.[21,26,68] Also contributing to the production of cerumen are hairs located in the external ear canal.[21]

2.7 / **2.** *What other clinical problems, if any, may this condition cause?*

In addition to loss of hearing and a feeling of fullness in the ear, impacted ear wax increases an athlete's risk of ear infections because it traps bacteria, and it may block the physician's vision of the inner ear structures, hiding other pathologies such as a ruptured tympanic membrane.[21]

2.7 / **3.** *Describe how Melanie was able to identify the yellowish substance packed in the ear canal and the technique she used.*

Melanie used a specialized light, known as an otoscope, with speculums of different sizes to look into the ear canal to identify the earwax. However, it should be noted that Figure 2.7.1 demonstrates the improper use of the device. When using the otoscope, hold the device like a pencil, allowing your hand to rest on the athlete's head. This is to avoid any sudden movements by the athlete. With the opposing hand, gently grasp the pinna away from the head by pulling back and up. If you are dealing with a child, pull back and down. Shine the scope's light into the opening to inspect the entrance to the ear canal, and then gently place the speculum into the athlete's ear canal observing for redness, irritation, and yellow discharge.

2.7 / **4.** *What neurological tests, if any, should Melanie have completed and documented?*

An assessment of cranial nerve VIII, the vestibulocochlear nerve, would have assessed Sunee's ability to identify sound and maintain balance. Sound can be assessed by snapping the clinician's finger next to the athlete's ear, while balance can be assessed by performing a Romberg Test, heel-to-toe walk, or finger-to-nose test.

2.7 / **5.** *What is the best approach to manage this clinical diagnosis?*

Impacted ear wax can be treated using a topical earwax medicine, irrigated using water- or oil-based preparations, or removed by trained medical professionals using specialized equipment. A systematic review of ear drops (either oil- or water-based) used to treat earwax found no particular drops could be recommended over any other.[11] According to Burton and Doree, "The review of trials found that ear drops (of any sort) can help to remove ear wax, but that water and saline drops appear to be as good as more costly commercial products. The quality of the trials was generally low, however, and more research is needed."

A review by Hand and Harvey found that water-based and oil-based preparations were equally effective in removing earwax and better than no treatment at all. They further found that water-based and oil-based preparations used in conjunction with syringing were equally effective, with an overall success rate around 97 percent.[24] When used long term, eardrops applied for 15 to 30 minutes followed by syringing appear to be as effective.

When applying over-the-counter eardrops, the patient must be placed in a side-lying position with the involved ear up. Syringing or irrigation must be done by a trained medical professional, and although it provides immediate relief, it does increase the risk of complications such as ear infection, ruptured tympanic membrane, and/or otitis externa.[57]

## CASE 2.8 Otitis Externa/Media

2.8 / **1.** *Based on the information presented in the case, determine the clinical diagnosis and its pathophysiology.*

The clinical diagnosis is otitis externa. Otitis externa most commonly results because of bacterial infections, fungal overgrowth in the ear canal, and a broad range of non-infectious dermatological conditions (e.g., psoriasis and acne).[8,68,75] Bacterial pathogens commonly associated with otitis externa include: *Pseudomonas aeruginosa, Staphylococcus epidermides, Staphylococcus aureus,* and *Streptococcus pyogenes.*[73,75] When the normal flora of the external auditory canal is disrupted, the warm, dark, moist environment provides excellent conditions for bacterial and fungal growth as excessive moisture removes cerumen and increases the pH.[75]

2.8 / **2.** *Define* otalgia *and* pruritus *and state the clinical diagnosis in laymen's terms.*

Otalgia means earache, and pruitus means itching. Otitis externa means inflammation of the outer ear and ear canal and is often known as "swimmers ear" or simply "an earache."

2.8 / **3.** *Identify three to five history questions Leisha could have asked to properly evaluate this condition.*

The answers will vary among students, but they could focus on:

a. The onset of symptoms
b. Pain characteristics
c. Mechanism of injury/nature of the illness
d. Past medical history and previous treatment
e. Use of earplugs as a swimmer
f. Questions regarding how the ears are cleaned

2.8 / **4.** *Traction of the pinna is used to differentiate between which two medical conditions?*

Normally traction of the pinna helps to differentiate between otitis externa (infection that occurs in the external auditory canal) and otitis media (inflammation of the middle ear, or tympanum). Pain with traction of the pinna indicates acute otitis externa.[68]

2.8 / **5.** *If the otorrhea presented as a bloody discharge, especially in the presence of granulated tissue, what medical condition would Leisha now be concerned about?*

The presence of blood from the ear may indicate the presence of chronic otitis externa rather than acute otitis externa.[75]

2.8 / **6.** *If, during the external auditory canal evaluation, Leisha visualized a tympanic membrane that appeared red and inflamed, what condition is potentially present?*

If the tympanic membrane appeared red and inflamed, the presence of otitis media should be suspected. The tympanic membrane, which separates the middle ear and external ear, is normally a translucent membrane.[55]

## CASE 2.9 Nasal Fracture

2.9 / **1.** *Sara is clearly suffering from a nasal fracture. However, she also presents with another injury. Please identify this potential injury and discuss the injury's MOI.*

Sara presents with signs and symptoms of a possible zygomatic arch fracture, which is often caused by a direct trauma to the cheek, such as being struck with a ball.[16]

2.9 / **2.** *What is the medical term for a bloody nose?*

The medical term for a bloody nose is *epistaxis,* and it is very common after nasal trauma.[89]

2.9 / **3.** *What is the difference between bright red blood and dark red blood when dealing with a nosebleed?*

In an anterior nosebleed, blood is usually seen running out of the nose. If the area of bleeding is close to the nostril, bright red blood can be seen. If the area of bleeding is deeper in the nose, the blood is usually dark red. Dizziness, rapid heartbeat, and shortness of breath can be experienced if a large amount of blood is lost.[30]

2.9 / **4.** *Why did Sara begin to have difficulty breathing?*

It is possible Sara was experiencing a deviated septum. A deviated septum is commonly caused by some type of impact trauma to the face, or it can be a congenital disorder. A deviated septum occurs when the top of the cartilaginous ridge shifts to the left or right, thereby obstructing oxygen flow. It is also responsible for nose bleeding because the deviated septum causes stretching and tearing of blood vessels.[89]

2.9 / **5.** *What tests, if any, should Samantha have performed?*

An athletic trainer can use an otoscope to assess the integrity of the septum, including septum hematomas. If left untreated, the condition can result in a saddle deformity of the septum, which will require surgical repair.[38]

2.9 / **6.** *Overall, do you believe that Samantha handled the situation appropriately? If not, what would you have done differently as the evaluating clinician?*

The answers for this question will vary among students. The evaluation was fine, except for returning Sara to play, which was inappropriate given the situation. As certified athletic trainers, we have an obligation to prevent and minimize further injury. Section 1.2 of the *Board of Certification Standards of Professional Practice* states: "Protects the patient from harm, acts always in the patient's best interests, and is an advocate for the patient's welfare." Therefore, Samantha should not have been intimidated into letting Sara play. Consider discussing the action of Samantha further as a class.

2.9 / **7.** *Using an algorithm, briefly outline the evaluation procedures you would take during an on-field and sideline assessment of the clinical diagnosis.*

This answer for this question will vary among students and should be discussed with the classroom instructor. In fact, this question is best answered via group discussion, because there is not necessarily only one correct answer.

## CASE 2.10 Throat Trauma

2.10 / **1.** *Based on the information presented in the case, determine the differential diagnoses.*

John is suffering from some type of throat trauma, possibly deviation of the trachea, hyoid fracture, and/or a throat contusion with rapid swelling.[68]

2.10 / **2.** *In addition to the throat, what other anatomical structures should Artie assess during the physical examination?*

Artie should have palpated the following structures (including but not limited to): the cricoid cartilage, thyroid cartilage, sternocleidomastoid, clavicle, mandible, cervical spine, and carotid pulse.

2.10 / **3.** *Define "dyspneic."*

Dyspneic or dyspnea can be defined as difficult, painful breathing or shortness of breath.

2.10 / **4.** *Had the puck struck the anterolateral neck, which anatomical structures should an athletic trainer be concerned about and why?*

If the puck struck the anterolateral neck, the athletic trainer should be concerned about the carotid sinus. When stimulated, the carotid sinus, which contains baroreceptors, causes slowing of the heart, vasodilation, and a fall in blood pressure causing an athlete to lose consciousness.[82] It is innervated primarily by the glossopharyngeal nerve.

2.10 / **5.** *During transport John began spitting up frothy blood. (a) Why was this not identified earlier in the assessment? (b) How could Artie have checked for blood in the throat during his primary assessment?*

a. Artie did not do a complete physical assessment that included evaluating the inside of the mouth, probably because John did not present with immediate signs of fluid in the oropharynx.

b. A penlight can be used on-field/on-ice to assess the mouth, looking for blood, loose or broken teeth, lacerations of the tongue or other soft tissue, or any unusual discoloration. There is also a possibility of trauma to the lungs; however, based on the mechanism of injury, it would be unlikely.

2.10 / **6.** *Did Artie appropriately manage the current situation? What if anything would you have done differently?*

Answers here will vary among students. It should be noted that the application of supplemental oxygen via a nasal cannula is not appropriate. Rather a non-rebreather or resuscitation mask should be applied at 15 L/min to a conscious patient.[4]

## CASE 2.11 Mandible Fracture

2.11 / **1.** *Based on the information presented in the case, determine (a) the differential diagnoses and (b) the clinical diagnosis. (c) What if any secondary trauma/condition may José be suffering concurrently?*

a. Differential diagnoses: temporomandibular joint dislocation, maxilla fracture, nasal trauma, facial soft tissue injury, cervical spine injury, and traumatic brain injury (i.e., concussion)

b. Clinical diagnosis: mandible fracture

c. José may also be suffering from shock and/or a possible concussion. It is also possible for mandible fractures to be associated with other facial fractures, broken teeth, and soft tissue damage.[6]

2.11 / **2.** *In addition to the mandible, what other bony anatomical landmarks should Amy have assessed/palpated during her physical examination?*

Amy should have palpated the following structures using personal protective equipment. These structures include but are not limited to: (1) maxilla, (2) TMJ (internal and external), (3) teeth, (4) facial bones (temporal, frontal, parietal, nasal), (5) orbits, (6) mastoid process, and (7) cervical spine and anterior neck.

2.11 / **3.** *If you were the evaluating clinician, what if anything would you have done differently?*

In the presence of an observable mandible deformity, an assessment of active jaw range of motion is not warranted, because of the increased risk of secondary injury and pain. A concussion assessment may be warranted based on the mechanism of injury and lack of intra-oral protection. However, because of the need to stabilize the jaw, this examination may be impossible.

2.11 / **4.** *Identify and describe how to perform a special test used to assist in determining the clinical diagnosis.*

The tongue blade test[47] or bite test[77] is used to assess for malocclusion and pain caused by a mandible fracture. With the patient in a sitting position, a tongue depressor is placed between the teeth. The clinician instructs the patient to bite down and hold the tongue depressor as the blade is twisted. Positive signs include the inability to maintain a firm bite, pain, and malocclusion of the jaw and teeth with biting.

2.11 / **5.** *What is the possible explanation for why Amy did not perform the special test identified in question 4, and what is the sensitivity of this test?*

Amy was unable to insert the tongue depressor into José's mouth because of the inability to move the jaw, pain, and probably joint guarding. Malhotra and Dunning[47] best practice evidence review calculated an overall sensitivity of the tongue blade test at 95.4 percent (confidence interval 84.5% to 99.4%) using data from Roberts.[70] They further suggest that the tongue blade test "is a useful screening tool in evaluating patients with mandibular fracture" but that the test "could not stand on its own as a single diagnostic tool in screening for mandibular fractures since missing these fractures can lead to serious long term complications."[47]

2.11 / **6.** *An athlete sustaining this type of injury is also at risk for developing a concussion. Discuss how and why concussion occurs and how a clinician can prevent concussion as well as the clinical diagnosis injury from occurring.*

A concussion in this case occurs as a result of direct or indirect impact forces being transmitted to the skull and brain through the mandibular condyles. Wearing a properly fitted athletic mouthguard places the mandibular condyles in an anterior position within the temporomandibular joint, decreasing the amount of superior and posterior displacement of the mandibular condyles in the fossa.[90,94] This reduction in mandibular displacement helps to protect the athlete against concussions and serious injuries to the neck and central nervous systems.[18] The mouthguard also acts as a shock absorber, decreasing force production by attenuating and spreading impact forces over a larger area at the temporomandibular joint.[7]

# CASE 2.12 Maxilla Fracture

2.12 / **1.** *Based on the information presented in the case, determine (a) the differential diagnoses and (b) the clinical diagnosis.*

a. Differential diagnoses: mandible fracture, nasal fracture, tooth intrusion and fracture, traumatic brain injury, cervical spine trauma

b. Clinical diagnosis: maxilla fracture

2.12 / **2.** *The trauma sustained to the facial structures in this case is classified using the LeFort system. Identify Sam's fracture type based on the information provided in the case above and your knowledge of the common mechanism of injury.*

LeFort fractures are typically the result of high-impact forces, and the incidence of these fractures is low in the athletic population[18] (Figure A2.12.1). Based on the signs and symptoms and the mechanism of injury in this case, a direct blow on the maxillary alveolar rim in a downward direction,[36] there is a high probability of a LeFort I fracture. LeFort I fractures extend across the lower portion of the maxilla but do not extend up into the medial canthal region (the angle at either end of the split between the eyelids).[63]

2.12 / **3.** *If Sam presented with pain and tenderness along the bridge of the nose and the zygomatic arch, bilateral subconjunctival hemorrhaging, abnormal skin sensitivity, and mobility of the maxilla, what further fracture classification is most likely to represent his signs and symptoms?*

If Sam presented with the above signs and symptoms, he could be suffering from a LeFort II fracture. A LeFort II fracture is a pyramidal-shaped fracture (due to the separation of the nasomaxillary complex from the upper face and skull) of the maxilla across the maxillary sinus posteriorly and laterally, extending laterally and inferiorly through the infra-orbital rims.[15]

FIGURE A2.12.1 LeFort fracture classification.

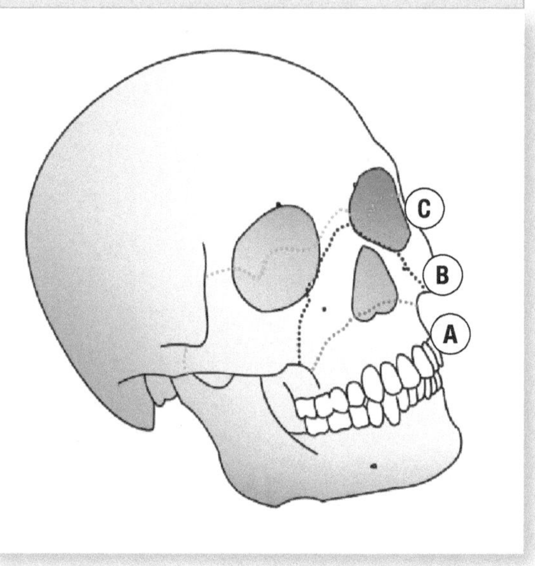


Key: (A) LeFort I fracture, (B) LeFort II fracture, (C) LeFort III fracture
*Source:* Wikimedia Commons.

2.12 / **4.** *If Sam reported a direct blow to the nasal bridge or upper maxilla and presented with facial elongation or flattening of the face, diplopia, movement of the facial bones in relation to the cranium, and positive halo sign, what further fracture classification is most likely to represent his signs and symptoms?*

He would be suffering from a LeFort III fracture.[74] LeFort III fractures extend posteriorly through the ethmoid bones and laterally through the orbits below the optic foramen.[92] This type of fracture is commonly known as a "floating fracture" because of the separation of facial bones from the cranium, and it often occurs in motor vehicle or motorcycle accidents. The separation is what causes the face to appear long and flat.[74] It should be noted that most cases do not produce one isolated fracture type, rather they produce combination fractures.

2.12 / **5.** *What if anything would you as the evaluating clinician have done differently in textbook Figure 2.12.2?*

Students should recognize that the clinician in textbook Figure 2.12.2 is not using personal protective equipment (i.e., gloves) to prevent the spread of blood-borne pathogens.

2.12 / **6.** *Formulate a plan to further analyze any other associated conditions that could affect the outcome of this case, including possible signs and symptoms.*

The answers for this question will vary among students and should be discussed with the classroom instructor, clinical instructor, and the approved clinical instructor. In fact, this question is best answered as a group discussion, because there is not necessarily only one correct answer. However, emphasis should be placed on managing the ABCs (airway, breathing, circulation) and treating for shock.

## CASE 2.13 Temporomandibular Dysfunction

2.13 / **1.** *Based on the information presented in the case, determine (a) the differential diagnoses and (b) the clinical diagnosis.*

a. Differential diagnoses: dental infections, gingivitis, periodontitis, otitis media, sinusitis, and Trigeminal neuralgia[62]
b. Clinical diagnosis: temporomandibular joint (TMJ) dysfunction

2.13 / **2.** *Identify three to five additional history questions you would have asked as the evaluating clinician in order to properly evaluate this condition.*

The answers to this question will vary among students but they should focus on:

a. Onset of symptoms
b. Pain, particularly in terms of onset, nature, intensity, site, duration, aggravating and relieving factors, and especially, how it relates to the other features such as joint noise and restricted mandibular movements
c. Mechanism of injury
d. Past medical history and previous treatment
e. Difficulty eating—chewing in particular, and
f. Clicking and popping sensations, particularly when chewing and yawning

A review of TMJ disorders suggests that the main complaints of a TMJ disorder include "orofacial pain, joint noises, restricted mouth opening, or a combination of these, in addition to other less-specific problems such as headache and tinnitus."[14]

2.13 / **3.** *Explain how Kim did assess, or could have qualitatively assessed, McKinley's TMJ movements.*

To adequately assess TMJ movement, a clinician must perform four different range-of-motion exams:

a. First is occlusion of the teeth, in which the athlete is asked to close her jaw to a position where the teeth are fully occluded.[12]
b. Next is depression of the mandible. Here the athlete is asked to open her mouth as the clinician observes any deviations of the mandible from the midline.[12] Functional ROM is evaluated by placing two to three knuckles between the upper and lower jaw.[12,82] A ruler can also be utilized to measure the distance between the upper and lower central incisor.[86] The normal maximum range of painless vertical opening is from 42 to 55 mm.[14]
c. This would be followed by protrusion of the mandible, whereby the athlete is asked to glide her jaw forward. The athlete should be able to protrude her lower teeth beyond her upper teeth.[12] Again this can be measured using a ruler.[86]
d. Finally, lateral deviation of the jaw occurs when the athlete glides her jaw to the right and left. This can be measured by picking two level points on the upper and lower teeth and measuring the distance between the two.

2.13 / **4.** *Kim referred McKinley for further medical care. (a) What type of specialist should McKinley see? (b) What do you believe was Kim's rationale for the referral, and what is considered to be the diagnostic gold standard for the above clinical diagnosis?*

a. McKinley could be referred to two types of physicians to manage this case: an oral surgeon or an otorhinolaryngologist/otolaryngologist—a head and neck surgeon. Otolaryngology is the branch of medicine specializing in the diagnosis and treatment of ear, nose, throat, and head and neck disorders.

b. According to Dimitroulis,[14] the "etiology of the most common types of temporomandibular disorders is complex and is still largely unresolved." He suggests that there "is a clear lack of substantial evidence" as to the nature of the condition and that trauma (as cited in this case), malocclusion, and psychogenic factors have also been implicated as possible—but are often considered as exacerbating—factors rather than the primary cause of temporomandibular disorders. It has been suggested that TMJ abnormalities cannot be reliably assessed from a clinical examination[91]; therefore, the decision to refer McKinley was an appropriate decision. Radiographs can prove to be useful in observing any gross pathological degenerative or traumatic changes[14]; however, magnetic resonance imaging technology is often required to identify joint abnormality.[41] Imaging findings include: joint fluid, internal disc derangement with a variety of pathologies, and disc deformation.[41]

2.13 / **5.** *What, if any, neurological tests should an evaluating clinician perform?*

Neurological testing in this case may not be warranted; however, a clinician should assess for areas of tenderness and trigger points, and patterns of pain-referral should be noted, bearing in mind that TMJ dysfunction is believed to cause headaches.[14,82]

# CASE 2.14 Temporomandibular Joint Dislocation

2.14 / **1.** *Based on the information presented in the case, determine the clinical diagnosis and the mechanism of injury.*

The clinical diagnosis is a TMJ dislocation. This injury is the result of a direct blow to the mandible, causing the mandibular condyle to be displaced from the mandibular fossa.[16] However, opening the mouth wide while yawning or eating, and spontaneous dislocation due to excessive laxity of the joint capsule and ligaments, have been reported in the literature.[48,79,84,85]

2.14 / **2.** *If Tina had been wearing a mouthguard, (a) would this injury have occurred? Why, or why not? (b) If not, identify two other possible injuries that may occur.*

a. The likelihood of a TMJ joint dislocation would have been lower had Tina been wearing her mouthguard. A mouthguard not only decreases the incidence of oral and soft tissue trauma to the mouth[3] but can also potentially decrease the risk of a concussion.[60,81] This information is, however, inconclusive at this point.[53] When applied properly, an athletic mouthguard acts as a shock absorber, decreasing the force production by attenuating and spreading impact forces over a larger area at the TMJ by placing the mandibular condyles in an anterior and inferior position rather than a posterior superior position.[7,54,60]

b. Had the dislocation not occurred, it is likely she would have suffered from some type of facial laceration, contusion, or even some level of TMJ dysfunction at a later date.

2.14 / **3.** *Why is there is no mention of Dale assessing Tina's ABCs prior to initiating her physical examination?*

It could be assumed that during the time Dale was summoned onto the field and his actual arrival he was observing the scene and performing his primary assessment. He could observe that Tina was conscious and that she was splinting her jaw and rolling around.

2.14 / **4.** *What, if anything, do you believe Dale omitted as part of his evaluation of Tina?*

The answers for this question will vary depending on a student's emergency response training. However, at a minimum, Dale should have removed any intra-oral devices or debris to ensure that Tina had an adequate airway. A cervical spine evaluation, including assessment of the distal extremities' circulation, sensation, and movement, should also have been performed. Furthermore, a thorough evaluation of the head, including possible use of the Standardized Assessment of Concussion (SAC) may have been done based on the MOI.[50–52] However, given the clinical diagnosis, this may be impractical and not warranted at the time.

2.14 / **5.** *During the application of the cervical collar, it was apparent the collar was the wrong size. (a) Do you believe the application of a cervical collar was appropriate given the clinical diagnosis? (b) Explain what alternative method may have been used to stabilize the jaw.*

a. The cervical collar was not appropriate. A rigid cervical collar increases the pressure applied to the TMJ dislocation, possibly increasing Tina's pain and increasing the risk of further trauma.

b. Because of the increased risk of secondary injury or a mandible fracture, Tina's jaw could have also been stabilized using a cravat, and the neck stabilized using sandbags or folded towels.[4,66] A soft cervical collar could also be used, assuming there is no compromise to the airway.[66]

2.14 / **6.** *Using an algorithm, briefly outline the evaluation procedures you would take during an on-field assessment and management of the injury.*

This answers for this question will vary among students and should be discussed with the classroom instructor. In fact, this question is best answered as a group discussion because there is not necessarily only one correct answer.

## CASE 2.15 Tooth Subluxation And Luxation

2.15 / **1.** *Based on the information presented in the case, determine the clinical diagnosis and the mechanism of injury.*

The clinical diagnosis is subluxation trauma to the lower left lateral and central incisor, luxation to the upper left central incisor, and soft-tissue damage to the lower lip. The mechanism of injury is typically a direct trauma to the teeth[16] caused by sporting equipment or opposing players.

2.15 / **2.** *Identify three to five additional history questions Adam could have asked to properly evaluate this condition.*

Answers will vary among students, but they should focus on:

a. Onset and mechanism of injury
b. Difficulty breathing
c. Pain, particularly as it relates to the elements
d. Past medical history and previous treatment
e. Questions related to a head trauma

2.15 / **3.** *In addition to the teeth, what other bony anatomical structures or landmarks should Adam have assessed for further trauma?*

In light of the mechanism of injury, Adam should be concerned about trauma to the following bony anatomical landmarks, including but not limited to: bilateral TMJs, mandible, maxilla, all remaining teeth, and possibly, the hyoid.

2.15 / **4.** *Discuss the differences between a tooth's three main components: enamel, dentin, and pulp.*

The enamel is "the hard, acellular, inert substance covering the tooth." Dentin is the "ivory forming the mass of the tooth," while the pulp is "a soft, moist, coherent solid" component of the tooth.[83]

2.15 / **5.** *What are the current recommendations for handling the avulsed tooth?*

Avulsed permanent anterior teeth can be replanted successfully in children under the age of 16 if the root apex is not formed.[71] Permanent teeth need to be replanted as soon as possible.[2] The clinician should hold the tooth by the crown, otherwise the periodontal ligament could be damaged.[71] If the tooth cannot be replanted within 5 minutes, the American Academy of Pediatric Dentistry recommends, based on a review of literature, that the avulsed tooth be transported in the following media (in order of preference): Viaspan, Hank's Balanced Salt Solution (tissue culture medium), cold milk, saliva (buccal vestibule), physiologic saline, or water.[2]

2.15 / **6.** *Discuss how you would have handled the above situation. Would you have done anything differently?*

The management steps will vary among students, according to their level of emergency response training; however, a discussion of management of the ABC's, assessing for a concussion, and referral to a dentist would be appropriate.

## CASE 2.16 Concussion

2.16 / **1.** *Based on the information presented in the case, determine the clinical diagnosis and the MOI.*

The clinical diagnosis is second-degree concussion according to the American Academy of Neurology grading scale.[1,23] According to the new Consensus Statement on Concussion in Sport Third International Conference on Concussion in Sport, the clinical diagnosis would be acute concussion.[53] The use of any other concussion grading scale could result in a different clinical diagnosis. The concussion was caused by a coup injury. A coup injury occurs as a result of a forceful blow to a resting head from a moving object that causes trauma at the point of cranial impact.[5]

2.16 / **2.** *According to the above case, a SAC evaluation was conducted on Lauren immediately after the injury and again at 15 minutes and 1 hour post injury. (a) What is a SAC assessment? (b) How would you have scored her initial SAC evaluation? (c) What is the clinical significance of the initial post-injury and baseline scores?*

a. The Standardized Assessment of Concussion (SAC) is an objective sideline measurement tool used to assess neurocognitive deficits in athletes immediately after an injury.[22,50–53] An examination of the efficacy of standardized mental status testing using the SAC tool immediately after a concussion found the tool to be 95 percent sensitive and 76 percent specific in accurately classifying injured and uninjured subjects on the sideline.[71]

b. Her initial assessment would be scored as a 23, which is 6 points below her preseason baseline score. This score is determined by summing the results of the orientation, immediate memory, concentration, and delayed recall sections.[52]

c. If the score on the SAC is lower than the baseline score, some type of cognitive impairment is indicated. However, a clinician should not rely solely on the findings of the SAC; it is intended only as a supplement to other methods of concussion assessment (e.g., neuropsychological evaluation, postural stability testing, etc.).[22]

2.16 / **3.** *What is the difference between the SAC and the Sport Concussion Assessment Tool 2 (SCAT2)?*

The SAC is an objective sideline measurement tool used to assess neurocognitive deficits in athletes immediately after an injury.[22,50–53] The SCAT2, which is now being advocated based on the new Consensus Statement on Concussion in Sport Third International Conference on Concussion in Sport, is a standardized clinical assessment tool used to evaluate and document an acute concussion.[53] The SCAT2, which still needs to be validated, supersedes the SCAT, which was published in 2005. One of the interesting features of the document is that it assists in the calculation of SAC scores and provides improved directions when assessing balance, using a modified version of the balance error scoring system (BESS).[53] A copy of the SCAT2 can be found in the Appendix, and the Consensus Statement on Concussion in Sport Third International Conference on Concussion in Sport can be located at www.ncbi.nlm.nih.gov/pmc/articles/PMC2707064/pdf/attr-44-04-434.pdf. Neither document is subject to copyright restrictions, and both can be integrated into any concussion prevention and assessment program.

2.16 / **4.** *How would you rate David's and Lisa's performances in the above evaluation? What would you have done differently in this situation, if anything?*

The answers to this question will vary among students, based on institutional and athletic department policies and procedures. In general they acted according to the National Athletic Trainers' Association Position Statement on the management of concussions.[22] Depending on institutional policy, it may be necessary to refer the athlete to a physician for further assessment and neuropsychological testing.

2.16 / **5.** *What is the significance of having a concussion policies and procedures document?*

A policy and procedure manual (PPM) is a crucial document both for clinicians and the individuals they serve. A policy is essentially a facility's or organization's rules and regulations regarding a specific point. Such policies often reflect the goals and objectives of the organization. A procedure describes how the policies are going to be met and/or carried out by the organization.[67] Therefore, the primary objective of the PPM regarding the management of a concussion should be to establish policies and procedures that will promote safety when providing care to athletes who have sustained a head injury.

2.16 / **6.** *The coach appeared more concerned with Lauren's continued participation in the game than about her health. What could David and Lisa have done to ensure that Lauren did not return to the game, if the athletic director had not intervened?*

In an effort to prevent Lauren from returning to play, David and Lisa could have taken away her field hockey sticks and mouthguards. In football, the helmet is commonly taken away from the injured player to prevent him from returning to play.

## CASE 2.17 Post-Concussion Syndrome

2.17 / **1.** *Based on the information presented in the case, determine (a) the differential diagnoses and (b) the clinical diagnosis.*

a. Differential diagnoses: depression and damage to the hypothalamus or the pituitary gland as a result of mild traumatic brain injury[32]

b. Clinical diagnosis: post-concussion syndrome (PCS)

2.17 / **2.** *(a) Do you believe Mary performed an adequate physical examination? (b) If not, what would you have done differently as the evaluating clinician?*

a. Mary chose to use only two neuropsychological tests as part of her evaluation process (i.e., Wechsler Digit Span Test and Stroop Color Word Test). A thorough assessment of PCS requires a complete assessment of an athlete's neurological functions, neuropsychological ability, and postural stability.[53] Neurological testing omitted in this case includes an assessment of cranial nerve function and spinal nerve roots (myotomes and dermatomes). There may have been accumulation of blood within the skull, even as a result of mild trauma, and this places pressure on the cranial nerves, altering their function. In the presence of a chronic subdural hematoma this alteration may take three weeks to manifest.[5]

b. Answers may vary among students, but they should note that Mary needed to perform more neuropsychological testing. Students should be able to list some of these additional tests. Assessing neuropsychological function/ability is now well established in the prevention and management of concussions and is used to contribute significant information during the clinical evaluation of a concussion, providing quantitative data to aid in making return-to-play decisions.[22,53,64]

Guskiewicz, et al,[23] also cite numerous studies demonstrating relationships among concussion, traumatic brain injuries, and reported problems with postural equilibrium. Postural stability testing is in fact a useful tool for "objectively assessing the motor domain of neurologic functioning and should be considered a reliable and valid addition to the assessment of athletes suffering from concussion, particularly when symptoms or signs indicate a balance component."[53] However, Mary did not assess P.J.'s postural equilibrium. Two common exams used both clinically and on the sideline to assess postural equilibrium disturbances are the stork stand and Romberg test.[22] Two exams that are most often used in a controlled clinical setting and as part of a pre-season baseline test include the BESS and Sensory Organization Test (SOT).

- The BESS assessment consists of 6 separate 20-second balance tests performed in different stances (i.e., double leg stance, single leg stance, and tandem stance) with the eyes closed and on different surfaces (i.e., firm versus hard), while the clinician measures postural stability under different testing conditions.[69,88] Errors include: (1) opening the eyes; (2) stepping, stumbling, and falling out of the test position; (3) lifting the hands off the iliac crests; (4) lifting the toes or heels; (5) moving the leg into more than 30° of flexion or abduction; and (6) remaining out of the test position for more than 5 seconds.
- According to Guskiewicz et al.,[22] the "Sensory Organization Test (SOT, NeuroCom International) is designed to disrupt various sensory systems, including the visual, somatosensory, and vestibular systems. The SOT consists of 6 conditions with 3 trials per condition, for a total of 18 trials, with each trial lasting 20 seconds."

Other neuropsychological tests, both in pen-and-paper and computer-based formats, include the Halstead-Reitan Neuropsychological Test Battery, Hopkins Verbal Learning Test, Penn State Cancellation Test, Stroop Test, Symbol Digit Modalities Test, Trail Making Test, Vigil Continuous Performance Test, Standardized Assessment of Concussion, and ImPACT Test Battery.[20,22,50,58]

2.17 / **3.** *What other history questions, if any, could Mary have asked P.J. in order to guide the evaluation?*

Answers will vary and may include:

a. Questions dealing with a past history of concussions
b. How P.J.'s head specifically hit the floor
c. Specific cognitive tasks that pose some difficulty
d. Balance problems or problems related to her cranial nerve function
e. Past medical history, including bouts of depression

2.17 / **4.** *(a) What is the relationship between the clinical diagnosis and depression? (b) Where should an athletic trainer refer an athlete who may be suffering from depression?*

a. Grant L. Iverson's examination of persistent PCS in patients with depression using the British Columbia Postconcussion Symptom Inventory[33] found "9 out of 10 patients with depression met liberal self-report criteria for a postconcussion syndrome and more than 5 out of 10 met conservative criteria for the diagnosis."[82] These findings are consistent with comparable studies reported in his work that suggest a moderate correlation between PCS-like symptoms and depression exits. Iverson further states that there is a "potential for misdiagnosing persistent postconcussion syndrome in patients with depression." Clinically this may be significant in athletic training, because athletes with a history of traumatic brain injury (TBI) may present with and meet the criteria for PCS, yet clinically they could also meet the criteria for depression. This may not be uncommon; depression can occur with traumatic brain injuries[37,53] and may manifest after the removal of the athlete from competition and exposure to teammates.
b. Referral to a mental health professional may be necessary when neurocognitive function and postural stability have returned to baseline while the athlete still presents with neuropsychological deficits.

2.17 / **5.** *(a) What if any decisions need to be made regarding the disqualification of P.J. from sports? (b) When should Mary allow P.J. to resume physical activity?*

a. Recommendation 24 of the *National Athletic Trainers' Association Position Statement* states:[22] "The decision to disqualify from further participation on the day of a concussion should be based on a comprehensive physical examination; assessment of self-reported postconcussion signs and symptoms; functional impairments, and the athlete's past history of concussions. If assessment tools such as the SAC, BESS, neuropsychological test battery, and symptom checklist are not used, a 7-day symptom-free waiting period before returning to participation is recommended. Some circumstances, however, will warrant even more conservative treatment (see recommendation 25)."
b. Recommendation 25 states: "Athletic trainers should be more conservative with athletes who have a history of concussion. Athletes with a history of concussion are at increased risk for sustaining subsequent injuries as well as for slowed recovery

of self-reported postconcussion signs and symptoms, cognitive dysfunction, and postural instability after subsequent injuries. In athletes with a history of three or more concussions and experiencing slowed recovery, temporary or permanent disqualification from contact sports may be indicated." When P.J.'s symptoms as defined by the PCS scale demonstrate a return to baseline neuropsychological status and diagnostic testing is negative, she may "resume a graded program of physical and mental exertion, without contact or risk of concussion, up to the point at which postconcussion signs and symptoms recur. If symptoms appear, the exertion level should be scaled back to allow maximal activity without triggering symptoms."[22]

## CASE 2.18 Subdural Hematoma

2.18 / **1.** *Based on the information presented in the case, determine (a) the differential diagnoses and (b) the clinical diagnosis.*

a. Differential diagnoses: epidural hematoma, subarachnoid hematoma, stroke, meningitis[5,59]

b. Clinical diagnosis: acute subdural hematoma (SDH)[5]

2.18 / **2.** *Identify the different ways to classify the clinical diagnosis.*

Subdural hematomas are classified according to the time course and volume of blood in the SDH. According to Bailes and Hudson,[5] there are two types of SDH: acute and chronic. An acute SDH presents within 48 to 72 hours after the injury; a chronic SDH presents three or more weeks after sustaining a traumatic head injury. A third category of subacute SDH refers to hematomas occurring between three and seven days after an injury. Additionally, SDH can be classified as either simple or complicated. Simple SDH presents without cerebral contusion or edema; complicated SDH consists of a contusion to the brain, with swelling or bleeding.[45,82]

2.18 / **3.** *What is the pathophysiology of the clinical diagnosis?*

An acute SDH often results from bleeding within the subdural space due to a stretching and tearing of the subdural veins.[5] The blood from these veins drains from the cerebral surface to the dura or dural sinuses, and because venous bleeding occurs at a lower pressure than arterial bleeding, blood in SDH has a chance to collect within the fissures and sulci of the cerebral surface.[5,82] Traumatic lacerations (e.g., falling from a great height) of the intracranial internal cranial artery may also cause SDH; however, this kind of SDH is often not reported.[59]

2.18 / **4.** *What if anything would you have done differently in handling this case?*

This answer will vary among students, depending on the student's education and clinical training, athletic training-room policies, and other experience. In fact, the question should be discussed with the classroom instructor. This question works well as a group discussion, because there is not necessarily only one correct answer.

2.18 / **5.** *Based on the information provided in the case, what if anything did Dennis do that helped to reduce his risk of liability?*

By providing Paul and his roommate with home instructions, he was able to alert both individuals to the possible complications that may arise after sustaining a head injury.

## CASE 2.19 Skull Fracture and Epidural Hematoma

2.19 / **1.** *Based on the information presented in the case, determine the clinical diagnosis.*

The clinical diagnoses is a skull fracture with a possible epidural hematoma.

2.19 / **2.** *Explain the series of events leading to Stephanie's current condition.*

The initial event was caused by Stephanie's fall off the stationary bike. This fall could have occurred for a variety of reasons, including a seizure, loss of equilibrium, and cardiac or respiratory distress. The seizure could be caused by epilepsy or other medical conditions. In this case, the head trauma occurred after the seizure. Striking the head upon falling most likely resulted in the skull fracture, which tore the middle meningeal artery[77] and caused blood to accumulate between the dura mater and skull (epidural hematoma).[4,5]

2.19 / **3.** *If Stephanie's seizure was caused by epilepsy, how could Curtis have possibly anticipated such an outcome?*

A thorough verbal or written history taken during the initial evaluation could have identified Stephanie's medical condition. There are red flags other than seizures to be found during a patient's history that should indicate the need for a follow-up[46]:

a. Persistent pain at night, constant pain anywhere in the body, loss of appetite, unwarranted fatigue (cancer)
b. Shortness of breath, dizziness, heaviness or pain in the chest, constant and severe arm pain (cardiac)
c. Changes in hearing, frequent headaches, changes in vision, fainting spells, sudden weakness (neurological)

2.19 / **4.** *Overall, how would you rate Curtis's and John's management of the above case? What would you have done differently in this situation, if anything?*

The answer for this question will vary among students. Students should recognize two major errors in this case. The first is the use of an intra-oral screw. Current first-aid guidelines do not recommend inserting anything into the mouth of a seizure patient. Second, when controlling bleeding for a skull fracture it is recommend to apply indirect instead of direct pressure to areas where a depression or soft spot in the skull is identified in order to minimize damage to the brain.

2.19 / **5.** *If this injury occurred during an athletic performance, describe the possible MOI for the clinical diagnosis.*

A common mechanism of injury in athletics is being struck in the head with a piece of sporting equipment such as a baseball or softball bat or ball while not wearing a helmet[77] or striking the skull on a stationary object such as a diving board while the head is traveling at a high velocity.[82] Skiers not wearing a helmet are also at risk for skull fractures as a result of falling or colliding with an object.[13]

## REFERENCES

1. American Academy of Neurology. Practice parameter: the management of concussion in sports (summary statement). Report of the Quality Standards Subcommittee of the American Academy of Neurology. *Neurology.* 1997;48:581–585.
2. American Academy of Pediatric Dentistry. *Guideline of Management of Acute Dental Trauma.* Chicago, IL: American Academy of Pediatric Dentistry; 2004.
3. American Dental Association. Using mouthguards to reduce the incidence and severity of sports-related oral injuries [electronic version]. *J Am Dent Assoc.* 2006;137: 1712–1720. Available from: http://jada.ada.org/cgi/content/abstract/137/12/1712. Accessed December 1, 2006.
4. American Red Cross. *Emergency response.* Yardley, PA: Staywell; 2001.
5. Bailes JE, Hudson V. Classification of sport-related head trauma: a spectrum of mild to severe injury. *J Athl Train.* 2001;36(3):236–243.
6. Bartkiw TP, Pynn BR. Close-up on mandible fractures. *Nursing.* 1993;23(12):45.
7. Berry DC, Miller MG. Athletic mouthguards and their role in injury prevention. *Athl Ther Today.* 2001;6(4):52–56.
8. Boustred N. Practical guide to otitis externa. *Aust Fam Physician.* 1999;28:217–221.
9. Brodsky M. Allergic conjunctivitis and contact lenses: experience with olopatadine hydrochloride 0.1% therapy. *Acta Ophthalmol Scand.* 2000;78:56–59.
10. Buglisi JA, Knoop KJ, Levsky ME, Euwema M. Experience with bandage contact lenses for the treatment of corneal abrasions in a combat environment. *Mil Med.* 2007;172(4):411–413.
11. Burton MJ, Doree C. Ear drops for the removal of ear wax. *Cochrane Database Syst Rev.* 2008;(2):CD004326.
12. Clarkson H. *Musculoskeletal Assessment: Joint Range of Motion and Manual Muscle Strength.* Philadelphia, PA: Lippincott Williams & Wilkins; 2000.
13. Diamond PT, Gale SD, Denkhaus HK. Head injuries in skiers: an analysis of injury severity and outcome. *Brain Inj.* 2001;15(5):429–434.
14. Dimitroulis G. Temporomandibular disorders: a clinical update. *Br Med J.* 1998;317(7152):190–194.
15. Frakes MA, Eva T. Evaluation and management of the patient with a LeFort facial fracture. *J Trauma Nurs.* 2004;11(3):95–102.
16. Gallaspy JB, May JD. *Signs and Symptoms of Athletic Injuries.* St. Louis, MO: Mosby; 1996.
17. Gariano RF, Kim CH. Evaluation and management of suspected retinal detachment. *Am Fam Physician.* 2004;69:1691–1698.
18. Greasley A, Karet B. Towards the development of a standard test procedure for mouthguard assessment. *Br J Sports Med.* 1997;31(1):31–35.
19. Grosse SJ, Lynch JM. Treating auricular hematoma: success with a swimmer's nose clip. *Physician and Sportsmed.* 1991;19(10):99–102.
20. Gualtieri CT, Johnson LG. Reliability and validity of a computerized neurocognitive test battery, CNS vital signs. *Arch Clin Neuropsychol.* 2006;21:623–643.
21. Guest JFG, Robinson AC, Smith AF. Impacted cerumen: composition, production, epidemiology, and management. *QJM.* 2004;97(8):477–488.
22. Guskiewicz KM, Bruce SL, Cantu RC, et al. National Athletic Trainers' Association Position Statement: management of sport-related concussion. *J Athl Train.* 2004;39(3):280–297.
23. Guskiewicz KM, Ross SE, Marshall SW. Postural stability and neuropsychological deficits after concussion in collegiate athletes. *J Athl Train.* 2001;36(3):263–272.
24. Hand C, Harvey I. The effectiveness of topical preparations for the treatment of earwax: a systematic review. *Br J Gen Pract.* 2004;54:862–867.
25. Harrahill M. (2005). Review of ruptured globe injuries: The case for early consult from ophthalmology. *J Emerg Nurs.* 31(3):40–410.
26. Hawke M. Update on cerumen and ceruminolytics. *Ear Nose Throat J.* 2002;81(8 Suppl 1):23–24.
27. Heimmel MR, Murphy MA. Ocular injuries in basketball and baseball: what are the risks and how can we prevent them? *Cur Sports Med Rep.* 2008;7(5):284–288.
28. Høvding G. Acute bacterial conjunctivitis. *Acta Ophthalmol.* 2008;86(1):5–17.
29. Huether SE. Pain, temperature, sleep, and sensory function. In Huether SE & McCance KL, Eds. *Understanding Pathophysiology.* New York: Elsevier; 2007:329–354.
30. Hui RC. Nosebleed (epistaxis) [electronic version]. *Hughston Health Alert, 10.* 1998;Spring. Available from: http://www.hughston.com/hha/a.nosebleed.htm. Accessed April 28, 2007.
31. Hyphema. *Review of Optometry,* 2005;142:30A–31A.
32. Iverson GL. *Misdiagnosis of the persistent postconcussion syndrome in patients with depression.* Arch Clin Neuropsychol. 2006;21(4):303–310.
33. Iverson GL, Gaetz M. Practical considerations for interpreting change following concussion. In: Lovell MR, Echemendia RJ, Barth J, Collins MW, eds. *Traumatic Brain Injury in Sports: An International Neuropsychological Perspective.* Netherlands: Swets-Zeitlinger; 2004:323–356.
34. Jones SEM, Mahendran S. Interventions for acute auricular haematoma. *Cochrane Database of Syst Rev.* 2008;(4):CD004166.
35. Khan FH, Silverberg MA. Corneal abrasion [electronic version]. *eMedicine.* 2009. Available from: http://www.emedicine.com/emerg/topic828.htm. Accessed December 29, 2009.
36. Kim DW, Egan KK. Facial trauma, maxillary, and Le Fort fractures [electronic version]. *eMedicine.* 2006. Available from: http://www.emedicine.com/plastic/topic481.htm. Accessed July 7, 2006.
37. Kreutzer JS, Seel RT, Gourley E. The prevalence and symptom rates of depression after traumatic brain injury: a comprehensive examination. *Brain Inj.* 2001;15:563–576.

38. Kucik CJ, Clenney T, Phelan J. Management of acute nasal fractures. *Am Fam Physician.* 2004;70(7):1315–1320.
39. Kwitko GM. Orbital fracture, floor [electronic version]. *eMedicine.* 2009. Available from: http://www.emedicine.com/oph/topic229.htm. Accessed May 15, 2009.
40. Lane SE, Rhame GL, Wrobble RL. A silicone splint for auricular hematoma. *Physician and Sportsmed.* 1998;26(9):77.
41. Larheim TA. Role of magnetic resonance imaging in the clinical diagnosis of the temporomandibular joint. *Cells Tissues Organs.* 2005;180(1):6–21.
42. Larkin G. Retinal detachment. *eMedicine.* 2008. Available from: http://www.emedicine.com/emerg/topic504.htm. Accessed July 25, 2009.
43. Lee D, Sperling N. Initial management of auricular trauma. *Am Fam Physician.* 1996;53(7):2339–2344.
44. Levine MR. How to manage orbital fractures. *Rev Ophthalmol.* 2000;7(3):70–73.
45. Logan SM, Bell G, Leonard JC. Acute subdural hematoma in a high school football player after 2 unreported episodes of head trauma: a case report. *J Athl Train.* 2001;36(4):433–436.
46. Magee DJ. *Orthopedic Physical Assessment* (5th ed.). Philadelphia, PA: WB Saunders; 2007.
47. Malhotra R Dunning J. The utility of the tongue blade test for the diagnosis of mandibular fracture [electronic version]. *Emerg Med J.* 2003;20:552–553. Available from: http://emj.bmj.com/cgi/content/full/20/6/552. Accessed April 28, 2007.
48. Mangi Q, Ridgway RF, Ibrahim Z, Evoy D. Dislocation of the mandible. *Surg Endosc.* 2004;18(3):554–560.
49. Marlin DS. Conjunctivitis, bacterial [electronic version]. *eMedicine.* 2009. Available from: http://emedicine.medscape.com/article/1191730-overview. Accessed July 19, 2009.
50. McCrea M. Standardized mental status testing on the sideline after sport-related concussion. *J Athl Train.* 2001;36(3):274–279.
51. McCrea M, Kelly J, Kluge J, Ackley B, Randolph C. Standardized assessment of concussion in football players. *Neurology.* 1997;48(3):586–588.
52. McCrea M, Kelly J, Randolph C. *Standardized Assessment of Concussion (SAC): Manual for Administration Scoring and Interpretation.* Waukesha, WI: CNS Inc.; 1996.
53. McCrory P, Meeuwisse W, Johnston K, Dvorak J, Aubry M, Cantu RC. Consensus statement on concussion in sport 3rd international conference on concussion in sport held in Zurich, November 2008. *J Athl Train.* 2009;44(4):434–448.
54. Miller MG, Berry DC, Gariepy GS, Tittler JG. Attitudes of high school ice hockey players toward mouthguard usage [electronic version]. *The Internet Journal of Allied Health Sciences and Practice.* 2006;4:1–6. Available from: http://ijahsp.nova.edu/articles/vol4num4/toc.htm. Accessed January 31, 2010.
55. Moore K, Dalley A. *Clinically Oriented Anatomy* (5th ed.). Baltimore, MD: Lippincott Williams & Wilkins; 2005.
56. National Collegiate Athletic Association. *2009–10 NCAA(r) Sports Medicine Handbook.* Indianapolis, IN: National Collegiate Athletic Association; 2009.
57. Neno R. Holistic ear care: cerum removal techniques. *J Community Nurs.* 2006;20(9):26–31.
58. Occupational Safety and Health Administration. Bloodborne pathogens.-1910.1030. Available from: http://www.osha.gov/pls/oshaweb/owadisp.show_document?p_table=STANDARDS&p_id=10051. Published 1997. Accessed July 19, 2009.
59. Oyama H, Nakamura S, Ueyama M, et al. Acute subdural hematoma originating from the lacerated intracranial internal carotid arteries: case report. *Neurol Med Chir (Tokyo).* 2006;46(2):84–87.
60. Padilla RR. A technique for fabricating modern athletic mouth-guards. *J Calif Dent Assoc.* 2005;33(5):399–408.
61. Parish KD, Cothran VE. Facial soft tissue injuries: treatment and medication [electronic version]. *eMedicine.* 2008. Available from: http://emedicine.medscape.com/article/84727-treatment. Accessed July 19, 2009.
62. Parnes J, Sinert RH, Heffer SM. Temporomandibular joint syndrome [electronic version]. *eMedicine.* 2009. Available from: http://emedicine.medscape.com/article/809598-overview. Accessed December 27, 2009.
63. Parsa T, Adamo A, Calderon Y. Initial evaluation and management of maxillofacial injuries [electronic version]. *eMedicine.* 2007. Available from: http://www.emedicine.com/med/topic3222.htm. Accessed July 19, 2009.
64. Patel DP, Shivdasani V, Baker RJ. Management of sport-related concussion in young athletes. *Sports Med.* 2005;35(8):671–684.
65. Petrigliano FA, Williams R. Orbital fractures in sport: a review. *Sports Med.* 2003;33(4):317–322.
66. Ranalli DN, Demas PN. Orofacial injuries from sport: preventive measures for sports medicine. *Sports Med.* 2002;32(7):409–418.
67. Ray R. *Management Strategies in Athletic Training* (3rd ed.). Champaign, IL: Human Kinetics; 2005.
68. Reynolds T. Ear, nose and throat problems in accident and emergency. *Nurs Stand.* 2004;18(26):47–55.
69. Riemann BL, Guskiewicz KM, Shields EW. Relationship between clinical and forceplate measures of postural stability. *J Sport Rehabil.* 1999;8:71–82.
70. Roberts A, Schwab MD, Robinson, WA. Clinical procedures of mandibular fractures. *Am J Emerg Med.* 1998;16:304–308.
71. Roberts G, Scully C, Shotts R. ABC of oral health: dental emergencies. *Br Med J.* 2000;321(7260):559–562.
72. Rodriguez JO, Lavina AM. Prevention and treatment of common eye injuries in sports. *Am Fam Physician.* 2003;67:1481–8,1494–6.
73. Roland P, Stroman D. Microbiology of acute otitis externa. *Laryngoscope.* 2002;112:1166–1177.
74. Rupp TJ, Karageanes S. Facial fractures [electronic version]. *eMedicine.* 2008. Available from: http://www.emedicine.com/sports/topic33.htm. Accessed July 19, 2009.
75. Sanders R. Otitis externa: a practical guide to treatment and prevention. *Am Fam Physician.* 2001;63:927–936,941–922.
76. Schatz P, Pardini JE, Lovell MR, Collins MC, Podell K. Sensitivity and specificity of the ImPACT Test Battery for concussion in athletes. *Arch Clin Neuropsychol.* 2006;(21):91–99.

77. Schultz SJ, Houglum PA, Perrin DH. *Examination of Musculoskeletal Injuries* (2nd ed.). Champaign, IL: Human Kinetics; 2005.
78. Sheppard JD, Crouch ER, Williams PB, Crouch ER, Rastogi S, Garcia-Valenzuela E. Hyphema [electronic version]. *eMedicine*. 2008. Available from: http://emedicine.medscape.com/article/1190165-overview. Accessed December 29, 2009.
79. Smally AJ, DelGross C. Spontaneous temporomandibular joint dislocation in an 80-year-old man. *J Fam Pract.* 1995;40(4):395–398.
80. Smith B, Regan W. Blowout fracture of the orbit: mechanism repair. *Am J Ophthalmol.* 1957;44:733–739.
81. Soporowski J. Fabricating custom athletic mouthguards. *J Mass Dent Soc.* 1994;43(4):25–27.
82. Starkey C, Ryan J. *Evaluation of Orthopedic and Athletic Injuries* (2nd ed.). Philadelphia, PA: FA Davis; 2002.
83. *Steadman's Medical Dictionary.* Philadelphia, PA: Lippincott Williams & Wilkins; 2001.
84. Tesfaye Y, Lal S. Hazard of yawning. *Can Med Assoc J.* 1990;142(1):15.
85. Tesfaye Y, Skorzewska A, Lal S. Hazard of yawning. *Can Med Assoc J.* 1991;145(12):1560.
86. Thurnwald PA. The effect of age and gender on normal temporomandibular joint movement. *Physiother Theory Pract.* 1991;7:209–221.
87. Torok PG, Mader TH. Corneal abrasions: diagnosis and management. *Am Fam Physician.* 1996;63(8):2521–2529.
88. Valovich McLeod TC, Barr WB, McCrea M Guskiewicz KM. Psychometric and measurement properties of concussion assessment tools in youth sports. *J Athl Train.* 2006;41(4):399–408.
89. Weller MD, Drake-Lee AB. A review of nasal trauma. *Trauma.* 2006;8(1):21–28.
90. Westerman B, Stringfellow PM, Eccleston JA. Forces transmitted through EVA mouthguard materials of different types and thickness. *Aust Dent J.* 1995;40(6):389–391.
91. Westesson PL, Yamamoto M, Sano T, Okano T. Temporomandibular joint. In PM Som & HD Curtis, eds. *Head and Neck Imaging.* St Louis, MO: Mosby; 2003:995–1053.
92. Widell T. Fractures, face [electronic version]. *eMedicine.* 2008. Available from: http://www.emedicine.com/emerg/topic192.htm. Accessed July 7, 2009.
93. Wilson SA, Last A. Management of corneal abrasions. *Am Fam Physician.* 2004;70(1):123–128.
94. Woodmansey KF. Athletic mouth guards prevent orofacial injuries. *J Am Coll Health.* 1997;45(4):179–182.

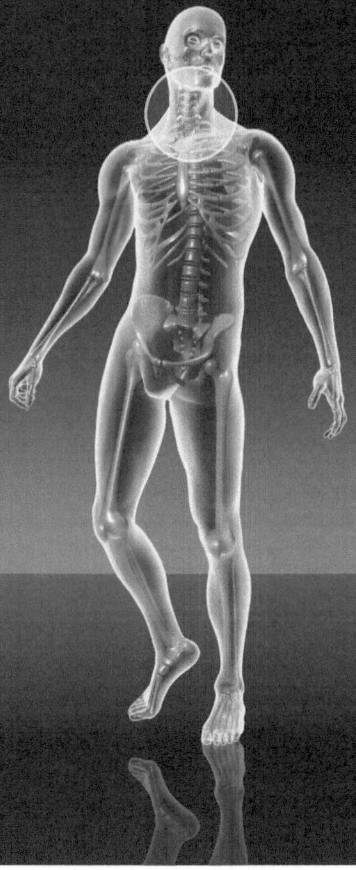

# CHAPTER 3 Cervical Spine

QUICK REFERENCE

CASE 3.1
**Vertebral Fracture with Spinal Cord Trauma (C5-C6)**

CASE 3.2
**Brachial Plexus Trauma**

CASE 3.3
**Intervertebral Disc Herniation**

CASE 3.4
**Atlano-Occipital Dislocation**

CASE 3.5
**Cervical Strain**

CASE 3.6
**Cervical Sprain**

# ANSWERS TO CASE QUESTIONS

## CASE 3.1 Vertebral Fracture with Spinal Cord Trauma (C5-C6)

3.1 / **1.** *Based on the information presented in the case, determine (a) the differential diagnoses and (b) the clinical diagnosis.*

a. Differential diagnoses: cervical spine dislocation, cervical strain, cervical sprain, spinal cord shock, spinal cord trauma, vertebral artery trauma

b. Clinical diagnosis: cervical fracture, possible secondary spinal cord trauma

3.1 / **2.** *Once Seth arrived at Hector's side and determined that the scene was safe, Seth should have immediately begun to assess what?*

After completing the scene survey, a primary assessment should be performed. This includes:

- Forming a general impression of the victim (i.e., CC, gender, and age)
- Assessing level of consciousness and/or mental status according to the AVPU scale or GCS
- Assessing the victim's airway, breathing, and circulation[2] and providing interventions as necessary, such as supplemental oxygen and, in this case, cervical stabilization

3.1 / **3.** *Based on the case, once a medic arrived on scene, she should have been responsible for performing what?*

Based on the MOI (i.e., fall over 15 ft or three times Hector's height), the rescuer(s) (Seth and medics) should have assumed a possible cervical spine trauma, and the second medic would have begun providing in-line stabilization in order to maintain stabilization of the cervical spine to limit secondary injury.

3.1 / **4.** *Discuss the difference between the AVPU scale and the Glasgow Coma Scale (GCS). If you were in this situation, which scale would you prefer to use and why?*

The acronym "AVPU" stands for Alert, Verbal, Painful, and Unresponsive and is a mnemonic used to determine a trauma patient's level of consciousness during an emergency. The Glasgow Coma Scale is a clinical scoring system for objectively assessing the consciousness of a patient (Table A3.1.1). Although the GCS is limited in predicting functional outcomes, the scale is useful when making decisions about management in the acute setting, particularly for patients with traumatic brain injuries. It is composed of three sections measuring the level of consciousness, each with a maximum and minimum point value based on a patient's eye-opening response (1–4), verbal response (1–5), and motor response (1–6). The sum of each section determines a patient's classification.[37] A severe traumatic brain injury has a GCS of 3 to 8, moderate traumatic brain injury 9 to 12, and slight traumatic brain injury ≥ 13.[40] "Patients who score less than 15 need imaging or observation, and patients with scores less than 9 need to be promptly considered for definitive airway management."[45]

A study examining the variability in agreement between ER physicians and nurses found a high level of inter-rater agreement.[11] However, in 10 of the 108 cases, some GCS

TABLE A3.1.1 Glasgow Coma Scale.

| | | |
|---|---|---|
| Eye-opening response | Spontaneous, open with blinking at baseline | 4 points |
| | Opens to verbal command, speech, or shout | 3 points |
| | Opens to pain, not applied to face | 2 points |
| | None | 1 point |
| Verbal response | Oriented | 5 points |
| | Confused conversation, but able to answer questions | 4 points |
| | Inappropriate responses, words discernible | 3 points |
| | Incomprehensible speech | 2 points |
| | None | 1 point |
| Motor response | Obeys commands for movement | 6 points |
| | Purposeful movement to painful stimulus | 5 points |
| | Withdraws from pain | 4 points |
| | Abnormal (spastic) flexion, decorticate posture | 3 points |
| | Extension (rigid) response, decerebrate posture | 2 points |
| | None | 1 point |

A GCS score ranges between 3 and 15 with the total score being the sum of the scores in three categories.

scores did differ more than 2 points. The authors suggest that although the agreement between the emergency room professionals was high, the disagreement indicates that clinical decisions should not be based solely on single GCS scores.

3.1 / **5.** *Discuss how you would have managed this situation from scene survey to packaging and transport of Hector.*

The answers to this question will vary among students, depending on level of training and clinical experience. However, the answers should be consistent with the recommendations established in the 2009 National Athletic Trainers' Association Position Statement on the acute management of cervical spine–injured athletes.[39] The answers should be discussed with the classroom instructor, clinical instructor, and/or approved clinical instructor. In fact, consider consulting with your athletic training medical staff and physician to determine whether this type of event has ever occurred and, if it has, how it was handled.

## CASE 3.2 Brachial Plexus Trauma

3.2 / **1.** *Based on the information presented in the case, determine (a) the differential diagnoses and (b) the clinical diagnosis.*

a. Differential diagnoses: cervical disc pathology, cervical spine sprain, cervical spine strain injuries, shoulder/AC joint dislocation, shoulder impingement, thoracic outlet syndrome[44]

b. Clinical diagnosis: brachial plexus trauma or what is commonly referred to as a "burner" or "stinger"[9,26]

3.2 / **2.** *Lisa asked several specific history questions to guide the physical examination. Based on the clinical diagnosis above, identify three to five additional history questions you may have asked as the evaluating clinician.*

These answers will vary among students. Overall, Lisa appeared to generate an adequate history; however, there are some specific questions that could have helped guide the physical examination. These include:

a. Any prior history of cervical trauma or brachial plexus injury?

b. What position was your head in while making the tackle?

c. Where specifically does the pain and numbness radiate down the arm?

d. Are you now suffering or did you ever suffer any changes in sensation?

e. Did you hear or feel any snapping or popping of the neck?

f. Are you now suffering or did you ever suffer any changes in muscle function?

3.2 / **3.** *If this injury was to persist during the athletic season, what type of physician would be best suited to manage Tom's case and why?*

Most clinicians would start with an orthopedic surgeon, but a neurologist would be preferred. A neurologist typically manages disorders of the nerves and nervous system, including the central nervous system and the peripheral nervous system (i.e., sensory and motor nerves throughout the body). In this situation, a neurologist would consider conducting an electromyography/nerve conduction velocity (EMG/NCV) tests to determine the extent of neurological damage to the brachial plexus.

A neurosurgeon may also be considered, depending on symptom severity and/or duration of symptoms. Lisa could assist the team physician in deciding which medical specialty is most appropriate for Tom's situation, based on her familiarity with the case and her medical documentation.

3.2 / **4.** *Based on the results of functional and neurological exams presented in this case, which nerve roots and peripheral nerves are most likely to be involved?*

A traction force applied to the cervical nerve roots can affect any level of the nerve roots; however, the lateral and posterior cords innervated by C5 and C6 are the most commonly affected (suprascapular, lateral pectoral, musculocutaneous, and axillary nerve). Forced abduction of the arm and lateral side bending involve the C8 and T1 nerve roots.[16,18,33,37] In this case, it is likely that the C5 to C7 nerve roots were affected, along with the axillary and suprascapular peripheral nerves.

3.2 / **5.** *Considering Tom's clinical diagnosis, identify the criteria Lisa should use in order to make a return-to-play decision.*

Based on the clinical diagnosis, Tom should present with full AROM of the neck and shoulder, normal upper extremity muscle strength including scapular stabilizers, paraspinal musculature (grip strength), and a normal neurological exam (i.e., peripheral nerves, dermatomes, myotomes, and deep tendon reflexes) before he is allowed to return to play. Returning with any deficits in ROM or muscular strength places Tom at risk of further injury. The athlete should be monitored closely for re-injury upon returning to play.

3.2 / **6.** *(a) What other special tests, if any, should Lisa perform to confirm her clinical diagnosis? (b) Identify how to perform these tests.*

a. Two tests commonly reported for assessing the brachial plexus are the brachial plexus traction and compression test and the Tinel's sign.[16,18,33,37]

b. To perform the brachial plexus traction and compression test, begin by placing the patient in a seated or standing position. Stand behind the patient, placing one hand on the side of the patient's head and the other over the ACJ of the ipsilateral side. Then passively laterally flex the patient's head to the contralateral side while applying a downward pressure over the ACJ (Figure A3.2.1). A positive finding may occur on either side of the neck. Pain and/or a reproduction of neurological symptoms on the side toward the flexed head indicate a compressive force, while pain and/or a reproduction of neurological symptoms on the side away from the stretch indicate a traction force.

To perform a Tinel's sign place the patient in a seated, standing, or supine position. Gently tap the cervical neck area near Erb's point (anterior to the transverse process of C6, 2 cm superior to the clavicle). A change in sensation in the upper extremity on the ipsilateral side is considered a positive finding.

FIGURE A.3.2.1

Brachial plexus traction test.

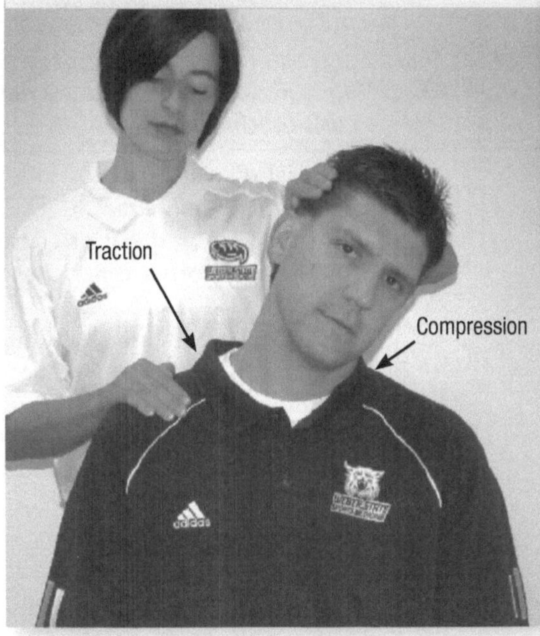

## CASE 3.3 Intervertebral Disc Herniation

3.3 / **1.** *Based on the information presented in the case, determine (a) the differential diagnoses and (b) the clinical diagnosis.*

a. Differential diagnoses: brachial plexus injury, cervical sprain, cervical strain, rotator cuff pathology, thoracic outlet syndrome, cervical facet syndrome, osteoarthritis,[7,8] and degenerative disc disease

b. Clinical diagnosis: intervertebral disc herniation with cervical radiculopathy

3.3 / **2.** *Overall, do you believe Nancy adequately evaluated Tim's condition? If not, what would you have done differently as the evaluating clinician and why?*

The answers to this question will vary among students. However, given the patient's history and the limited physical examination, Nancy should have included a more thorough assessment of Tim's neurological status. It would appear from the facts in the case that Nancy did not adequately assess the dermatomes, myotomes, and/or deep tendon reflexes of the upper extremity.[1,27] This is necessary to determine the extent of neurological involvement, considering that Tim is complaining of pain radiating down his arm.

3.3 / **3.** *Which nerve root or roots are involved in this condition and how and why did you come to this conclusion?*

"Cervical disc disease most often involves the C4-C5, C5-C6, and C6-C7 interspaces, singly or in combination."[34] The radiculopathy signs and symptoms (reported numbness and decreased muscular strength) presented in this case suggest a compression on the fifth and sixth cervical nerve roots from a pathology (by the intervertebral disc in this case) at the C4-C5 and C5-C6 levels, respectively. Radiculopathy of the fifth and sixth cervical nerve presents with numbness over the superolateral aspect of the arm, extending laterally down to the midpart of the arm and down the lateral arm and forearm into the thumb and index finger. Profound weakness of the deltoid and weakness of the supraspinatus and infraspinatus are possible with a fifth cervical nerve root compression. Motor deficits are best elicited in the wrist extensors and in elbow flexion; however, supination weakness and pronator muscle weakness may be present.[1,27]

3.3 / **4.** *Complete Table 3.3.2, which lists the location of sensory and motor deficits associated with nerve root involvement at each cervical spine level and upper extremity peripheral nerve.*

A completed version of textbook Table 3.3.2 is provided in Table A3.3.1.

3.3 / **5.** *An individual's sensory perception arises from a variety of afferent receptors located within the skin that relay information to the CNS. Given the findings from the case, how and what should be assessed in order to measure Tim's sensory perception?*

In order to best assess Tim's sensory function, a clinician could assess a variety of receptors, including mechanical (light touch, pressure), thermal (temperature), and noxious (pain) stimuli[33] by checking the cutaneous distribution of the various peripheral and cervical nerve roots. Superficial tactical sensation is tested with light touch using a cotton ball or brush, while a pinwheel or safety pin is used to assess superficial pain.[18] Temperature can be assessed using a test tube filled with hot and cold water. Assessing the various cervical nerve roots and their associated peripheral nerves requires the patient to

**TABLE A3.3.1 Sensory and motor deficits in association with nerve root involvement at individual cervical spine levels and upper extremity peripheral nerves.**

| DISC LEVEL | LOCATION OF DERMATOME/PERIPHERAL NERVE SENSORY SYMPTOMS | MOTOR DEFICIT |
|---|---|---|
| C5 | Deltoid patch, lateral upper arm | Shoulder abduction (deltoid), elbow flexion (biceps) |
| C6 | Lateral forearm, radial side of hand, first and second phalanges | Elbow flexion (biceps, supinator), wrist extension |
| C7 | Posterior lateral arm and forearm, third phalange | Elbow extension (triceps), wrist flexion |
| C8 | Medial forearm, ulnar border of hand, fourth and fifth phalanges | Ulnar deviation, thumb extension, finger flexion and abduction |
| T1 | Medial elbow, arm | Finger abduction (hand intrinsic) |
| Median | Distal radial aspect, second phalange | Thumb pinch, opposition, and abduction |
| Ulnar | Distal ulnar side of fifth phalange | Abduction, fifth phalange (abductor digiti minimi) |
| Radial | Dorsal web space between the first and second phalanges | Wrist extension and thumb extension |

have his eyes closed while the clinician assesses bilaterally, marking out any changes in sensory perception.

3.3 / **6.** *During the assessment it is determined that the grip strength is decreased by 50 percent. (a) Why is grip strength assessed? (b) Should the non-dominant hand equal the dominant hand? (c) What is the reliability of dynamometers for measuring grip strength?*

a. Grip strength testing is performed in order to identify functional limitations associated with trauma,[18] document functional changes during rehabilitation,[13] and determine the patient's effort level.[10]

b. The non-dominant hand normally presents with a 10 to 15 percent deficit compared with the dominant hand.

c. Furthermore, grip dynamometers themselves have demonstrated acceptable levels of inter-instrument reliability and concurrent validity when referenced against known weights.[4,20,21]

3.3 / **7.** *What, if any, other special tests could Nancy have performed to assist in determining the clinical diagnosis?*

The most common cause of cervical radiculopathy is cervical disc herniation, followed by cervical spondylosis.[1] However, the diagnostic criteria for determining the presence of radiculopathy are unknown.[32,34] Rubinstein[32] conducted a systematic review of the diagnostic accuracy of provocative tests of the neck for diagnosing cervical radiculopathy and concluded that a positive Spurling's maneuver, traction/distraction test, and/or a Valsalva in conjunction with a consistent history and physical findings might indicate cervical radiculopathy. Shah and Rajshekhar[34] found an overall sensitivity of 92 percent and a specificity of 95 percent for the Spurling's test when compared against surgical or MRI findings. They further found that the Spurling's test had a "positive predictive value of 96.4% and negative predictive value of 90% in predicting a diagnosis of soft lateral cervical disc prolapse."

However, Rubinstein disagrees with the findings of Shah and Rajshekhar. During their systematic review, Rubinstein, et al. found that the categorization used by Shah and Rajshekhar was incorrect because they considered the soft disc prolapse found on MRI as a positive finding and considered the presence of an osteophyte as negative even though the root canal diameters on the symptomatic and asymptomatic sides were equal. They suggest that the osteophyte could have caused radiculopathy via nerve root impingement. The recalculation of the Spurling's test revealed a sensitivity of 52.9 percent and specificity of 93.8 percent.

Deep tendon reflexes can also be performed for the biceps tendon (C5), the brachioradialis tendon (C6), and the triceps tendon (C7).

## CASE 3.4 Atlano-Occipital Dislocation

3.4 / **1.** *Based on the information presented in the case, (a) what is the likely clinical diagnosis? (b) What is the typical MOI?*

a. Given the information presented in the case, the athlete probably suffered an atlanto-occipital dislocation (AOD).

b. An AOD is believed to occur as a result of cervical hyperextension with disruption of the tectorial membrane (a broad, strong band covering the odontoid process and its ligaments) and/or excessive lateral flexion or hyperflexion.[12,23] This commonly occurs in motor vehicle accidents and can also occur from falls or direct trauma. In athletics, axial loading occurs when the head and neck are flexed approximately 30°, as in a head-first tackle (commonly referred to as spearing). In this position, the normal lordotic curve of the cervical spine disappears, which removes the energy-absorbing elastic component of the region[40] and does not allow for proper distribution of force to the thorax.[3]

3.4 / **2.** *The athlete in this case went into respiratory arrest. Given the information provided in the case, why did this occur?*

Disruption of supporting structures (i.e., apical and alar ligaments and tectorial membrane) allows the cranium to move in relation to the cervical spine. The displacement of the atlas and cranium leaves the medulla oblongata vulnerable to injury, including transection.[23] The medulla oblongata is part of the brainstem, connecting the brain to the spinal cord. It is responsible for governing autonomic functions such as breathing, heart rate, and swallowing. Victims of AOD are therefore at increased risk for cardiorespiratory arrest, which explains the high mortality associated with this injury.[12,23]

3.4 / **3.** *(a) Pat was unconscious; so how did Joel gather any history information? (b) Had the athlete been conscious, identify three to four history questions you, as the evaluating clinician, would have asked to guide the physical examination.*

a. In emergency situation where a victim is unresponsive, the history or SAMPLE information is normally gathered from family members or bystanders. In this case, other athletes, coaches, and officials may assist in providing information such as the athlete's behavior prior to the trauma, mechanism of injury, and immediate response after sustaining the trauma.

b. According to the clinical diagnosis, there are several history questions a clinician could ask to assist in guiding a physical examination of a conscious patient. Some of these questions include:

- What happened?
- What position was your head in while making the tackle or when you got hurt?
- Do you have any numbness or tingling and/or other altered sensations in your neck or extremities?
- Can you wiggle your fingers and toes?

3.4 / **4.** *Overall, do you believe Joel appropriately managed the current situation? If not, what would you have done differently as the evaluating clinician, and why?*

According to the clinical presentation and the action performed by Joel, it would appear he did not appropriately manage the current situation. There are two obvious errors built within this case. First, when establishing the airway, Joel used a head-tilt chin-lift, which should be used only in situations where there is no potential trauma to the spine. A better option would have been a jaw thrust (without extension). This maneuver limits the overall movement of the cervical spine. Secondly, removing only two of the four helmet loop straps is not consistent with the current standard of care. According to the Inter-Association Task Force for Appropriate Care of the Spine-Injured Athlete[15] and the NATA Position Statement on Acute Management of the Cervical Spine–Injured Athlete,[39] the facemask should be removed before transporting an athlete, regardless of current respiratory status, using whatever tools are available and offer the least amount of cervical spine movement.[38] Failure to remove the complete face mask may affect the EMT's ability to properly intubate and ventilate the athlete, which in this case was necessary en route to the hospital.

3.4 / **5.** *Based on the clinical presentation, the football equipment was not removed until Pat's arrival at the emergency department. If you were in Sean's place, discuss how you would have removed the football equipment in the emergency room.*

Both the Inter-Association Task Force and the NATA position statement on acute management of the cervical spine–injured athlete recommend the removal of athletic equipment such as helmet and shoulder pads be delayed until the athlete has been transported to an emergency medical facility, except under specifically appropriate circumstances. Removal should be done in a controlled environment after radiographs have been obtained and only by qualified medical personnel with proper training.[15,39] For further information on the current recommendations, please see *National Athletic Trainers' Association Position Statement: Acute Management of the Cervical Spine–Injured Athlete.*[39]

- Removing the helmet:
  - (1) One person should stabilize the head, neck, and helmet while another person cuts the chin strap.
  - (2) Accessible internal helmet padding, such as cheek pads, should be removed, and air padding should be deflated before removal of the helmet, while a second assistant manually stabilizes the chin and back of the neck, in a cephalad direction, making sure to maintain the athlete's position.
  - (3) The cheek pads are removed through the insertion of a tongue depressor or a similar stiff, flat-bladed object between the snaps and helmet shell to pry the cheek pads away from their snap attachment.
  - (4) If an air cell-padding system is present, deflate the air inflation system by releasing the air at the external port with an inflation needle or large-gauge hypodermic needle. The helmet should slide off the occiput with slight forward rotation of the helmet.
  - (5) In the event the helmet does not move, slight traction can be applied to the helmet, which can then be gently maneuvered anteriorly and posteriorly, although the head/neck unit must not be allowed to move.
  - (6) The helmet should not be spread apart by the ear holes, because this maneuver serves only to tighten the helmet on the forehead and occiput region.
- Removing the shoulder pads (Note: The Inter-Association Task Force recommends that shoulder pads be removed only in conjunction with the athlete's helmet and only when removal is warranted.)
  - (1) Cut jersey and all other shirts from the neck to waist and from the midline to the end of each arm sleeve.

(2) Cut all straps used to secure the shoulder pads to the torso. Attempts to unbuckle or unsnap any fasteners should be avoided because of the potential for unnecessary movement.

(3) Cut all straps used to secure the shoulder pads (and extenders) to the arms.

(4) Cut laces or straps over the sternum. A consistent manufactured characteristic of shoulder pads is the mechanism to attach the two halves of the shoulder pad unit on the anterior aspect. This lace or strap system allows for quick and efficient access to the anterior portion of the chest.

(5) Cut and/or remove any and all accessories such as neck rolls or collars, so they can be removed simultaneously with the shoulder pads. The shoulder pads can now be released with full access to chest, face, neck, and arms. The posterior portion of the shoulder pads helps to maintain spinal alignment when the helmet and shoulder pads are in place.

(6) A responder maintains cervical stabilization in a cephalad direction by placing her forearms on the athlete's chest while holding the maxilla and occiput. This is a skilled position that requires personnel who are practiced in this technique.

(7) With responders at each side of the athlete, their hands are placed directly against the skin in the thoracic region of the back.

(8) Additional support is placed at strategic locations down the body as deemed appropriate in consideration of the size of the athlete.

(9) While the athlete is lifted, the individual who was in charge of head/shoulder stabilization should remove the helmet and then immediately remove the shoulder pads by spreading apart the front panels and pulling them around the head.

(10) All shirts, jerseys, neck rolls, extenders, and so on should be removed at this time.

(11) The athlete is lowered to the starting position.

# CASE 3.5 Cervical Strain

3.5 / **1.** *Based on the information presented in the case, determine (a) the differential diagnoses and (b) the clinical diagnosis.*

a. Differential diagnoses: atlanto-axial injury and dysfunction, brachial plexus pathology, cervical disc pathology and radiculopathy, cervical facet syndrome, myofascial pain[19]

b. Clinical diagnosis: cervical strain

3.5 / **2.** *Based on the results of the physical examination in this case scenario, why would AROM be limited, but PROM be within functional limits?*

Active range of motion is designed to assess a patient's ability and willingness to move an injured extremity or joint through its available motion allowing a clinician to assess the quality and quantity of contractile tissue.[33] Passive range of motion, on the other hand, assesses the status of a patient's inert tissue, such as the joint capsule and ligaments. The primary structures involved in this case are muscular (SCM, anterior, middle, and posterior scalenes, and cervical extensors); therefore, Kyla presents with muscular weakness within the active contractile tissue that caused her pain and limited motion. However, pain may be noted at the end range of the movements opposite the involved muscles, because they are passively lengthened.

3.5 / **3.** *Overall, do you believe Josh adequately evaluated Kyla's condition given the provided information? If not, what would you have done differently as the evaluating clinician and why?*

The answers to this question will vary among students. Given the patient's history and physical examination, Josh completed a relatively thorough evaluation. He may have considered reflex testing of C5, C6, C7. Josh could have considered screening Kyla for a head injury because she was involved in a golf cart accident; however, this should have been ruled out at the ER. Conditions such as subdural hematoma do take a period of time to manifest, however, and may be considered as part of the differential diagnosis when there are obvious neurological deficits or changes.

3.5 / **4.** *(a) What other anatomical structures, if any, should Josh have palpated to help determine the clinical diagnosis? (b) When Josh noted cervical extension strength to be a 3/5, which structures were specifically being assessed? (c) Which structure(s) were specifically involved in the clinical diagnosis, and which other structures could have been traumatized?*

a. Josh should have also assessed the following structures, including but not limited to the thyroid cartilage, cricoid cartilage, trachea, SC joint, clavicle, first rib, suboccipital muscular structures, vertebral bodies and spinous processes, facet joints, trapezius, levator scapula, and others.

b. The primary movements occurring at the AOJ allow the cranium to move independently relative to the atlas, that is, nodding of the head (i.e., flexion and extension of the head on the cervical spine),[40] which accounts for about half of the total cervical ROM. The remaining ROM occurs in the lower cervical spine (in combination with the upper cervical spine) through a combined action of superficial and deep muscles working together bilaterally. The superficial layer is composed of the splenius cervicis and splenius capitis. Deep muscles include the iliocostalis cervicis, longissimus cervicis, spinalis cervicis, semispinalis cervicis, and rotators.

c. The primary structures involved in the clinical diagnosis were the SCM and cervical extensor muscle group. However, given the MOI, a longitudinal ligament (anterior and posterior) sprain, facet joint dislocation, cervical trauma (bony avulsion, compression, or subluxation), and TMJ trauma are all possible.[14]

3.5 / **5.** *Based on the clinical diagnosis presented in this case, describe the MOI and provide other examples of how the injury may occur.*

Given the information provided in the case study, the MOI could be classified as an acceleration-deceleration mechanism. Diving accidents can also cause this kind of "whiplash" injury[6] when the head is suddenly forced backward and forward. The concept of whiplash was introduced by Harold Crow in 1928 and was not seen in the literature until 1945.[36] The original description by Crow in 1928 defined *whiplash* "as the effects of sudden acceleration-deceleration forces on the neck and upper trunk due to external forces exerting a 'lash-like effect'."[29] Crow emphasized that term *whiplash* "describes only the manner in which a head was moved suddenly to produce a sprain in the neck." In many athletic training textbooks, the term *whiplash* is still commonly used to denote trauma sustained to the cervical ligaments.[9,26,33] However, in 1995 the Quebec Task Force on Whiplash Associated Disorders redefined *whiplash* to include: "Whiplash is an acceleration-deceleration mechanism of energy transfer to the neck which may result from rear-end or side impact, predominantly in motor vehicle collisions, but also from diving accidents, and from other mishaps. The energy transfer may result in bone or soft tissue injuries (whiplash injury) which in turn may lead to a wide variety of clinical manifestations (whiplash associated disorder)."[36] Whiplash injuries are often associated with regional neck pain and stiffness, headaches, and shoulder pain, which may become persistent and eventually be termed as chronic whiplash associated disorder (WAD).

Answers to the second half of the question will vary among students. However, in athletics, acceleration-deceleration injuries may occur in sports such as ice hockey and football, where an athlete is struck from behind, causing the head to forcefully move backward and forward. Although the force is not as great as those suffered by individuals in a motor vehicle accident, an abnormal rotation of the vertebra may result from lack of a posterior restraint to the head and neck.[39,41]

3.5 / **6.** *After completing the physical examination, Josh documented his findings electronically for Kyla's file. Using your athletic training room's computer tracking software, document your findings electronically as if you were the treating clinician. If the case did not provide information you believe is pertinent to the clinical diagnosis, please add this to your documentation. If you do not have access to injury-tracking software, consider downloading a trial version from CSMI Solutions (Sportsware) by going to www.csmisolutions.com/cmt/publish/service_software_dl.shtml and following the on-screen directions.*

Answers will vary. Students should consider writing a SOAP note (see textbook Appendix B) using the ABCD format when writing the short- and long-term goals.

## CASE 3.6 Cervical Sprain

3.6 / **1.** *Based on the information presented in the case, determine (a) the differential diagnoses and (b) the clinical diagnosis.*

a. Differential diagnoses: atlanto-axial injury and dysfunction, cervical disc pathology and radiculopathy, cervical facet syndrome, and cervical fracture/dislocation

b. Clinical diagnosis: cervical sprain, possible concomitant cervical strain

3.6 / **2.** *Overall do you believe Jared handled the situation correctly? Would you have handled it the same way?*

The answers to this question may vary among students; however, if in this situation an athlete were to present with point tenderness directly over the cervical spine and pain in AROM, the clinician should stop the physical examination. Cervical spine precautions should be taken immediately, and the athlete should be stabilized with an adequate airway, transported, and evaluated for possible cervical trauma (fractures, discolorations), and the like.[39]

3.6 / **3.** *Given the information presented in the case, there are two very possible clinical diagnoses that are very similar and present nearly identically. What are the diagnoses, and what would lead you to determine one clinical diagnosis over the other?*

Sprains to the cervical spine display many of the same signs of as a strain to the cervical spine. However, a cervical sprain may present with little pain initially, which gradually increases over time and remains symptomatic for a longer period of time. A patient with a cervical sprain will also present with more localized pain over the spinous and transverse processes.[26] The ROM will also be restricted and painful in the direction that stresses the injured ligament, while muscular structures are affected when moved into the opposite direction.

3.6 / **4.** *According to the case study, Tyler did not appear to perform any stress or special tests. (a) Why? (b) How can a clinician adequately assess and establish the clinical diagnosis?*

a. There are no specific ligamentous stress tests or special tests that are used to assess the general stability of the ligamentous structures supporting the cervical spine.

b. Magee[18] does provide several tests for assessing instability of the upper cervical spine (i.e., atlanto-axial articulation). The end range of PROM, in the absence of muscle tightness or contractions can provide clinicians with a general sense of the function of the cervical spine ligaments.[37] For example, passively moving the head into forward flexion places stress on the posterior longitudinal ligament, ligamentum nuchae, interspinous ligament, and ligamentum flavum. Passively moving the cervical spine into extension assesses the anterior longitudinal ligament, and passive rotation assesses the interspinous ligament and ligamentum flavum.

3.6 / **5.** *(a) How would you manage the injury? (b) What instructions would you have given the athlete for weekend management?*

a. Immediate, short-term management of a cervical sprain typically includes: RICE (rest, ice, compression, elevation) and, depending on the severity of the injury, a soft cervical collar to help reduce muscle spasm (P, for protection; added to acronym makes PRICE). Complete rest and avoidance of normal neck movement are not often recommended when dealing with a cervical sprain or strain, because prolonged rest and loss of movement can result in a "disuse syndrome,"[35] further promoting disuse atrophy and soft tissue tightness.[5,14] Instead, the athlete's activities should be modified (reduction in intensity and frequency of activity). More recently an "active" approach to patient care has been shown to be more beneficial in the management of pain and range of motion than complete rest and the use of soft cervical collars.[22,24,29–31] Other more conservative forms of treatment may include anti-inflammatory medicine to manage pain, electrical stimulation, and ultrasound.

b. Instructions to Jared could include icing his neck 15 to 20 minutes 2 to 3 times per day to assist with inflammation control and AROM as tolerated, to assist in preventing disuse, and to improve mobility. Tyler may want to instruct Jared to perform the active motion in a supine position to reduce the work of the cervical musculature while the muscles are no longer working to keep the head in an erect posture. Tyler may also want to give Jared instructions about when to seek medical attention if necessary.

3.5 / **6.** *If Jared's signs and symptoms progressed to the point where Tyler needed to initiate cervical spine mobilization techniques to treat the injury, (a) which screening test should Tyler employ to rule out any contraindicating pathologies, and (b) is this test really necessary?*

a. Tyler would probably use a vertebral artery test (cervical quadrant test). This test places the head and neck into extension and side flexion for a period of 30 seconds[18,25] and is often used to assess the relative risk of injury to the vertebral artery, particularly vertebrobasilar insufficiency, before performing any spinal manipulative therapy or mobilizations. This position causes compression/stretching of the arteries with the contralateral/ipsilateral cervical spine rotation occurring at the AAJ.[25] Positive findings may include dizziness, vertigo, nystagmus, light headedness, nausea, diplopia, and unilateral facial numbness.[43]

b. Recently, the diagnostic accuracy of the test has come into question. Ritcher and Reinking[28] examined the literature to determine the diagnostic accuracy of the test, particularly as it influences the teaching of the test, and concluded that "the strength of the evidence for VA testing is weak. In spite of the common clinical recommendations to use the VA test for VBI we found only one study that reported diagnostic accuracy for the test." Thiel and Rix[43] also believe that pre-manipulation of the cervical spine should not be performed and is unlikely to provide any useful additional diagnostic information.

# REFERENCES


1. Abbed KM, Coumans JCE. Cervical radiculopathy: pathophysiology, presentation, and clinical evaluation. *Neurosurgery.* 2007;60(Suppl 1):S-28–S-34.
2. American Red Cross. *Emergency Response.* Yardley, PA: Staywell; 2001.
3. Bailes JE, Petschauer M, Guskiewicz KM, Marano G. (2007). Management of cervical spine injuries in athletes. *J Athl Train.* 2007;42(1):126–134.
4. Bellace JV, Healy D, Besser MP, Byron T, Hohman L. Validity of the Dexter Evaluation System's Jamar dynamometer attachment for assessment of hand grip strength in a normal population. *J Hand Ther.* 2000;13(1):46–51.
5. Clark S. Organizing the approach to musculoskeletal misuse syndrome. *Nurse Pract.* 2001;26(7):11–25.
6. Day C, Stolz U, Mehan T, Smith G, McKenzie L. Diving-related injuries in children <20 years old treated in emergency departments in the United States: 1990–2006. *Pediatrics.* 2008;122:e388–e394.
7. Furman MB, Puttiliz KM, Pannullo R, Simon J. Spinal stenosis and neurogenic claudication [electronic version]. *eMedicine.* 2006. Available from: http://www.emedicine.com/pmr/TOPIC133.HTM. Accessed June 9, 2009.
8. Furman MB, Simson J, Puttlitz KM, Falco F. Cervical disc disease [electronic version]. *eMedicine.* 2009. Available from: http://www.emedicine.com/pmr/topic25.htm. Accessed June 6, 2009.
9. Gallaspy JB, May JD. *Signs and Symptoms of Athletic Injuries.* St. Louis, MO: Mosby; 1996.
10. Hildreth DH, Breidenbach WC, Lister GD, Hodges AD. Detection of submaximal effort by use of the rapid exchange grip. *J Hand Surg.* 1989;14(4):742–745.
11. Holdgate A, Ching N, Angonese L. Variability in agreement between physicians and nurses when measuring the Glasgow coma scale in the emergency department limits its clinical usefulness. *Emerg Med Australas.* 2006;18(4):379–384.
12. Houle P, McDonnell DE, Vender J. Traumatic atlanto-occipital dislocation in children. *Pediatr Neurosurg.* 2001;34:193–197.
13. Janda DH, Geiringer SR, Hankin FM, Barry DT. Objective evaluation of grip strength. *J Occup Med.* 1987;29(7): 569–571.
14. Jaye C. Managing whiplash injury. *Emerg Nurse.* 2004;12(7):28–33.
15. Kleiner DM, Almquist JL, Bailes J, Burrusss P, Feuer H, Griffin LY. Prehospital care of the spine-injured athlete: A document from the Inter-Association Task Force for Appropriate Care of the Spine-Injured Athlete. 2001;1–31. Retrieved from: http://www.nata.org/statements/index.htm. Accessed May 9, 2007.
16. Konin JG, Wiksten D, Isear JA, Brader H. *Special Tests for Orthopedic Examination* (3rd ed.). Thorofare, NJ: Slack; 2006.
17. Levangie PK, Norkin CC. *Joint Structure and Function: A Comprehensive Analysis.* Philadelphia, PA: FA Davis; 2001.
18. Magee DJ. *Orthopedic Physical Assessment* (5th ed.). Philadelphia, PA: WB Saunders; 2007.
19. Malanga GA, Mehnert MJ, Kim D. Cervical spine sprain/strain injuries [electronic version]. *eMedicine.* 2008. Available from: http://www.emedicine.com/sports/topic24.htm. Accessed June 4, 2009.
20. Mathiowetz V. Comparison of Rolyan and Jamar dynamometers for measuring grip strength. *Occup Ther Int.* 2002;9(3):201–209.
21. Mathiowetz V, Vizenor L, Melander D. Comparison of baseline instruments to the Jamar dynamometer and the B & L engineering pinch gauge. *Occup Ther J Res.* 2000;20:147–62.
22. McKinney L, Doman J, Ryan M. The role of physiotherapy in the management of acute neck sprains following road-traffic accidents. *Arch Emerg Med.* 1989;6:27–33.
23. McKenna DA, Roche CJ, Lee WK, Torreggiani WC, Duddalwar VA. Atlanto-occipital dislocation: case report and discussion. *Can J Emerg Med.* 2006;8(1):50–53.
24. Mealy K, Brennan H, Fenelon G. Early mobilization of acute whiplash injuries. *BMJ.* 1986;292:656–657.
25. Mitchell J, Keene D, Dyson C, Harvey L, Pruvey C, Phillips R. Is cervical spine rotation, as used in the standard vertebrobasilar insufficiency test, associated with a measureable change in intracranial vertebral artery blood flow? *Man Ther.* 2004;9(4):220–227.
26. Prentice WE. Arnheim's Principles of Athletic Training: A Competency-Based Approach (13th ed.). Boston, MA: McGraw Hill Publishing; 2009.
27. Rao R. Neck pain, cervical radiculopathy, and cervical myelopathy. *J Bone Joint Surg.* 2002b;84-A(10):1872–1881.
28. Richter RR, Reinking MF. Evidence in practice. How does evidence on the diagnostic accuracy of the vertebral artery test influence teaching of the test in a professional physical therapist education program? *Phys Ther.* 2005;85(6):589–599.
29. Rosenfeld M, Gunnarsson R, Borenstein P. Early intervention in whiplash-associated disorders: a comparison of two treatment protocols. *Spine.* 2000;25(5):1782–1787.
30. Rosenfeld M, Gunnarsson R, Borenstein P. Early intervention in whiplash-associated disorders: a comparison of two treatment protocols. *Spine.* 2001;25(4):1782–1787.
31. Rosenfeld M, Seferiadis A, Carlsson J, Gunnarsson R. Active intervention in patients with whiplash-associated disorders improves long-term prognosis: a randomized controlled clinical trial. *Spine.* 2003;22:2491–2498.
32. Rubinstein S, Pool J, Tulder M, Riphagen I, Vet H. A systematic review of the diagnostic accuracy of provocative tests of the neck for diagnosing cervical radiculopathy. *Eur Spine J.* 2007;16(3):307–319.
33. Schultz SJ, Houglum PA, Perrin DH. *Examination of Musculoskeletal Injuries* (2nd ed.). Champaign, IL: Human Kinetics; 2005.
34. Shah KC, Rajshekhar V. Reliability of diagnosis of soft cervical disc prolapse using Spurling's test. *Br J Neurosurg.* 2004;18(5):480–483.
35. Sizer Jr PS, Poorbaugh K, Phelps V. Whiplash associated disorders: pathomechanics, diagnosis, and management. *Pain Pract.* 2004;4(3):249–266.

36. Spitzer WO, Skovron ML, Salmi LR, Cassidy JD, Duranceau J, Suissa S. Scientific monograph of the Quebec Task Force on whiplash-associated disorders: redefining "whiplash" and its management. *Spine.* 1995;20(8 Suppl):1S–73S.

37. Starkey C, Ryan J. Evaluation of Orthopedic and Athletic Injuries (2nd ed.). Philadelphia, PA: FA Davis; 2002.

38. Swartz EE. Efficient football helmet face-mask removal. *Athl Ther Today.* 2007;12(2):21–24.

39. Swartz EE, Boden BP, Courson RW, Decoster LC, Horodyski M, Norkus S. National Athletic Trainers' Association Position Statement: acute management of the cervical spine–injured athlete. *J Athl Train.* 2009;44(3):306–311.

40. Swartz EE, Floyd RT, Cendoma M. Cervical spine functional anatomy and the biomechanics of injury due to compressive loading. *J Ath Train.* 2005;40(3):155–161.

41. Swartz EE, Nowak J, Shirley C, Decoster LC. A comparison of head movement during back boarding by motorized spine-board and log-roll techniques. *J Athl Train.* 2005;40(3):162–168.

42. Teasdale G, Jennett B. Assessment of coma and impaired consciousness. a practical scale. *Lancet.* 1974;2(7872):81–84.

43. Thiel H, Rix G. Is it time to stop functional pre-manipulation testing of the cervical spine? *Man Ther.* 2005;10(2):154–158.

44. Trojian TH, Vaca FE, Young O. Brachial plexus injury [electronic version]. *eMedicine.* 2006. Available from: http://www.emedicine.com/sports/topic13.htm. Accessed April 30, 2007.

45. Wiese MF. British hospitals and different versions of the Glasgow coma scale: telephone survey. *BMJ.* 2003;327(7418):782–783.

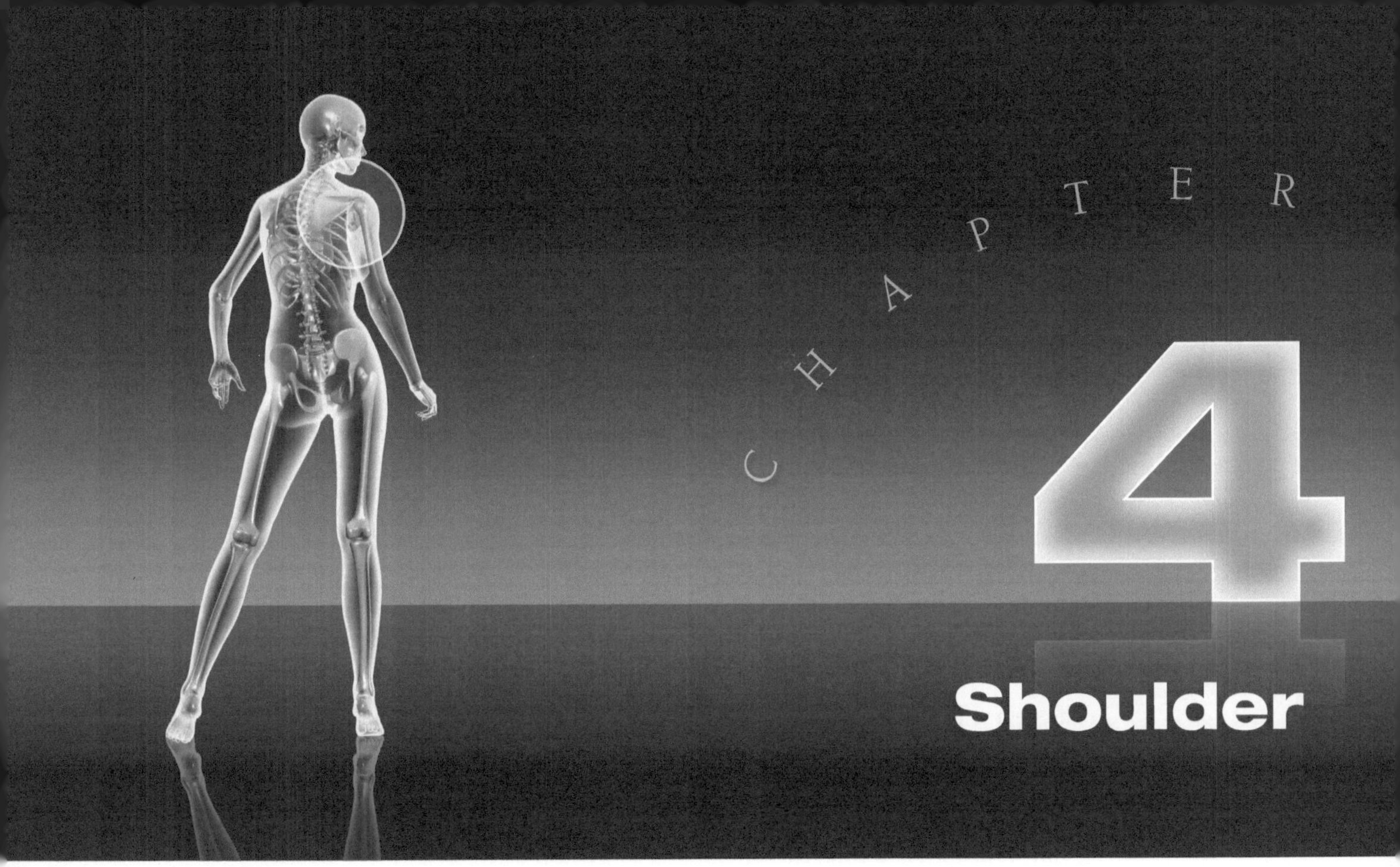

# Chapter 4 Shoulder

## QUICK REFERENCE

CASE 4.1
**Acromioclavicular Sprain/Separation**

CASE 4.2
**Sternoclavicular Sprain/Separation**

CASE 4.3
**Multi-Directional Shoulder Instability**

CASE 4.4
**Transverse Humeral Ligament Sprain, Concomitant Bicipital Subluxation**

CASE 4.5
**Bicipital Tendonitis/Strain**

CASE 4.6
**Rotator Cuff Strain with Possible Shoulder Impingement**

CASE 4.7
**Anterior Glenohumeral Dislocation**

CASE 4.8
**Distal Clavicle Fracture**

CASE 4.9
**Scapula Fracture**

CASE 4.10
**Axillary Nerve Injury**

CASE 4.11
**Long Thoracic Nerve Injury**

CASE 4.12
**Rotator Cuff Impingement**

CASE 4.13
**Subacromial Bursitis**

CASE 4.14
**Thoracic Outlet Syndrome**

# ANSWERS TO CASE QUESTIONS

## CASE 4.1 Acromioclavicular Sprain/Separation

4.1 / **1.** *Based on the information presented in the case, determine (a) the differential diagnoses and (b) the clinical diagnosis.*

a. Differential diagnoses: clavicular fracture, rotator cuff pathology, shoulder dislocation, labrum lesion, deltoid contusion[42]

b. Clinical diagnosis: AC joint sprain/separation

4.1 / **2.** *Based on the clinical diagnosis, describe the common grading scale used to quantify this injury.*

The degree of clavicular displacement depends on the severity of injury to the AC joint capsule, ligaments, and supporting muscles of the shoulder. Rockwood's classification quantifies AC joint injuries into six grades[38]:

- Grade or Type I: minor sprain of AC ligament, intact joint capsule, intact CC ligament, intact deltoid and trapezius
- Grade or Type II: rupture of AC ligament and joint capsule, sprain of CC ligament but CC intact, minimal detachment of deltoid and trapezius
- Grade or Type III: rupture of AC ligament, joint capsule, and CC ligament; clavicle elevated (up to 100% displacement); detachment of deltoid and trapezius
- Grade or Type IV: rupture of AC ligament, joint capsule, and CC ligament; clavicle displaced posteriorly into the trapezius; detachment of deltoid and trapezius
- Grade or Type V: rupture of AC ligament, joint capsule, and CC ligament; clavicle elevated (>100% displacement); detachment of deltoid and trapezius
- Grade or Type VI (rare): rupture of AC ligament, joint capsule, and CC ligament; clavicle displaced behind the tendons of the biceps and coracobrachialis

4.1 / **3.** *Based on the clinical diagnosis, identify the ligaments that may be affected and their location.*

Ligamentous structures that may be affected include the inferior and superior AC ligaments and the CC ligament, specifically the conoid and trapezoid. The AC ligaments arise from between the medial facet of the acromion process of the scapula and attach to the distal clavicle; the CC ligaments attach from the coracoid process of the scapula to the inferior surface of the clavicle.

4.1 / **4.** *What would be the appropriate short-term management plan for treating this type of injury?*

The most appropriate management plan for an acute AC joint injury includes applying a sling and swath to support the weight of the arm to lessen stress on the AC joint. Refer the athlete for diagnostic tests to rule out fractures and to determine the degree of displacement or laxity of the AC joint.[46]

4.1 / **5.** *Overall, do you believe Tony adequately evaluated Rob's condition given the information presented in the case? If not, what would you have done differently as the evaluating clinician?*

The answers to this question will vary among students. Given the MOI and initial presentation, Tony should have noted a step deformity and completed ligamentous stress testing to confirm the clinical diagnosis before referring him to a physician. Ligamentous stress testing to confirm an AC joint sprain includes the piano key sign, AC joint compression test, and AC joint distraction/traction test.[7,20,26,41]

- Step deformity: obvious displacement of the clavicle from the acromion, resulting in a gap or separation
- Piano key: pressing on the distal end of the clavicle that results in pushing the clavicle downward and springing back up when let go
- AC joint traction test: applying downward traction on the humerus, resulting in a step deformity or pain
- AC joint compression test: placing both hands on either side of the AC joint, squeezing together to compress the joint, causing pain or joint movement is a positive result

4.1 / **6.** *Based on the clinical diagnosis, what are some potential complications (short or long term) as a result of the injury?*

Potential complications of AC joint sprains are based on the severity of the MOI. These complications include: (1) wound abrasions or lacerations, (2) arthritis resulting from grade II or III separation, (3) development of thoracic outlet syndrome (TOS), (4) neurovascular alterations (i.e., paresthesia over the shoulder or upper arm, trapezius weakness), (5) brachial plexus injury,[39] and (6) subacromial space stenosis (SAS). Therefore, a complete examination of the shoulder joint is necessary even in the presence of an easily recognizable injury.

## CASE 4.2 Sternoclavicular Sprain/Separation

4.2 / **1.** *Based on the information presented in the case, determine (a) the differential diagnoses and (b) the clinical diagnosis.*

a. Differential diagnoses: clavicle fracture and dislocation, rib fracture, sternal fracture[39]

b. Clinical diagnosis: anterior sternoclavicular joint sprain/separation

4.2 / **2.** *Describe the classification of ligamentous injuries commonly associated with this type of injury.*

The degree of sternoclavicular displacement depends on the severity of injury to the SC joint capsule, ligaments, and supporting muscles of the shoulder. There are three types of SC joint injuries.

- Type 1: ligaments (anterior and posterior SC and interclavicular ligaments) are intact with the patient usually experiencing pain and swelling of the joint
- Type 2: rupture of the above ligaments with pain and swelling and anterior deformity
- Type 3: complete rupture of the above ligaments and joint dislocation and asymmetry. The head may also be titled to the affected side, and the patient will experience pain, swelling, and difficulty moving the arm of the affected side.[4]

4.2 / **3.** *The evaluating clinician should palpate several bony and soft tissue landmarks in order to determine the correct clinical diagnosis. Based on the clinical diagnosis above, identify the bony and soft tissue landmarks you should/would have palpated to guide the physical examination.*

The exact anatomical structures palpated will depend on the extent of the athlete's pain and apprehension. Given the information presented in the case, you would have been wise to palpate, at a minimum, the following bony structures: the jugular notch, the sternum, the SC joint, the clavicle, the acrominion process, and the AC joint (Figure A4.2.1).

FIGURE A4.2.1 Bony landmarks of the shoulder.

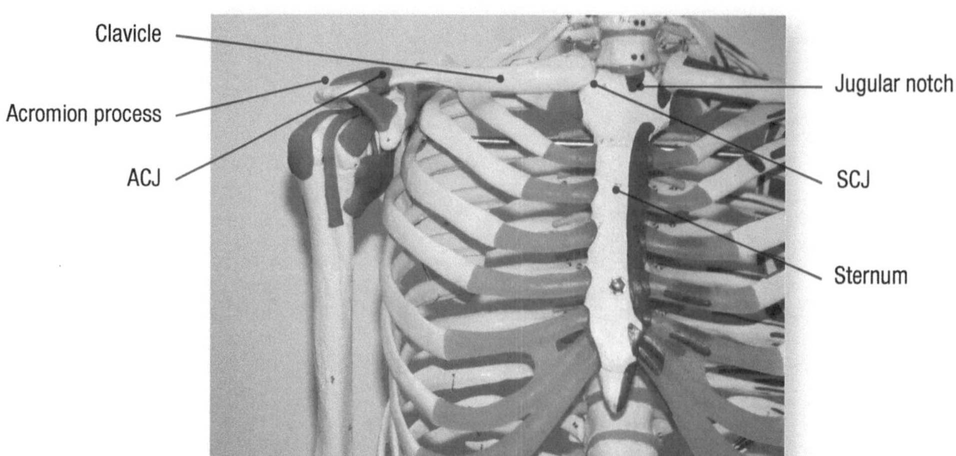

It would also be wise to palpate the following soft-tissue areas: the interclavicular, sternoclavicular, and costoclavicular ligaments, the pectoralis major and minor, the SCM, the scalene (anterior and middle), and the deltoid.

Instructors may wish to add additional structures based on their learned injury-evaluation approach.

4.2 / **4.** *If this injury were a posterior dislocation as opposed to an anterior one, the injury would be classified as a potential medical emergency. Why?*

A posterior SC joint dislocation can result in a life-threatening respiratory obstruction with dyspnea, particularly in younger patients.[4,26] This occurs because of trauma to the trachea as the clavicle moves in a posterior direction and places pressure on the structure. Many times, patients with a posterior dislocation can complain of neurovascular conditions in the upper extremity (numbness, weakness, lack of blood flow), difficulty breathing, or difficulty swallowing.[4,46] Other associated complications include haemopneumothorax, tracheal damage or rupture, laceration, damage to the larynx and superior vena cava, and occlusion of the subclavian artery and/or vein.[24,39]

4.2 / **5.** *As the evaluating clinician, describe how you would initially manage this injury?*

The answer to this question may vary among students. However, students should recognize the need to place the athlete in a sling or figure-8 harness. Medical referral is required to rule out potential life-threatening complications. The athlete should initially avoid exercises or movements that cause or increase pain. The application of cryotherapy and NSAIDs (assuming no contraindication) for pain and swelling will be warranted. If the patient has a Type 3 SC joint sprain, surgical intervention may be necessary.

## CASE 4.3 Multi-directional Shoulder Instability

4.3 / **1.** *Based on the information presented in the case, determine (a) the differential diagnoses and (b) the clinical diagnosis.*

a. Differential diagnoses: AC separation, supraspinatus/bicipital tendonitis, rotator cuff pathology, bursitis
b. Clinical diagnosis: multidirectional instability of the glenohumeral joint

4.3 / **2.** *Identify any other possible pathologies occurring secondary to this kind of injury.*

Because of general instability to the shoulder, a patient may also present with secondary injuries such as, but not limited to:

- Shoulder impingement and subacromial bursitis
- Rotator cuff tendonitis and impingement
- Labral tear, SLAP lesion
- Axillary nerve palsy
- Hill-Sachs or Bankart lesions as a result of shoulder instability

4.3 / **3.** *Figure 4.3.2 demonstrates a positive ligamentous stress test. What is the name of this test, and what important step is necessary to ensure a proper clinical decision?*

Textbook Figure 4.3.2 demonstrates a sulcus sign at 0°. To perform the test, the athlete is seated, with the arms resting in the lap, while the clinician stands with one hand grasping the subject's scapula (superiorly) and the other hand grasping the subject's elbow. Stabilizing the scapula, apply an inferior force with the hand grasping the elbow. A positive finding includes excessive inferior humeral head translation with a visible/palpable "sulcus" deformity inferior to the acromion.[20] When performing a sulcus sign, the scapula must be stabilized in order to allow the GH ligament to be appropriately stressed. The AC joint distraction test is performed similarly to the sulcus sign; however, distraction or downward movement of the scapula is necessary to assess the stability of the AC joint.

4.3 / **4.** *What other special tests could be used to make the clinical diagnosis?*

Numerous techniques, including tests for shoulder laxity and tests that reproduce some of the symptoms of GH joint laxity, can be used when assessing an unstable shoulder.[34] These tests include, but are not limited to:

- Load and shift test
- Protzman test for anterior instability
- Leffert's test
- Dugas' test
- Anterior and posterior drawer
- Feagin test
- Rowe test
- Neer impingement
- Hawkins-Kennedy impingement
- Relocation test
- Apprehension and Jobe's test

When assessing for multi-directional instability, it is recommend to begin with the sulcus sign, followed by a load and shift test, and then an O'Brien's test when possible.[30,31]

4.3 / **5.** *What management options would you use to treat this condition?*

Management options for this case include anti-inflammatory medication, strengthening of the scapulothoracic and rotator cuff muscles and deltoids, PNF patterns of the upper arm, avoiding overhead positions that cause pain, and surgical repair if the athlete does not respond to conservative rehabilitation.

4.3 / **6.** *After completing the physical examination, Kari documented her findings and sent a copy of the report over to the athletic administration office. Please document your findings as if you were the treating clinician. If the case did not provide information you believe is pertinent to the clinical diagnosis please feel free to add this information to your documentation.*

Answers will vary. Students should consider writing a SOAP note (see textbook Appendix B) using the ABCD format when writing the short- and long-term goals.

## CASE 4.4 Transverse Humeral Ligament Sprain, Concomitant Bicipital Subluxation

4.4 / **1.** *Based on the information presented in the case, determine (a) the differential diagnoses and (b) the clinical diagnosis.*

a. Differential diagnoses: impingement syndrome, rotator cuff strain, bicipital strain or tendonitis, pectoralis strain

b. Clinical diagnosis: transverse humeral ligament sprain with concomitant bicipital subluxation

4.4 / **2.** *What anatomical structures provide support for the long head of the biceps in the bicipital groove?*

The transverse humeral ligament, which extends from the lesser tuberosity to the greater tuberosity of the humerus, secures the long head of the biceps within the intertubercular (bicipital) groove. It can be noted that research has shown that the superficial collagen fibers of the subscapularis tendon transverse across the long head of the biceps and insert into the greater tuberosity. The deep fibers attach to the lesser tuberosity just medial to the long head of the biceps. Fibers within the floor of the groove create a "sling" around the biceps tendon.[14] The research also found no distinct structure as identifiable as the transverse humeral ligament.

4.4 / **3.** *Figure 4.4.2 demonstrates a positive special test performed on Manuel. (a) What is the name of this test, and (b) did it appear to be performed correctly?*

a. Figure 4.4.2 demonstrates the Speed's test. The Speed's test was originally designed to assess for pathology of the long head of the biceps, including tendonitis, muscular strain, and lesions related to the biceps/labral complex.[6] In Bennett's examination of the specificity of the Speed's test, he examined 46 shoulders in 45 patients. Results demonstrate that the Speed's test was positive in 40 shoulders when correlated with biceps/labral pathology by direct arthroscopic visualization; however, biceps/labral complex pathology was present in only 10 of these patients. Therefore, the calculated specificity was 13.8 percent and sensitivity 90 percent. Bennett concluded that the Speed's test was a nonspecific but sensitive test for macroscopic biceps/labral pathology.

b. The procedure in Figure 4.4.2 is in fact incorrect. Julie should have performed the test with Manuel's elbow extended, humerus elevated between 60° and 90°, and the forearm supinated, rather than pronated.

4.4 / **4.** *(a) What is the purpose of the Yergason's test? (b) Why is the hand of the examiner placed over the bicipital groove?*

a. Both the Yergason's and Speed's tests examine the integrity of the long head of the biceps and transverse humeral ligament as it relates to maintaining the long head of the biceps within the bicipital groove.

b. If you apply pressure with your fingers over the bicipital groove, you may feel a slight subluxing of the long head of the biceps. Also, by placing your thumb over the groove, you keep the long head in the groove, which may help decrease the discomfort. However, studies have questioned the extent of damage to the transverse humeral ligament by noting that many subluxations or dislocations of the long head of the biceps are a result of avulsion or tearing of the deep fibers of the subscapularis tendon, allowing the biceps to move out of the groove while the transverse humeral ligament appears intact. It has been postulated that the coracohumeral ligament and superior GH ligaments may be the main stabilizers against dislocations of the tendon of the long head of the biceps brachii.[44]

4.4 / **5.** *Why would performing a lat pull-down cause this type of injury?*

In most cases, when a patient uses an overhead pronated grip, the force of pulling down an object (in this case the weight of the machine) places stress on the anterior portion of the shoulder. The biceps tendon is being stretched from the origin on the glenoid to the insertion on the radius. This pressure pulls the tendon upward and forward, placing stress over the connective tissue that keeps it in the bicipital groove.

## CASE 4.5 Bicipital Tendonitis/Strain

4.5 / **1.** *Based on the information presented in the case, determine (a) the differential diagnoses and (b) the clinical diagnosis.*

a. Differential diagnoses: capsulitis, supraspinatus or infraspinatus tear, transverse humeral ligament rupture, biceps tendon rupture[49]

b. Clinical diagnosis: bicipital tendonitis/strain

4.5 / **2.** *Based on the physical examination, Alexis clearly forgot to perform ligamentous or special shoulder tests. List and describe at least three special tests you as the evaluating clinician may have performed in order to guide the physical examination. Explain why each test will assist in making the clinical diagnosis.*

Possible special tests include:

- Yergason's test: The elbow is placed at 90° of flexion and full pronation at the side of the patient's trunk. Resist the patient while she is performing supination and at the same time laterally rotating her shoulder. Place your fingers in the bicipital groove to feel for sensations such as popping or clicking. This test will examine the integrity of the transverse humeral ligament.[20,23]
- Speed's test: One method of performing this test is to apply a resistive force to shoulder flexion while the forearm is supinated. A second method is to place the shoulder in 90° flexion and complete forearm supination. The patient then resists against an extension movement, both supinated and pronated. Positive tests will reveal pain or tenderness in the bicipital groove. This test elicits a good response because the humerus slides along the tendon over a longer ROM than the Yergason's test.[6,20,23]
- Ludington's test: The patient places both hands over his head and interlocks his fingers together. Instruct the patient to contract and relax the biceps muscles while the examiner palpates the biceps tendon.[20,23] A positive finding for a longhead biceps tendon rupture is the inability to feel the muscle contraction.
- Gilchrest's sign: Have the patient lift a 2 to 3 kg weight overhead with the shoulder in lateral rotation. This places stress in and around the bicipital groove and tendon. The patient may experience a snapping or popping feeling, especially between 90° and 100° of abduction.[20,23]
- Lippman's test: The patient stands while you hold the patient's shoulder in 90° of flexion. With the examiner's other hand, the biceps tendon is located about 7 to 8 cm below the GH joint and moved back and forth. A positive finding is pain.

4.5 / **3.** *Besides forgetting the ligamentous and special tests to the shoulder, do you feel that Alexis assessed the injury adequately enough? If you were the evaluating clinician, what if anything would you add to the evaluation? What might you expect to find clinically?*

The answers to this question may vary among students. Given the results of the ROM testing in Table 4.5.1, it would appear that Alexis did not perform PROM testing. Had she performed the same passive tests as active tests in Table 4.5.1, she may have found minimal-to-no discomfort with shoulder flexion or abduction. However, when the biceps tendon is placed on stretch it would be likely that shoulder extension would have caused an increase in end-range pain.

4.5 / **4.** *Why does Alexis need to speak with Doreen's mother?*

Doreen is a minor. All injuries and illnesses need to be reported to a minor's parents or guardian. Had Doreen suffered a life-threatening injury, such as a pneumothorax, while playing tennis, then consent to treat the minor is implied; however, valid attempts to contact the parents or guardians need to be made.[1]

4.5 / **5.** *If you were the evaluating clinician, how would you rehabilitate this injury during the next month?*

Medical referral to an orthopedic physician, because of her age, is warranted to determine whether anti-inflammatory medication (NSAIDs) or any other therapeutic modality techniques (iontophoresis or phonophoresis) are necessary. Application of cryotherapy and rest from activity for several days are prudent measures to take. Functional exercises can include shoulder elevation and biceps curls, and eccentric actions of the above two exercises are suggested, along with massage (i.e., deep friction) of the shoulder and biceps muscles.

## CASE 4.6 Rotator Cuff Strain with Possible Shoulder Impingement

**4.6 / 1.** *Based on the information presented in the case, determine (a) the differential diagnoses and (b) the clinical diagnosis.*

a. Differential diagnoses: brachial plexus injury, cervical disc pathology, peripheral nerve injury (e.g., long thoracic nerve), subacrominal and/or bicipital bursitis, bicipital and/or supraspinatus tendonitis, subscapular weakness

b. Clinical diagnosis: rotator cuff strain with possible shoulder impingement

**4.6 / 2.** *Identify three to four additional history questions you may have asked in order to differentiate between the above condition and other shoulder pathologies.*

The answers will vary among students; however, they may include examples such as:

- What is your occupation?
- Do you remember a single traumatic event that caused your pain to worsen?
- Have you changed your work or recreational routine?
- When is your pain the worst: before, during, or after use of the shoulder?
- Do you have pain lifting overhead, such as when reaching into an overhead cabinet?
- What limitations or changes in activities of daily living have you noticed?

**4.6 / 3.** *Answer the following questions about the palpation portion of the physical examination: (a) What are the bony and soft tissue structures that should have been palpated as part of the physical examination? (b) Based on the clinical diagnosis, where would one expect the patient to be point tender? (c) When should the palpation portion of the physical examination be conducted?*

a. The bony structures are the acromion process, coracoid process, clavicle, bicipital groove, greater and lesser tuberosity, and spine of the scapula. The soft tissue structures are the deltoid, supraspinatus, infraspinatus, teres minor, biceps tendon, latissimus dorsi tendon, and subacromial bursa.

b. Tenderness is most probable over and around the acromion process, in the subacromial space, and at the insertion of the supraspinatus into the greater tuberosity.

c. Palpation usually follows a thorough history and visual inspection of the area. However, whenever palpation may produce an increase in pain that limits the ability to further examine the shoulder, the clinician may chose to perform this step near the end of the evaluation.[10]

**4.6 / 4.** *What type of functional active ROM testing could a clinician perform to determine an overall sense of the patient's shoulder function? Describe the test and what motions the test assesses.*

To get a general sense of patient's functional ROM, three variations of the Apley's scratch test could be performed (Figure A4.6.1). To perform the exam, instruct the patient to: (1) touch the opposite shoulder bilaterally, (2) reach overhead and reach behind the neck bilaterally, and (3) reach to the small of the low back and then reach up as far as possible bilaterally.[20] Positive findings in position 1 are indicative of limited GH adduction, internal rotation, and horizontal flexion. Positive findings in position 2 are indicative of limited GH abduction, external rotation, scapular upward rotation, and elevation.

FIGURE A4.6.1 Apley's scratch test.

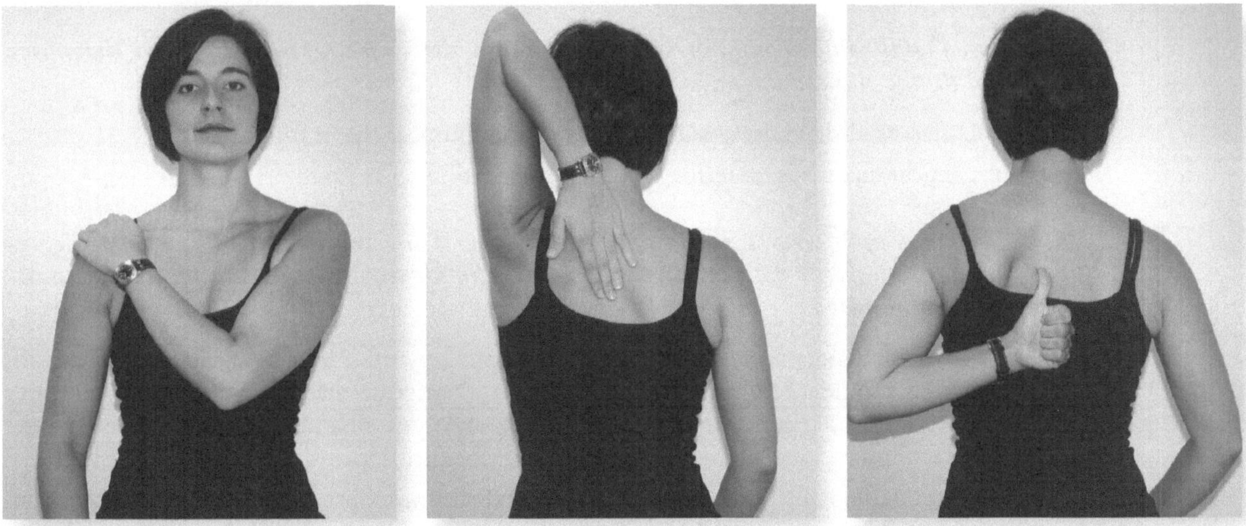

Position 1 Position 2 Position 3

Positive findings in position 3 are indicative of limited GH adduction, internal rotation, scapular retraction, and downward rotation.

4.6 / **5.** *Identify a second special test other than the commonly used empty can test that a clinician may use to identify the specific rotator cuff pathology in this case. What makes this test useful for clinicians?*

Another test used to evaluate the shoulder could be the drop arm test. The subject is placed in a seated or standing position. The clinician passively abducts the involved shoulder to 90° and then instructs the patient to slowly lower the arm to the side. A positive finding occurs when the patient is unable to slowly return the arm to the side and/or has significant pain when attempting to perform the task.[20] When the drop arm test is used in conjunction with the painful arc sign and infraspinatus muscle test, there is a 91 percent probability of detecting full thickness rotator cuff tears.[33]

4.6 / **6.** *When trauma occurs to the involved structure, as in this case, it may result in two types of tears: partial thickness and full thickness. (a) Identify the difference between the two types. (b) Compare and contrast the signs and symptoms using an evidenced-based approach that allows a clinician to discriminate between the two conditions during a clinical evaluation.*

a. Partial-thickness tears are short, longitudinal lesions that develop in the superficial or mid-substance of the tendon. A full-thickness tear is a complete tear of the tendon and may result from partial-thickness tears that are left untreated or from a single traumatic event.[46]

b. Students should prepare a comparison chart that examines the differences between partial and full thickness rotator cuff tears. Some of the criteria used may include: (1) history, onset, and mechanism of injury; (2) observation; (3) active, passive, and resistive movements; (4) special test (including sensitivity and specificity); (5) diagnostic imagining.

## CASE 4.7 Anterior Glenohumeral Dislocation

4.7 / **1.** *Based on the information presented in the case, determine (a) the differential diagnoses and (b) the clinical diagnosis.*

a. Differential diagnoses: AC joint separation, humeral head fracture

b. Clinical diagnosis: anterior GH joint dislocation

4.7 / **2.** *The injury in this case scenario can occur in several directions. (a) Identify the most common directions for the clinical diagnosis, and (b) identify which anatomical structures are compromised.*

a. Anterior dislocations account for approximately 90–98% of all acute dislocations to the shoulder,[5] followed by posterior and inferior dislocations. In fact, anterior dislocations account for approximately 90–98% of all acute dislocations seen in the ER, followed by posterior (3%)[45] and inferior dislocations (.5%).[22]

b. Anterior GH dislocation from forced abduction, external rotation, and extension[3] moves the head of the humerus forward and inferior to the glenoid fossa, resting approximately at or under the coracoid process and resulting in medical complications.[47] In an anterior dislocation, the anterior capsule can be torn. The glenoid labrum can be torn, predisposing the athlete to more recurrent dislocations (does not heal adequately and comprises the integrity of the shoulder joint). The greater tuberosity can also be fractured. Stretching or compressing the axillary nerve (if the humeral head lies in the quadrangular space) can occur. Musculocutaneous and median nerves can be compromised. Possible rotator cuff tear, Hill-Sachs lesion, and biceps tendon pathology can also occur. Posterior dislocations (1%–2% of all shoulder dislocations) occur when the arm is forced backward while it is in a flexed position. The head of the humerus can be felt at the posterior deltoid region, and the deltoid could be flat. The coracoid process may be more prominent. In most instances, the shoulder may appear to look normal. The athlete may experience pain when moving the extremity medially and decreased lateral rotation and elevation range of motion.

4.7 / **3.** *What is the proper short-term management of this injury?*

To manage an anterior GH dislocation, begin by removing/cutting clothing away from the injury site, being careful not to move or cause further pain or damage. Initial immobilization of a shoulder dislocation should be accomplished with a soft splint and a sling and swathe or the clinician's splint of choice. A sling/swathe immobilization is probably the method of choice for most athletic trainers. Place ice around the injury to help control pain and swelling. Refer to appropriate medical personnel for diagnostic imaging to rule out fractures of the humerus or glenoid.

If you are experienced in reducing shoulders and have been APPROVED by medical oversight, apply gentle pressure internally and externally with distraction, if there are no apparent neurological implications (be careful to avoid damaging the axillary nerve).[48] Linear traction will allow the humeral head to clear the anterior and inferior portion of the glenoid fossa to aid in reduction and most likely will not exacerbate a proximal humerus fracture.[3] The athlete may try a reduction herself by sitting on the ground and interlocking the fingers around the knee, applying a steady linear force by leaning backward and extending the hip.[2]

Note that the axillary nerve is most commonly affected with anterior shoulder dislocation and results in loss of sensation over the lateral upper arm and muscle function of the deltoid.[5] Damage to the axillary artery is also possible if the joint spontaneously reduces or has been reduced incorrectly. Because of the risk of neurovascular damage, it is recommended the athlete be stabilized and immediately transported to the nearest medical facility.

4.7 / **4.** *Explain why the structural integrity of the joint predisposes athletes to this injury.*

The GH joint is a ball-and-socket joint, allowing increased mobility of the shoulder in all directions and planes. The humeral head articulates with the glenoid fossa and is secured by the GH ligament and a thick but weak capsule that blends with the muscles of the rotator cuff and is reinforced by the coracohumeral ligament. Joint stability is increased through the glenoid labrum, by doubling the joint's articular surface area.[25,27] Dynamic stability of the humeral head within the glenoid fossa, particularly in the mid-range, is provided by the supraspinatus, infraspinatus, teres minor, and subscapularis (rotator-cuff) muscles. In fact, dynamic EMG studies have shown that the rotator cuff works in a combined synergistic action to create a compressive force at the GH joint during shoulder movement to provide joint stability.[18,21]

4.7 / **5.** *Kyla provided basic first-aid care on the field. What are some basic rehabilitation strategies or techniques a clinician may use for this injury?*

The strategies or techniques that a clinician may use to manage anterior GH dislocation vary depending on the stage.

- Initial stage: ice, rest, sling for approximately five to ten days, NSAIDs for pain and swelling; isometric exercises of the rotator cuff, biceps, and scapular muscles; ROM exercises; avoidance of abduction and forward flexion above 90°
- Intermediate stage: therapeutic modalities including ice, electrical stimulation, diathermies, and ultrasound as swelling subsides; isotonic exercises for the rotator cuff muscles, biceps, deltoid, and other scapular muscles; ROM exercises such as Codman's, with or without equipment to hold during the movements; stretching of the muscles of the shoulder
- Advanced stage: increase strengthening exercises with tubing, dumbbells, and weight machines for the shoulder muscles; PNF patterns, catching and throwing exercises with a ball, functional exercises based on sport requirements; upper body plyometrics; closed kinetic chain exercises

4.7 / **6.** *If you were the evaluating clinician in this case, how would you determine if the athlete is ready to return to competition?*

The answers to this question may vary among students. Generally, an athlete who is ready to return to play should meet the following criteria:

- Full shoulder ROM with no pain
- Equal and bilateral strength in all shoulder muscles
- Overhead shoulder motion activities with no pain
- No neurological abnormalities of the affected side
- Consider the use of shoulder bracing to reduce the likelihood of reinjury

## CASE 4.8 Distal Clavicle Fracture

4.8 / **1.** *Based on the information presented in the case, determine (a) the differential diagnoses and (b) the clinical diagnosis.*

a. Differential diagnoses: AC joint sprain, SC joint sprain, GH joint dislocation, humerus fracture, rotator cuff pathology, and rib fracture[8]

b. Clinical diagnosis: distal clavicle fracture

4.8 / **2.** *Based on the information presented in the case, what should Jon do next?*

Jon should begin to stabilize the shoulder and affected arm while another individual contacts EMS. Because it appears that Paul has a fractured clavicle, Jon should use a sling to stabilize the involved shoulder, using either a commercial or improvised sling. After applying the sling, Jon would need to assess the distal pulse and check for any abnormal sensations or movement. If normal, Jon would apply a swath to support the arm against the body and alleviate the effects of gravity and arm weight to be more comfortable for Paul. After stabilizing the injured site, Jon would wait for the EMS and transport Paul to the appropriate medical facility for treatment, monitoring Paul's airway, breathing, and circulation.

4.8 / **3.** *Jon asked a couple of history questions to guide his physical examination. Based on the clinical diagnosis above, identify three to five additional history questions you may have asked as the evaluating clinician.*

These answers will vary among students, but there are some specific questions or requests that could have helped guide the physical examination:

- Describe the onset of pain.
- Were there any unusual sounds or sensations?
- Do you have any neck or arm pain?
- Tell me more about your previous history of injury.

4.8 / **4.** *Jon identified several signs and symptoms related to the injury. If you were the evaluating clinician what other signs and symptoms associated with the injury would you be looking to identify?*

The answers will vary among students. Common signs and symptoms for a clavicle fracture include pain, point tenderness at the fracture site, limited ROM mostly because of pain and possible malalignment of the structures, loss of sensation from disruption of the brachial plexus, and diminished pulse if the subclavian artery is occluded. In the case of a distal fracture, skin bulging over fracture site (acromion) is typical; a middle fracture causes the athlete to splint the affected limb against the body to immobilize joint; and a proximal fracture results in the affected shoulder presenting in a downward and slightly forward position.[13]

4.8 / **5.** *Overall, do you believe Jon adequately evaluated Paul's condition, considering the information provided? If not, what would you have done differently as the evaluating clinician?*

The answers to this question will vary among students. Students should note that even in light of the athlete's history and physical exam, Jon did not assess Paul's neurovascular status. If a clavicle fracture is suspected, clinicians need to carefully manage the injury to limit secondary damage to the neurovascular structures (i.e., the brachial plexus) posterior to the clavicle.[27] Early immobilization and referral to appropriate medical personnel also assists in limiting secondary trauma such as a posterior displacement of the clavicle against the trachea and pneumothorax and subclavian artery and vein injury, internal jugular vein injury, and axillary artery injury.

# CASE 4.9 Scapula Fracture

4.9 / **1.** *Based on the information presented in the case, determine (a) the differential diagnoses and (b) the clinical diagnosis.*

a. Differential diagnoses: rotator cuff tendonitis, impingement syndrome, labral tear, shoulder dislocation

b. Clinical diagnosis: scapula fracture

4.9 / **2.** *If you were the evaluating clinician, what would lead you to the clinical diagnosis?*

A scapula fracture would probably not be top on the list, because these injuries usually require high-energy trauma. While direct trauma can lead to fractures of the scapula, the force required is usually related to motor-vehicle accidents or falls from a height. The amount of force generated by a collision in the sport of football, combined with shoulder padding protection, generally makes a fracture to the scapula a rarity. Rotator cuff strain, or a complete tear, would be the most common injury and should be suspected first. However, in this case, because of the significant pain and disability present in and around the shoulder, the team physician is likely to order an x-ray. Often the definitive diagnosis cannot be made until the fracture is seen on plain films.

4.9 / **3.** *After reviewing the X-ray with the team physician, the clinical diagnosis is clear. What are the common types/locations and the mechanisms of injury associated with this injury?*

The common types/locations and mechanisms of injury include:[43]

- Spine, usually a direct blow over the area
- Body, usually a direct blow over the area
- Acromion process, usually a direct blow, or fall on the point of the shoulder
- Glenoid neck, an anterior or posterior direct force to the shoulder; usually associated with fracture or dislocation of the humerus; if displaced, risk of nonunion, malunion, or chronic arthritis
- Glenoid, may be a direct blow, a fall on an out-stretched hand, or associated with GH dislocation; subtyped, requiring referral to an orthopedic surgeon
- Coracoid process; may be direct trauma to the coracoid process or a violent contraction of the coracobrachialis

4.9 / **4.** *What is/are the treatment options for the clinical diagnosis?*

In general the scapula is covered with large, strong muscles that support and otherwise stabilize it. Fractures involving the glenoid can affect shoulder function. Fractures involving the spine or body should be immobilized for two weeks using a sling for comfort.

Introduce early ROM at two weeks as tolerated. With acromion process fractures ROM can be initiated early if the fracture is non-displaced. An Open Reduction Internal Fixation (ORIF) is necessary if the scapula is displaced and/or the scapula and clavicle are injured. Fractures to the glenoid neck do well with early mobilization and may progress as tolerated if non-displaced, but glenoid fractures require immobilization and consultation with an orthopedic surgeon.

4.9 / **5.** *Given the clinical diagnosis, when can the athlete return to play?*

Working in conjunction with the physician, the athlete may normally return to play within six to eight weeks. Once no sling or bracing is necessary, the athlete can begin ROM as tolerated. The team physician may choose to repeat x-rays at two weeks. If healing has begun, rotator cuff strengthening can begin. The athlete may return when pain-free ROM is returned and strength is 90 percent of the uninvolved arm.

## CASE 4.10 Axillary Nerve Injury

4.10 / **1.** *Based on the information presented in the case, determine (a) the differential diagnoses and (b) the clinical diagnosis.*

a. Differential diagnoses: deltoid contusion/strain, humeral head fracture, brachial plexus pathology

b. Clinical diagnosis: axillary nerve injury

4.10 / **2.** *How does a blunt trauma cause this type of injury? Is there another MOI that a clinician should be aware of?*

a. A blunt trauma from being hit by an external piece of equipment (e.g., helmet, shoulder pads) or from direct contact can cause a compression of the axillary nerve between the humerus and external forces.[35,36]

b. Trauma caused by a shoulder dislocation can cause the axillary nerve to stretch over the humeral head and occurs 19%–55% of the time with anterior shoulder dislocation.[9,51]

4.10 / **3.** *Describe the anatomical landmarks as the structure involved in the injury traverses through the shoulder area.*

The axillary nerve originates at the C5 and C6 levels from the posterior cord of the brachial plexus. The axillary nerve is found lateral to the radial nerve and posterior to the axillary artery. It travels just below the coracoid process and through the quadrilateral space. The nerve then travels around the posterolateral humeral neck and branches into an anterior and posterior portion.

4.10 / **4.** *Based on the findings of the physical examination, ligamentous testing was WNL. What other special or neurological tests may be used to help differentiate this condition?*

The answers to this question will vary among students. Some suggestions about how to rule out differential diagnoses include:

- Assessment of vascular signs/symptoms, including: examination of skin color and temperature, capillary refill, and heaviness of the arm.
- Assessment of dermatomes and myotomes of the upper extremity as compared with the unaffected side.
- Special tests to rule out compromises to the neurovascular structures, including: Adson's test for thoracic outlet syndrome of the medial cord of the brachial plexus and subclavian artery and vein, Allen test for compression of the brachial plexus from pectoralis minor tightness/pathology, and costoclavicular test indicating subclavian artery blockage from costoclavicular structures.

4.10 / **5.** *If Sadie had been a male, would anything need to change in the clinical evaluation?*

Yes, it would not be wise for Samuel to bring Samantha, a minor, to a private location without another adult present. Even Sadie's actions could be questionable, considering that she asked Samantha to remove her shirt.

# CASE 4.11 Long Thoracic Nerve Injury

4.11 / **1.** *Based on the information presented in the case, determine (a) the differential diagnoses and (b) the clinical diagnosis.*

a. Differential diagnoses: cervical disk pathology, brachial plexus pathology, rotator cuff pathology, GH joint instability, thoracic outlet syndrome

b. Clinical diagnosis: long thoracic nerve injury

4.11 / **2.** *How does the injury in this case occur with repetitive use?*

Injury to the long thoracic nerve usually occurs from a traction (stretch) of the long thoracic nerve when the head is tilted away from the affected side and the arms are overhead.[15] Traction also may occur to the nerve when the shoulder is depressed and the neck is bent. Direct contact or compression can also cause the nerve to be damaged. Anatomical locations for a compression injury are: (1) within the scalene muscle and superior aspect of the serratus anterior,[40] (2) approximately one inch proximal to the first rib, and (3) between the second rib and the clavicle or coracoid process.[11,12,16]

4.11 / **3.** *What other sports or activities may predispose the athlete to this injury?*

Overhead sports/activities, such as baseball, softball, tennis, archery, golf, or gymnastics, and contact sports, such as football, ice hockey, and rugby, can make an athlete susceptible to the development of a long thoracic nerve injury.

4.11 / **4.** *Describe the anatomical landmarks associated with the clinical diagnosis as the structure traverses through the shoulder region.*

The long thoracic nerve arises from the C5 through C7 nerve roots and passes through the scalenus muscle (middle portion). The nerve then passes below the clavicle and under the first or second rib. It travels along the chest wall of the serratus anterior muscle. The entire length of the long thoracic nerve is approximately 22 to 24 cm.[12,19]

4.11 / **5.** *Identify the myotomes an athletic trainer should assess to accurately determine the clinical diagnosis.*

The answers will vary among students because several muscles and muscle actions can be assessed. The following are the ones we have chosen to represent:

- C4: resisted scapular elevation, assesses scapular elevators (trapezius, levator scapulae)
- C5: resisted shoulder abduction, assesses middle deltoid, supraspinatus and infraspinatus, teres minor
- C6: resisted elbow flexion and wrist extension, assesses biceps brachii, brachialis, brachioradialis, extensor carpi radialis longus and brevis, extensor digitorum communis, extensor digiti minimi, extensor carpi ulnaris
- C7: resisted elbow extension and wrist flexion, assesses triceps, anconeus, pronator teres, flexor carpi radialis, palmaris longus, flexor digitorum superficialis
- C8: resisted thumb extension and ulnar deviation, assesses flexor pollicis longus and brevis, extensor carpi ulnaris, flexor carpi ulnaris
- T1: resisted finger abduction/adduction, assesses abductor pollicis brevis, abductor digiti minimi, and dorsal interossei

4.11 / **6.** *Identify the dermatomes an athletic trainer should assess to accurately determine the clinical diagnosis.*

The answers will vary among students because dermatome patterns vary slightly among authors. The following are the ones we have chosen to represent:

- C4: back of neck, side of neck to clavicle and over to acromion
- C5: deltoid patch, lateral upper arm
- C6: lateral forearm, radial side of hand, first and second phalanges
- C7: posterior lateral arm and forearm, third phalange
- C8: medial forearm, ulnar border of hand, fourth and fifth phalanges
- T1: medial elbow, arm
- T2: inner side of axilla, pectoral
- T3: axilla (underneath)
- T4: upper chest from axilla to sternum
- T5: upper chest from axilla to sternum about 1 inch from nipple line
- T6: axilla to sternum just above or over nipple line

4.11 / **7.** *What are some special tests available to an athletic trainer to help with the differential diagnoses?*

- Neurological signs/symptoms: examine for numbness, tingling, or paresthesia of arm, hands, and fingers
- Adson's test: assesses for thoracic outlet syndrome of the medial cord of the brachial plexus and the subclavian artery and vein
- Allen test: compresses the brachial plexus via pectoralis minor tightness/pathology
- Costoclavicular test: indicates subclavian artery blockage from costoclavicular structures
- Scapula protraction test: causes winging of the scapula if the long thoracic nerve is involved

## CASE 4.12 Rotator Cuff Impingement

4.12 / **1.** *Based on the information presented in the case, determine (a) the differential diagnoses and (b) the clinical diagnosis.*

a. Differential diagnoses: bicipital tendonitis, labral tear, GH joint laxity, rotator cuff strain

b. Clinical diagnosis: rotator cuff impingement

4.12 / **2.** *Figure 4.12.2 demonstrates a positive special test. What is the name of this test? Why did only this test reveal discomfort and not the Neer test?*

a. Figure 4.12.2 demonstrates a Hawkins-Kennedy impingement test.

b. While both the Hawkins-Kennedy and Neer tests are used for diagnosing shoulder impingement, research through MRI testing has shown in eight normal subjects that the Hawkins-Kennedy produces contact of either the supraspinatus or infraspinatus against the subacromion space and is more sensitive for indentifying rotator cuff impingement than the Neer test.[32]

4.12 / **3.** *As the evaluating clinician, what other concerns or issues should you be concerned about? Identify some of the main causes of this injury.*

The answers to this question will vary among students. They should recognize that rotator cuff impingement is a syndrome. Syndromes are a collection of signs and symptoms that characterize a specific disease or condition in a patient. In this case, a variety of intrinsic and extrinsic factors need to be considered in primary and secondary impingement. These include:

- Primary impingement, intrinsic causes
  - i. Narrowing of the subacromial space
  - ii. Rotator cuff degeneration
  - iii. Subacromial bursitis
  - iv. Long head of biceps inflammation
- Primary impingement, extrinsic causes (acromion morphology)
  - i. Type 1 (flat)
  - ii. Type II (curved)
  - iii. Type III (hooked)
- Secondary impingement caused by
  - i. Glenohumeral instability
  - ii. SLAP lesions
  - iii. Posterior capsule tightness

4.12 / **4.** *Describe the stages of Neer's classification system used in the clinical diagnosis.*

Neer describes three stages of rotator cuff impingement.[29] They include the following:

- Stage 1: acute bursitis and edema, point tenderness around the greater tuberosity and anterior edge of the acromion, painful arc (abduction) between 60° and 120° of abduction

- Stage 2: presents with same signs and symptoms as Stage 1 with cuff tendonitis, thickening or fibrosis of subacromial bursa, rotator cuff partial thickness tear, possible clicking or catching while lowering the arm from 100° of abduction
- Stage 3: presents as a bone spur and/or tendon rupture, long head of biceps lesions

4.12 / **5.** *What rehabilitation techniques are indicated for Rosa?*

Rehabilitation options for Rosa should include:[28]

- Pain and inflammatory reduction
- Posterior capsule joint mobilizations
- Posterior cuff stretching
- GH and scapular muscle strengthening exercises
  - i. Push-ups
  - ii. Shoulder shrugs (scapula elevation)
  - iii. Biceps curls
  - iv. Shoulder flexion, external rotation
  - v. Rowing
  - vi. Functional exercises (this would be based on sport)

4.12 / **6.** *Clearly, Marge has placed herself in a difficult position by initially agreeing not to share the results of her physical examination with the coach. If you were the evaluating clinician, how would you have handled this situation? Would you have agreed to keep the information quiet?*

The answers will vary among students. This is a difficult situation and one that many athletic trainers will find themselves in. Ethically, Marge is bound to respect the rights of the athlete's confidentiality. To breach an athlete's confidentiality breaks the bonds between both parties and may jeopardize the establishment of further bonds. The coach, however, may need to be aware of her athlete's condition to make appropriate personnel decisions. There are typically three reasons to breach the rule of confidentiality, and these include: (1) when the athlete is in clear and imminent danger, (2) when other person(s) are in clear and imminent danger, or (3) when legal requirements demand the release of confidential information.[37] Marge should not have agreed to keep the information between her and Rosa. Refer to your University/College's policy and procedure manual to determine what action would be the most appropriate.

## CASE 4.13 Subacromial Bursitis

4.13 / **1.** *Based on the information presented in the physical examination, determine (a) the differential diagnoses and (b) the clinical diagnosis.*

a. Differential diagnoses: shoulder impingement, degenerative joint disease of the distal AC joint, rotator cuff tendonitis, labral tear

b. Clinical diagnosis: subacromial bursitis

4.13 / **2.** *How did you arrive at the clinical diagnosis?*

The history of increased shoulder activity and pain with overhead activities, insidious pain, and no previous shoulder pathology are consistent with subacromial bursitis. The physical examination reveals no obvious rotator cuff weakness or findings of shoulder instability. However, the physical examination does reveal palpable crepitus over the bursa of the right shoulder.

4.13 / **3.** *Impingement syndrome can lead to many of the same shoulder pain symptoms as the clinical diagnosis. How can you, as a practicing clinician working in conjunction with a physician, make an accurate diagnosis?*

Generally, bursitis is a diagnosis of exclusion. Impingement syndrome can have several causes. The most common in an older population is hypertrophy of the distal clavicle. Younger patients may have a down sloping acromion. Overuse of the rotator cuff can lead to a functional impingement. Over time, impingement can lead to calcifications in and along the tendons, or calcific tendinosis. Further work-up with plain x-rays can identify and rule out many primary causes of impingement. Shoulder bursitis and impingement often respond well to injection. For this reason, early referral to a physician can be very beneficial.

4.13 / **4.** *Why is treatment in the form of rest, oral medication, therapeutic modalities, and possibly even a shoulder injection so important?*

This is an overuse injury. As the pain and symptoms progress, throwing mechanics can change and other structures like the rotator cuff, biceps tendon, and labrum can become injured. Throwers will often notice a decrease in performance in terms of velocity earlier than the coach or athletic trainer and should report these changes immediately to the medical staff. It should also be noted that even lower-extremity injuries or core weakness can lead to significant changes in throwing mechanics. Therefore, an athletic trainer should evaluate the athlete for other injuries and core weakness.

## CASE 4.14 Thoracic Outlet Syndrome

**4.14 / 1.** *Based on the information presented in the case, determine (a) the differential diagnoses and (b) the clinical diagnosis.*

a. Differential diagnoses: cervical nerve root impingement, nerve impingement, upper extremity DVT, fourth rib dysfunction

b. Clinical diagnosis: thoracic outlet syndrome

**4.14 / 2.** *Based on the information presented in the case, explain how you determined the clinical diagnosis.*

Thoracic outlet syndrome can be associated with various nerve impingement syndromes, and a complete neurological examination of the upper extremity, including sensation, motor, and reflex testing, should help identify the specific nerve(s) involved.[17] The absence of symptoms with Spurling's test makes it less likely that this is a nerve root injury. Since nerve root injuries are common, this should be ruled out first. Usually with an upper extremity DVT, there will be a history of trauma or overuse throwing. Swelling is almost always present and obvious. Shoulder dislocations are often associated with directional apprehension upon physical examination. Fourth rib dysfunction will be associated with abnormal rib motion upon inspiration and/or expiration.

**4.14 / 3.** *Explain at least three different physical examination maneuvers that may help an evaluating clinician determine the clinical diagnosis.*

Possible physical examination maneuvers include:

- Adson's test: Palpate the radial pulse, and monitor for any changes as the athlete extends and rotates his head to the same side (as if looking over his shoulder). As he is extending his neck and rotating his head, extend and externally rotate the involved shoulder (keeping the elbow near extension). Ask the athlete to take and hold a deep breath. Continue palpating the radial pulse. A positive finding occurs when the pulse diminishes or becomes absent or neurological symptoms are reproduced[41] secondary to compression of the neurovascular bundle by the scalene muscles.
- Costoclavicular maneuver (military brace test or position, costoclavicular syndrome test, Eden's test): The athletic trainer locates the radial pulse and draws the athlete's shoulder down and back into extension with the elbow extended. The athlete lifts his chest into an exaggerated "chest out or military stance" position as the shoulder is put into hyperextension with lateral rotation. The athlete is instructed to rotate the head and neck to the contralateral side[41] or hyperextend the neck and head.[46] A positive test is indicated by a diminished or absent radial pulse as the neurovascular bundle is compressed between the first rib and clavicle.
- Wright's test: The athlete's shoulder is hyper-abducted and externally rotated while the athletic trainer palpates the pulse and compares to uninvolved arm. The test is positive if the pulse is diminished or absent, or paresthesias develops[40] as a result of pectoralis minor involvement.
- Roos stress test: The athlete is positioned with both shoulders in abduction and external rotation of 90 degrees with the elbows flexed at 90 degrees (as if they were "giving up"). The athlete opens and closes his hands slowly for 3 minutes. A positive test is indicated by pain, fatigue, arm weakness or numbness and tingling of the hand.[40]

- Allen test: Palpate the radial pulse, and monitor for any changes as the athletic trainer flexes the athlete's elbow to 90 degrees while the shoulder is horizontally abducted to 90 degrees and laterally rotated (mimicking a throwing motion).[41,46] Ask the athlete to rotate the head away from the involved arm. If the radial pulse is diminished or disappears as the head is rotated, the test is considered positive secondary to compression of the neurovascular bundle by the pectoralis minor.

These special tests, however, are known to have high rates of false-positive and false-negative and should be interpreted with caution.

4.14 / **4.** *What are the treatment options for this condition?*

If the athlete experiences only intermittent neurological symptoms (i.e., numbness, paresthesia, tingling, etc.), a course of conservative treatment is appropriate. If the athlete presents with persistent neurological problems or weakness, then further work-up with MRI and EMG can be beneficial in directing possible surgical management. If the athlete presents with vascular compromise, then blood-flow studies of the upper extremity should be performed with thoracic outlet positioning. Athletes with documented vascular compromise respond well to first rib resection.[50]

4.14 / **5.** *Given her condition, when can Jean begin swimming again?*

The athlete should be evaluated for full ROM and strength in the upper extremity and may resume her swimming activities when her symptoms have resolved.

# REFERENCES


1. American Red Cross. *Emergency Response.* Yardley, PA: Staywell; 2001.
2. Aronen J. Anterior shoulder dislocations in sports. *Sports Med.* 1986;3(3):224–234.
3. Aronen J, Chronister R. Anterior shoulder dislocations: easing reduction by using linear traction techniques. *Physician Sportsmed.* 1995;23(10):65–69.
4. Asplund C. Posterior sternoclavicular joint dislocation in a wrestler. *Mil Med.* 2004;169:134–136.
5. Baykal B, Sener S, Turkan H. Scapular manipulation technique for reduction of traumatic anterior shoulder dislocations: experiences of an academic emergency department. *Emerg Med J.* 2005;22:336–338.
6. Bennett W. Specificity of the Speed's test: Arthroscopic technique for evaluating the biceps tendon at the level of the bicipital groove. *J Arthroscop Related Surg.* 1998; 14(8):789–796.
7. Bergfeld J, Andrish P, Clancy W. Evaluation of the acromioclavicular joint following first and second degree sprains. *Am J Sports Med.* 1978;6:153–159.
8. Brilliant L. Fracture, clavicle [electronic version]. *eMedicine.* 2007. Available from: http://emedicine.medscape.com/article/824564-overview. Accessed June 4, 2009.
9. DeLaat E, Visser C, Coene L, Pahlplatz P, Tavy D. Nerve lesions in primary shoulder dislocations and humeral neck fractures: a prospective clinical and EMG study. *J Bone Joint Surg Br.* 1994;76-B:381–383.
10. Demont R. The place for palpation. *Athl Ther Today.* 2003; 8(2):42–43.
11. Disa J, Wang B, Dellon A. Correction of scapular winging by supraclavicular neurolysis of the long thoracic nerve. *J Reconstr Microsurg.* 2001;17:79–84.
12. Foo C, Swann M. Isolated paralysis of the serratus anterior: a report of 20 cases. *J Bone Joint Surg Br.* 1983;65-B:552–556.
13. Gallaspy JB, May JD. *Signs and Symptoms of Athletic Injuries.* St. Louis, MO: Mosby; 1996.
14. Gleason P, Beall D, Sanders T, Bond J, Ly J, Holland L, et al. The transverse humeral ligament: a separate anatomical structure or a continuation of the osseous attachment of the rotator cuff? *Am J Sports Med.* 2006;34(1):72–77.
15. Gregg J, Labosky D, Harty M. Serratus anterior paralysis in the young athlete. *J Bone Joint Surg Am.* 1979;61-A: 825–832.
16. Horwitz M, Tocantins L. An anatomic study of the role of the long thoracic nerve and the related scapular bursae in the pathogenesis of local paralysis of the serratus anterior. *Anat Rec (Hoboken).* 1938;71:375–385.
17. Hutchins C. Thoracic outlet syndrome. In: Sponseller PD, ed. *The 5-Minute Orthopedic Consult.* Philadelphia, PA: Lippincott Williams & Wilkins; 2001:22–323.
18. Itoi E, Newman S, Kuechle D, Morrey B, An K. Dynamic anterior stabilisers of the shoulder with the arm in abduction. *J Bone Joint Surg Br.* 1994;76-B(5):834–836.
19. Kauppila L. The long thoracic nerve: possible mechanisms of injury based upon autopsy study. *J Elbow Surg.* 1993; 2:244–248.
20. Konin JG, Wiksten D, Isear JA, Brader H. *Special Tests for Orthopedic Examination* (3rd ed.). Thorofare, NJ: Slack; 2006.
21. Kronberg M, Brostrom L. Electromyographic recordings in shoulder muscles during eccentric movements. *Clin Orthop Relat Res.* 1995;314:143–151.
22. Kumar K, O'Rourke S, Pillay J. Hands up: a case of bilateral inferior shoulder dislocation. *Emerg Med J.* 2001;18(5):404–405.
23. Magee DJ. *Orthopedic Physical Assessment* (5th ed.). Philadelphia, PA: WB Saunders; 2007.
24. Marker L, Klareskov B. Posterior sternoclavicular dislocation: an American football injury. *Br J Sports Med.* 1996;30:71–72.
25. Mazoue C, Andrews J. Injuries to the shoulder in athletes. *South Med J.* 2005;97(8):784–754.
26. Mirza A, Alam K, Ali A. Posterior sternoclavicular dislocation in a rugby player as a cause of silent vascular compromise: a case report [electronic version]. *Br J Sports Med.* 2005;39:e28–e30. Available from: http://www.bjsportmed.com/cgi/content/full/39/5/e28. Accessed June 4, 2009.
27. Moore K, Dalley A. *Clinically Oriented Anatomy* (5th ed.). Baltimore, MD: Lippincott, Williams, & Wilkins; 2005.
28. Myers JB. Conservative management of shoulder impingement syndrome in the athletic population. *J Sport Rehabil.* 1999;8:230–253.
29. Neer C. Impingement lesions. *Clin Orthop Relat Res.* 1983;173:70–77.
30. Neer C, Foster C. Inferior capsular shift for involuntary and multidirectional instability of the shoulder. *J Bone Joint Surg Am.* 1980;62-A(6):897–908.
31. O'Brien S, Pagnani M, Fealy S, et al. The active compression test: a new and effective test for diagnosing labral tears and acromioclavicular joint abnormality. *Am J Sports Med.* 1999;2(5):610–643.
32. Pappas G, Blemker S, Beaulieu C, McAdams T, Whalen S, Gold G. In vivo anatomy of the Neer and Hawkins sign positions for shoulder impingement. *J Shoulder Elbow Surg.* 2006;15:40–49.
33. Park H, Yokota A, Gill H, Rassi G, McFarland E. Diagnostic accuracy of clinical tests for the different degrees of subacromial impingement syndrome. *J Bone Joint Surg Am.* 2005;87-A(7):1446–1455.
34. Paxinos A, Walton J, Tzannes A, Callanan M, Hayes K, Murrell GAC. Advances in the management of traumatic anterior and atraumatic multidirectional shoulder instability. *Sports Med.* 2001;31(11):819–828.
35. Perlmutter G, Leffert R, Zarins B. Direct injury to the axillary nerve in athletes playing contact sports. *Am J Sports Med.* 1997;25:65–68.

36. Petrucci F, Morelli A, Raimondi P. Axillary nerve injuries: 21 cases treated by nerve graft and neurolysis. *Journal of Hand Surgery [Am]*. 1982;7:271–278.
37. Ray R. *Management Strategies in Athletic Training* (3rd ed.). Champaign, IL: Human Kinetics; 2005.
38. Rockwood C, Young D. Disorders of the acromioclavicular joint. In: Rockwood C, Matsen F, eds. *The Shoulder.* Philadelphia, PA: WB Saunders; 1990:413–476.
39. Rudzki J, Matava M, Paletta G. Complications of treatment of acromioclavicular and sternoclavicular joint injuries. *Clin Sports Med.* 2003;22:387–405.
40. Safran M. Nerve injuries about the shoulder in athletes, part 2. *Am J Sports Med.* 2004;32(4):1063–1076.
41. Schultz SJ, Houglum PA, Perrin DH. *Examination of Musculoskeletal Injuries* (2nd ed.). Champaign, IL: Human Kinetics; 2005.
42. Seade E, Bartz R, Josey R. Acromioclavicular joint injury [electronic version]. *eMedicine.* 2008. Available from: http://emedicine.medscape.com/article/92337-overview. Accessed June 4, 2009.
43. Simon RR, Koenigsknecht SJ. The scapula. In: *Emergency Orthopedics.* Stamford, CT: Appleton & Lange; 1996:207–215.
44. Slatis P, Aalto K. Medical dislocation of the tendon of the long head of the biceps brachi. *Acta Ophthalmol Scand.* 1979;50(1):73–77.
45. Spencer EJ, Brems J. A simple technique for management of locked posterior shoulder dislocations: report of two cases. *J Shoulder Elbow Surg.* 2005;14(6):650–652.
46. Starkey C, Ryan J. *Evaluation of Orthopedic and Athletic Injuries* (2nd ed.). Philadelphia, PA: FA Davis; 2002.
47. Summers A. Shoulder dislocation: reduction without sedation in the emergency department. *Emerg Nurse.* 2007;5(1):24–28.
48. Sutherland T. Shoulder injuries. In: Andrews J, Clancy W, Whiteside J, eds. *On-field Evaluation and Treatment of Common Athletic Injuries.* St. Louis: Mosby; 1997:215–224.
49. Tsur A, Gillson S. Brachial biceps tendon injuries in young female high-level tennis players. *Clin Sciences.* 2000;41(2):84–185.
50. Vanti C, L Natalini, A Romeo, D Tosarelli, P Pillastrini. Conservative treatment of thoracic outlet syndrome: a review of the literature. *Euro Medicophys.* 2007;43(1):55–70.
51. Visser C, Coene L, Brand R, Tavy D. The incidence of nerve injury in anterior dislocation of the shoulder and its influence on functional recovery: a prospective clinical and EMG study. *J Bone Joint Surg Br.* 1999;81-B:679–685.

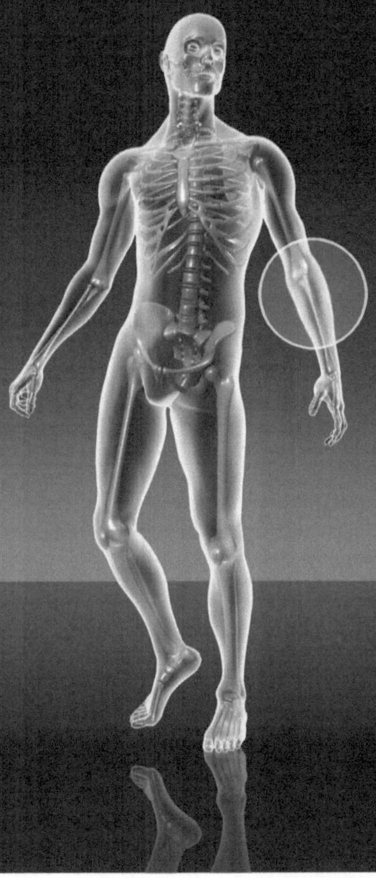

# CHAPTER 5

# Elbow and Forearm

## QUICK REFERENCE

CASE 5.1
**Ulnar Collateral Ligament Sprain**

CASE 5.2
**Radial Collateral Ligament Sprain**

CASE 5.3
**Triceps Tendon Partial Avulsion**

CASE 5.4
**Wrist Flexor and Pronator Strain**

CASE 5.5
**Distal Biceps Tendon Rupture**

CASE 5.6
**Posterior Humeroulnar Dislocation**

CASE 5.7
**Radial Head Fracture**

CASE 5.8
**Isolated Ulnar Shaft Fracture**

CASE 5.9
**Supracondylar Fracture**

CASE 5.10
**Forearm Fracture with Acute Volar Compartment Syndrome**

CASE 5.11
**Pronator Teres Syndrome—Median Nerve**

CASE 5.12
**Cubital Tunnel Syndrome—Ulnar Nerve**

CASE 5.13
**Olecranon Bursitis**

CASE 5.14
**Lateral Epicondylitis**

CASE 5.15
**Medial Epicondylitis**

CASE 5.16
**Condylar, Epicondylar, or Intercondylar Fracture**

# ANSWERS TO CASE QUESTIONS

## CASE 5.1 Ulnar Collateral Ligament Sprain

5.1 / **1.** *Based on the information presented in the case, determine (a) the differential diagnoses and (b) the clinical diagnosis.*

a. Differential diagnoses: cervical disc or nerve root pathology, flexor pronator muscle tear, ulnar neuritis/ulnar nerve entrapment, medial epicondyle fracture, medial epicondylitis, valgus extension overload, medial triceps subluxation, olecranon osteophytes[40,54]

b. Clinical diagnosis: medial (ulnar) collateral ligament injury (sprain) with ulnar neuritis (caused by a traction force)

5.1 / **2.** *Sean asked several history questions to guide the physical examination. Based on the information presented in the case, (a) do you believe Sean took an adequate history? If not, (b) what questions would you have asked as the evaluating clinician?*

a. According to the clinical diagnosis, there are several other questions the evaluating athletic trainer should have inquired about. Specifically, these questions should have addressed changes in training regimens or any changes in the athlete's accuracy, velocity, stamina, and strength.[17,44,54] An athletic trainer should be asking about a gradual decrease in velocity and accuracy which may be explained by a decrease in wrist flexor/pronator EMG[54] from the increased stress placed on these structures in providing stability to the medial elbow joint complex.[17]

b. Other history questions given the case should focus around changes in the neurovascular status of the athlete, including but not limited to, numbness and tingling, stiffness or heaviness in the arm, tendency to drop objects, and cold intolerance.

5.1 / **3.** *The injury in this case presents as a chronic condition with an insidious onset. What piece of information obtained as part of the history could have led Sean to believe that the injury was acute in nature?*

Athletes suffering from an acute ulnar collateral ligament sprain of the elbow can normally pinpoint the exact day and pitch thrown when the injury occurred.[6] They will often report hearing and/or feeling a "pop" during the throwing phase.[44,57]

5.1 / **4.** *(a) Identify the dynamic and static stabilizers of the medial elbow joint. (b) Identify the location of the static stabilizers. (c) Which structures were specifically involved in the injury and why?*

a. The static stabilizers of the medial elbow joint are the anterior bundle, posterior bundle, and transverse ligament of the ulnar collateral ligament. The dynamic stabilizers include the flexor-pronator muscle mass (particularly the flexor carpi ulnaris), flexor digitorum superficialis, triceps, anconeus, and internal rotators of the shoulder.

b. The anterior bundle of the ulnar collateral ligament originates on the inferior medial epicondyle and inserts onto the medial aspect of the coronoid process. The anterior band of the anterior bundle serves as the primary restraint to a valgus force between 30° and 90°, increasing its contribution to valgus stability as the angle increases[18,44,84]

## CASE 5.2 Radial Collateral Ligament Sprain (RCL)

5.2 / **1.** *Based on the information presented in the case, (a) what is the likely clinical diagnosis? (b) What makes this clinical diagnosis unique?*

a. Clinical diagnosis: radial collateral elbow sprain

b. Isolated injury to the radial collateral ligament complex is rare. Because the body protects the medial aspect of the elbow, there is less chance for a direct traction or for varus forces to be applied to the elbow.[76,85] Significant trauma, such as elbow dislocations and fracture dislocations, increase the risk of soft-tissue disruption to the radial collateral ligament[52] and insufficiency of the lateral soft tissue[22]; isolated injuries occur with forearm supination and elbow hyperextension.[76]

5.2 / **2.** *Don asked several specific history questions to guide the physical examination. However, there was one question that may have assisted in narrowing down the clinical diagnosis, which he either did not ask or which may not have been answered appropriately because of a translation error. Can you identify this question?*

Don did not determine the specific MOI for this case. He determined that Natsuko fell backwards as she was backpedaling, but he never identified the position of the arm and hand when she landed. This information may have revealed that she fell with her elbow extended and forearm supinated versus extended and pronated, suggesting isolated trauma to the radial collateral ligament.

5.2 / **3.** *If Natsuko presented with the same clinical findings from the case but also had weakness with wrist extension, (a) would your clinical diagnosis possibly change? (b) What would cause you to make this change?*

a. Given this information, the clinical diagnosis may now be acute posterolateral rotatory instability of the elbow. This condition occurs when a patient experiences a combination of axial compression, external rotation, and valgus force applied to the elbow, which causes a disruption of the lateral restraints and muscle origins from the lateral epicondyle.[22]

b. The lateral ulnar collateral and annular ligaments are the primary restraints against rotatory instability. With this injury, if left unchecked or misdiagnosed, gaping at the humeroulnar articulation occurs from ligamentous damage and the inability of the secondary static and dynamic stabilizers to support the joint. This leads to the development of chronic posterolateral rotatory instability.

5.2 / **4.** *Do you believe Don adequately evaluated Natsuko's condition? If not, what would you have done differently as the evaluating clinician?*

The answers to this question will vary among students. However, students should recognize that Don performed one inappropriate test and failed to perform several others. He performed posteromedial rotatory instability when he should have performed a posterolateral rotatory instability test. There was no mention of a varus stress test or a radioulnar joint test. A varus stress test is used to assess the integrity of the radial collateral ligament. This test, similar to a valgus test, should be performed in extension and again at approximately 20° to 25° of flexion. A varus stress test in full extension with the forearm supinated is resisted by the radial collateral ligament (15%), anterior capsule (30%), and the articular surface (50%).[87] When flexed, the articular surface now resists 75 percent of the load, and the radial collateral 10 percent.[87] The radioulnar stress test assesses the integrity of the annular ligament, which shares the same insertion point as the radial collateral ligament on the proximal ulna and functions to bind the radius and ulna together, preventing proximal radioulnar joint dislocations and subluxations.

Don's instructions for the use of cryotherapy also seemed to be incomplete. He does not suggest whether a layer of insulation should be placed between the skin and the physical agent. Depending on these instructions, the treatment time may need to be varied.

5.2 / **5.** *In this case, a language barrier existed. Fortunately, a translator was able to assist Don during the physical examination. If you were placed in a situation in which you were unable to communicate with a patient because of a language barrier, how would you handle the situation?*

When placed in a language-barrier situation, several strategies could be employed. These include, but are not limited to, the following:

- Begin by identifying those individuals on your staff who have knowledge of the language, and use them as interpreters.
- If the patient has brought a friend who may be able to interpret, and the patient consents, use the intermediary.
- When an interpreter is not present, speak slowly and carefully in terms as simple as possible. Do not use technical jargon or terms that convey value judgments.
- Remember to ask for permission to physically examine the patient, and do not touch the patient until granted permission.
- If you work in the area where this language barrier is encountered often, consider learning the necessary key phrases and terms.
- When possible, provide simple, illustrated printed materials to allow the patient to describe her situation. For example, use pain charts or images of patients falling on the ground or being struck with an object.

Good patient communication is a necessary component of a successful physical examination. Being able to interact and engage with the patient involves recognizing and responding to the patient as a whole person. When communication between the clinician and patient is unhampered, the patient feels a sense of value, and this helps improve patient satisfaction and clinical outcomes that ultimately affect the productivity and appearance of the facility. There are several models that clinicians can employ in their practices to improve clinician-patient communication. One area in need of development is cultural competency. In many parts of the country, clinicians must learn to effectively communicate with non–English speaking patients. When dealing with a non–English speaking patient, remember to be aware of your own cultural biases and preconceptions, and respect the patient's cultural beliefs. In some situations, the patient's view of you may be defined by ethnic or cultural stereotypes, so do not take things personally.

## CASE 5.3 Triceps Tendon Partial Avulsion

5.3 / **1.** *Based on the information presented in the case, determine (a) the differential diagnoses and (b) the clinical diagnosis.*

a. Differential diagnoses: olecranon fracture, medial humeral condyle fracture, medial epicondyle avulsion fracture, lateral epicondyle avulsion fracture, and olecranon bursitis[25,89]

b. Clinical diagnosis: partial avulsion of the triceps tendon

5.3 / **2.** *The MOI in this case study was a fall on the outstretched hand with the elbow in mid-flexion. During Eugene's fall, what specific action was being performed by the tissue involved in the injury?*

The triceps were eccentrically contracting to control the descent to the floor. In this case, the partial avulsion of the triceps tendon occurred as a result of the fall on an outstretched hand with the elbow in mid-flexion. This is considered a typical MOI.[77,82] Another common MOI is eccentric stress on the triceps during a blow to the posterior aspect of the elbow.[29]

5.3 / **3.** *If you were the evaluating clinician, what "general information" would you have gathered at the beginning of the history?*

The answers to this question will vary among students. However, given the clinical diagnosis and work-setting, questions as to age, job responsibility, history of cortisone injection, and history of physical activity are all warranted. Other cited factors contributing to complete triceps ruptures include drug use (anabolic steroids), secondary hyperparathyroidism, hypertension, diabetes mellitus, and chronic renal failure.[82] This suggests that a thorough past medical history is necessary.

5.3 / **4.** *In addition to the clinical observations presented in the case, what other signs or symptoms may be presented depending on how old the injury is?*

The answers to this question will vary among students. However, depending on when the injury occurred, a patient may present with bruising, and swelling into the forearm and/or hand, to name a few.

5.3 / **5.** *If you were in Monica's position, (a) discuss how you would have assessed Eugene's muscular strength against gravity. (b) Why was he still able to extend the elbow?*

a. To assess muscle strength of the triceps, place the patient in a supine position with the shoulder internally rotated and flexed to 90° and the elbow bent to 90°. Screen the patient by asking him to extend his elbow. Inability to actively extend the elbow would require placing the patient in a seated position to assess the triceps in a gravity-eliminated position.

b. Eugene was still able to extend the arm for two possible reasons. The triceps may have been only partially avulsed, and the anconeus also assists in the extending the elbow.

## CASE 5.4 Wrist Flexor And Pronator Strain

5.4 / **1.** *Based on the information presented in the case, determine (a) the differential diagnoses and (b) the clinical diagnosis.*

a. Differential diagnoses: medial head of the triceps strain, ulnar collateral ligament sprain, ulnar nerve trauma, medial epicondylitis, and medial epicondyle apophysitis[17,54]

b. Clinical diagnosis: wrist flexor-pronator strain

5.4 / **2.** *McKinley asked several history questions to guide the physical examination. Based on the information presented in the case, do you believe she took an adequate history? If not, what questions would you have asked as the evaluating clinician?*

The answers to this question will vary among students. According to the information presented in the case, there appeared to be a previous history of elbow trauma. Therefore, a complete past medical history would be warranted in this case. Because Tabatha is a throwing athlete, she is predisposed to the development of several medial elbow pathologies, including ulnar collateral ligament injury or insufficiency, ulnar neuritis, medial epicondylitis, osseous, and intra-articular changes.[4,27,30] Compounding the problem is difficulty in distinguishing a proximal flexor-pronator strain from acute tendonitis or epicondylitis,[76] which is why a thorough past and present history, particularly in a throwing athlete, can help to define the etiology of the medial elbow pain.[30]

5.4 / **3.** *McKinley assessed AROM and muscle strength but failed to assess PROM. If you were the evaluating clinician, how would you assess PROM, and what would you expect to find?*

Elbow flexion and extension passive range could be assessed with Tabatha in a supine or sitting position. McKinley should stabilize the humerus proximally, while grasping the distal radius and ulna. Slight traction is applied through the distal hand while moving the elbow through flexion and extension (Figures A5.4.1 and A5.4.2), applying overpressure at the end range of each motion.

Pronation and supination are performed with Tabatha in a seated position with her arm at the side and elbow flexed 90°. McKinley should stabilize the humerus proximally, while grasping the distal radius and ulna in a neutral forearm position. The distal hand rotates the hand downward and upward to the end range.[21]

FIGURE A5.4.1 PROM elbow flexion.

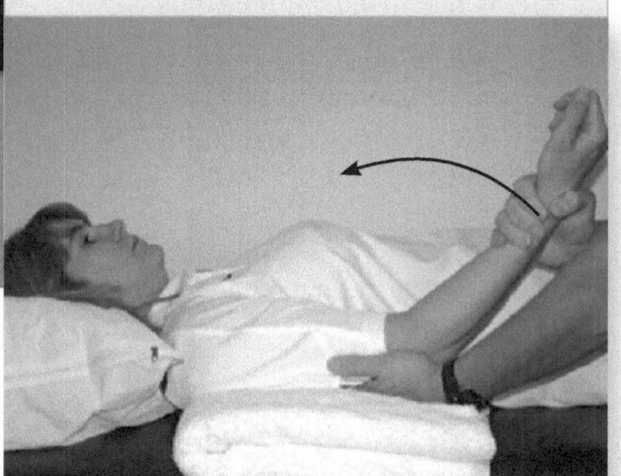

FIGURE A5.4.2 PROM elbow extension.

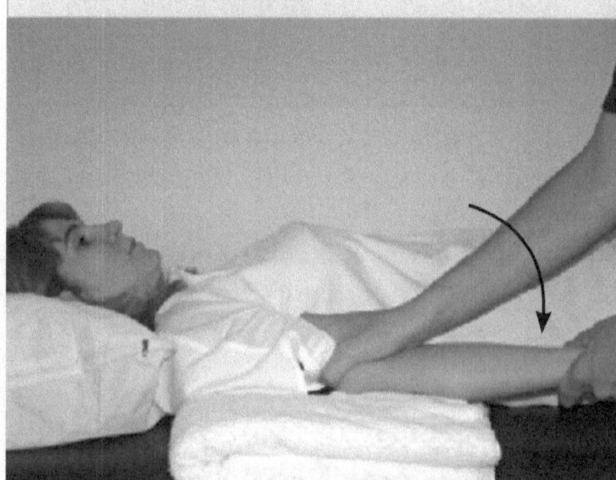

Given the clinical diagnosis, complaints of pain should occur when the traumatized tissue is placed on stretch (wrist extension and forearm supination).

5.4 / **4.** *(a) What is ketorolac tromethamine? (b) Is this an appropriate course of action?*

a. Ketorolac tromethamine is the generic name for Toradol®, an NSAID used to relieve moderate to severe acute pain. It is administered intravenously, intramuscularly, or orally and inhibits the synthesis of prostaglandins, acting peripherally as an analgesic.[63]

b. Medication to reduce inflammation and pain is often used as an adjunct to other therapies. However, injecting an athlete to return to play immediately after sustaining an injury is a controversial issue with no agreed-upon right or wrong answer. Consult your state practice act, standard operating procedures, policy and procedure manual, and athletic training medical staff to determine if this practice is acceptable.

5.4 / **5.** *If you were the evaluating clinician, what if anything would you do regarding the coach's actions?*

The answer to this question will vary among students. Certainly, the coach's action demonstrates either a lack of confidence in McKinley's decision or a potential lack of concern for the athlete's best interests. Regardless of the reason, athletic trainers in this situation need to have administrative support regarding the decisions they make about allowing athletes to return to play. When an athletic trainer's decision is undermined, it not only places the athlete at risk but it also places the athletic trainer in a position where her decisions are always subject to question by the coach and athletes. Consult your athletic training medical staff, including your physician, to determine whether this type of event has ever occurred, and if it has, how it was handled.

## CASE 5.5 Distal Biceps Tendon Rupture

5.5 / **1.** *Based on the information presented in the case, determine (a) the differential diagnoses and (b) the clinical diagnosis.*

a. Differential diagnoses: humeral fracture, shoulder dislocation/instability, radial head fracture (distal), avulsion fracture (radial tuberosity)[12]

b. Clinical diagnosis: distal biceps tendon third-degree strain

FIGURE A5.5.1 Retracted biceps brachii secondary to tendon rupture.

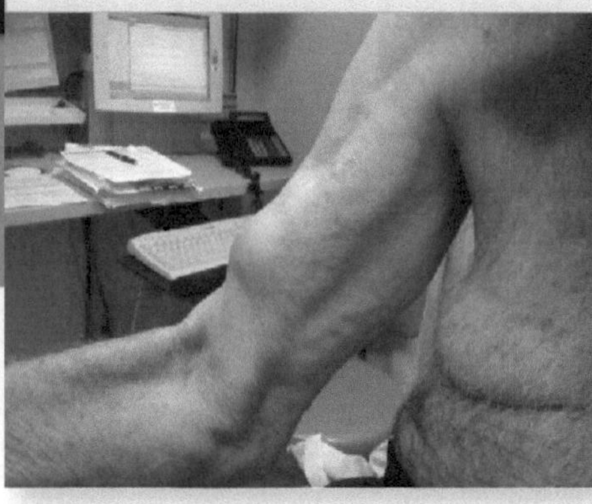

5.5 / **2.** *What, if any, other signs should Sam have observed during the physical examination that may have helped to guide his clinical diagnosis?*

Patients with a complete distal biceps tendon tear will typically present with proximal retraction of the ruptured tendon (Figure A5.5.1), creating a palpable defect of the distal biceps tendon.[34] Comparison of the contralateral limb is also helpful in identifying the deformity.

5.5 / **3.** *Based on the clinical diagnosis, (a) what component of the physical examination did Sam forget? (b) What is the clinical significance of omitting this part of the physical examination?*

a. Sam forgot to assess muscle strength using muscle strength testing. The patient should have been tested for elbow flexion and extension strength and forearm supination and pronation.

b. Clinically, a distal biceps tendon rupture will present with significant weakness with supination.

"Electromyographic (EMG) analysis of the contribution of the muscles of the arm to elbow motion found that the brachialis is the main flexor of the elbow and is active in all elbow positions. The contribution of the biceps to elbow flexion is minimal when the forearm is pronated, and much more significant when the forearm is supinated. EMG studies also showed that the amount of elbow flexion determines the relative contribution of different muscles to forearm rotation. With the elbow fully extended, the supinator is largely responsible for forearm supination. The biceps becomes the primary supinator of the forearm with progressive flexion of the elbow."[34]

5.5 / **4.** *According to the case report, the special tests were positive. Based on your clinical diagnosis, (a) name at least one test that you feel could have been positive. (b) Describe how to perform the test.*

a. The Ludington's test could have been positive. Tests such as the Speed's and Yergason's can be used in situations in which a patient is suspected of having a proximal partial tear or may be predisposed to a future rupture.[12]

b. In the Ludington's test, the patient's hands are clasped behind the head, and biceps muscles are flexed. The clinician feels for active contraction of the long head of the biceps.

5.5 / **5.** *Would radiographic studies be useful in this case? Why, or why not?*

a. Yes, radiographs would prove useful.

b. These would need to be ordered by Paul's referring physician, but radiographs help to rule of out concomitant fractures or other joint pathology.[34] They may also reveal hypertrophic spurring or bony irregularities[12] that may have been contributing factors to the injury, particularly in older individuals with a previous history.

## CASE 5.6 Posterior Humeroulnar Dislocation

5.6 / **1.** *Based on the information presented in the case, determine (a) the differential diagnoses and (b) the clinical diagnosis.*

a. Differential diagnoses: medial or lateral collateral ligament sprain, anterior capsule rupture, supracondylar or intercondylar distal humerus fracture, osteochondral fractures, radial head fractures, coronoid fracture, capitellar or trochlear fracture, olecranon fracture, or any combination[42]

b. Clinical diagnosis: posterior humeroulnar elbow dislocation with brachial artery compression

5.6 / **2.** *Based on the clinical diagnosis above, identify three to five additional history questions you may have asked as the evaluating clinician.*

These answers will vary among students, but they may include the following:

- Any prior history of elbow injury or trauma?
- Any heaviness in the arm as a result of vascular trauma?
- Is the hand cold?
- Any changes in sensation in the forearm or hand?
- Any sounds or sensations aside from the popping?

5.6 / **3.** *Do you believe Jeff and Sue adequately evaluated Adam's condition? If not, what would you have done differently as the evaluating clinician?*

The answers to this question will vary among students. However, given the athlete's history and physical exam, Jeff should have included a more thorough assessment of Adam's neurovascular status. If a simple or complex elbow dislocation is suspected, athletic trainers need to carefully manage the injury to limit damage to the neurovascular structures such as the brachial artery and ulnar and median nerves.[8,41] The ulnar nerve crosses the elbow's joint line medially and is relatively superficial. Damage to the ulnar nerve will result in numbness and tingling into the little finger. The median nerve crosses over the anterior elbow joint, following the same path as the brachial artery, and may become entrapped within the joint once the elbow is reduced. Any change in the neurovascular status is considered a medical emergency requiring immediate immobilization and transportation. Any change in the athlete's neurovascular status, such as a diminished pulse, cold hands, numbness, or loss of distal limb function requires immediate medical attention to restore normal function.

5.6 / **4.** *Given the clinical diagnosis, describe the exact MOI and which, if any, other structures may have been injured.*

Posterior elbow dislocations occur when the elbow is forced into hyperextension and the olecranon process of the ulna impinges on the olecranon fossa of the humerus, forcing the forearm away from the distal arm, rupturing the support structures, and driving the humerus in an anterior direction.[8] This is what happened in Adam's case. In a simple elbow dislocation, there are no concomitant fractures about the elbow; however, a rupture of the anterior capsule and collateral ligaments,[8] particularly the lateral collateral ligament,[76] does occur. A complex dislocation results in concomitant injuries (e.g., elbow dislocation with a radial head fracture).

Elbow dislocations are classified according to the direction of movement of the radius and ulna (posterior, anterior). It is the second most commonly dislocated joint after shoulder dislocations.[60]

5.6 / **5.** *If you were the athletic trainer in this case, would you have provided the same type of immediate care? Why, or why not? Describe the steps you would have used.*

The answers to this question will vary among students. However, immobilization of an elbow dislocation does commonly require the use of a rigid splint or vacuum splint to stabilize the joint in the position found. The rigid splint could be applied using a dorsolateral board splint or a posterior SAM SPLINT with the elbow in the position it was found and so that the radial pulse is still accessible. These should be followed with a sling and swathe. Students should remember to include steps that involve checking for signs of circulation, sensation, and movement before and after immobilization of the extremity. All open wounds should be covered with sterile dressings; apply cryotherapy to decrease edema formation if warranted and available.[2]

## CASE 5.8 Isolated Ulnar Shaft Fracture

5.8 / **1.** *Based on the information presented in the case, determine the clinical diagnosis.*

The clinical diagnosis is isolated ulna shaft fracture.

5.8 / **2.** *What is the colloquial term for this clinical diagnosis?*

The colloquial term is "nightstick fracture" because isolated ulna fractures occur from a direct blow to the ulna, such as from a policeman's nightstick or baton.[1,46]

5.8 / **3.** *Shane asked a couple of history questions to guide his physical examination. Based on the clinical diagnosis above, identify three to five additional history questions you may have asked as the evaluating clinician.*

The answers will vary among students, but they should focus on questions about the general health of the athlete and questions such as:

- When was the onset of pain?
- What worsens or relieves the symptoms?
- Were there unusual sounds or sensations?
- Do you have any elbow or wrist pain?

5.8 / **4.** *Do you believe Shane adequately evaluated Justin's condition? If not, what would you have done differently as the evaluating clinician?*

The answers for this question will vary among students. It would appear that Shane did not complete a neurovascular physical examination. This examination is important from an immobilization viewpoint because of the risk of injury to the deep branch of the radial nerve[36] and because of the risk of concomitant trauma to the elbow and wrist. Therefore, it is necessary to thoroughly evaluate these joints.

5.8 / **5.** *Discuss how you as the evaluating clinician would have managed this situation once the physical examination has been completed.*

The answers will vary among students, depending on the level of training and their clinical experience. However, they should focus on providing immediate care such as rest, ice, compression, elevation, and immobilization. Immobilization of the forearm can be accomplished using a variety of immobilization devices such as a rigid board splint, SAM SPLINT, or a vacuum splint. Regardless of the technique, it will be necessary to immobilize the joints above and below the fracture site (i.e., elbow and wrist). The following are two methods of immobilizing a forearm fracture.

Immobilizing trauma to the radius and/or ulnar is best accomplished using a sugar tong splint.

1. Stabilize and support the extremity.
2. Assess the distal neurovascular status.
3. Fold a 36-inch SAM SPLINT in half, creating two 18-inch halves.
4. To correctly fit the splint, place the folded splint around the elbow running from the dorsal metacarpophalangeal (MCP) joint to the proximal interphalangeal (PIP) joint volarly. Any extra material should be folded over on the volar side.

5. Fold a C-curve into distal 2/3 of the dorsal and volar halves of the splint.
6. Using the athletic trainer's arm as a model, shape the splint to the approximate dimensions.
7. Pad any bony prominences, such as the radial styloid process, to avoid pressure points. Fit the splint to the athlete, and secure it using the wrap of choice.
8. Secure the extremity to the chest by applying a sling and swath with the forearm in a slightly elevated position if comfortable.
9. Place a gauze pad between the sling and swathe knots for comfort.
10. Reassess the distal neurovascular status, and document findings.

Immobilization may also be achieved by using a rigid volar splint.

1. Stabilize and support the extremity.
2. Assess the distal neurovascular status.
3. Place a padded rigid splint on the volar surface of the involved forearm.
4. Place a roller bandage in the athlete's hand so the hand assumes a position of function.
5. Secure the splint using the bandage of choice (e.g., elastic wrap, cravat, roller bandage).
6. When dealing with a trauma to the bone, be sure to immobilize the wrist to limit flexion and extension.
7. Provide additional support by applying a sling and swathe with the forearm in a slightly elevated position if comfortable.
8. Place a gauze pad between the sling and swathe knots for comfort.
9. Reassess the distal neurovascular status, and document findings.

5.8 / **6.** *After completing the physical examination, Shane documented his findings and sent a copy of the report to the administration office. Please document your findings as if you were the treating clinician. If the case did not provide information you believe is pertinent to the clinical diagnosis, please feel free to add this information to your documentation.*

Answers will vary. Students should consider writing a SOAP note (see textbook Appendix B) using the ABCD format when writing the short- and long-term goals.

# CASE 5.9 Supracondylar Fracture

5.9 / **1.** *Based on the information presented in the case, determine the clinical diagnosis.*

The clinical diagnosis in this case would be a supracondylar humerus fracture with neurovascular compromise. A fracture-dislocation of the humeroulnar joint is certainly possible. However, given the age of the patient, a supracondylar fracture is most likely. In fact, supracondylar fractures are the most common type of elbow fracture in children, accounting for 58 to 75 percent of all injuries affecting children age 5 to 10 years.[38,43,88,90]

5.9 / **2.** *Sherrie was able to determine the MOI by questioning the patient, in this case falling on an outstretched hand with the elbow extended. If you were the evaluating clinician, do you believe you would have been able to arrive to the same conclusion? Why or why not?*

Obtaining an exact account of the injury is difficult in this age population.[88] It is possible for an evaluating clinician to obtain the information necessary to determine the exact MOI. However, getting an exact account of the MOI normally depends on a reliable adult who has witnessed the accident. Clinicians need to remember when they are communicating and interacting with school-aged children (6–12 yrs) to avoid talking down to them, avoid using large words or complex questions,[2] and approach them on their own level (e.g., kneeling or sitting rather than standing).[24] Even when parents are present, it is still necessary to avoid talking down and using large words and complex questions, because parents are often facing some type of emotional distress regarding their injured child.

5.9 / **3.** *(a) Identify the bony and soft tissue structure Sherrie should have palpated as part of her evaluation specific to the elbow. (b) Identify the neurological and vascular structures at greatest risk, based on the clinical diagnosis. (c) Identify the anatomical landmarks in textbook Figures 5.9.2 and 5.9.3 (repeated on p. 103).*

a. Given the information presented in the case, Sherrie would have been wise to palpate the humerus, radius, ulna, olecranon, epicondyles, triceps, elbow flexors, and pronator teres. The exact anatomical structures that can be palpated will depend on the extent of the patient's pain and apprehension. Increased pain associated with palpation makes completing a thorough evaluation more difficult because children regress when in pain. In the case of pediatric patients, palpation is also more challenging because pain tolerance is low.

b. Supracondylar fractures pose an increased risk for development of both neurological and vascular deficits. The most common neurological impairment is neuropraxia, which often resolves over time.[59,90] The neurological structures at greatest risk include the radial, ulnar, and median nerves because of trauma or swelling.[59,64,83,88] The brachial artery, which crosses anterior to the cubital fossa before splitting into the radial and ulnar arteries, is also vulnerable to trauma from sharp bony fragments or displacement of the humerus.[43,64,66,88] Lack of adequate blood flow further increases the risk of compartment syndrome and Volkmann's ischemic contractures,[90] making a compromise to the radial or ulnar artery a medical emergency.

c. In Figure 5.9.2, A is *ulna,* B is *medial epicondyle,* C is *humerus,* D is *lateral supracondylar ridge,* E is *olecranon fossa,* F is *lateral epicondyle,* and G is *radial head.*

In Figure 5.9.3, H is *radius,* I is *radial tuberosity,* J is *capitulum,* and K is *olecranon process.*

5.9 / **4.** *According to the case, Sherrie notes a deficit in grip strength and the inability to extend the wrist on the involved side. What does this indicate?*

The deficit in grip strength and inability to extend the wrist would indicate damage to the radial nerve. The radial nerve runs distally down the posterior upper arm, crossing laterally over the lateral supracondylar ridge and lateral epicondyle before passing between the brachioradialis and the brachialis muscles. It further divides into motor and sensory branches, of which the motor branch provides innervation to the wrist extensors and several thumb muscles.

5.9 / **5.** *Given the age of the patient in this case, would you have handled the situation any differently? If so, why?*

The answers to this question will vary among students, depending on how they analyze the case. One issue to be concerned about is the questionable lack of Sherrie's obtaining parental consent. Because Sherrie was acting as an emergency medical responder and not as an athletic trainer, she had no formal duty to act and therefore needed to obtain consent in order to assess Jeremy. If Jeremy were over 18 years of age and conscious, Sherrie would have needed to acquire express consent from Jeremy himself. If he were unconscious, implied consent is assumed. But because he is conscious and under 18 years of age, parental assent is required. What becomes challenging is the question: at what point do you begin care for a child who is conscious but in obvious distress? One way to alleviate this problem is for all organized sports to have a permission-to-treat form that provides the sponsoring organization with parental consent to treat children in the event of an accident.

FIGURE 5.9.2 Adult elbow in extension.

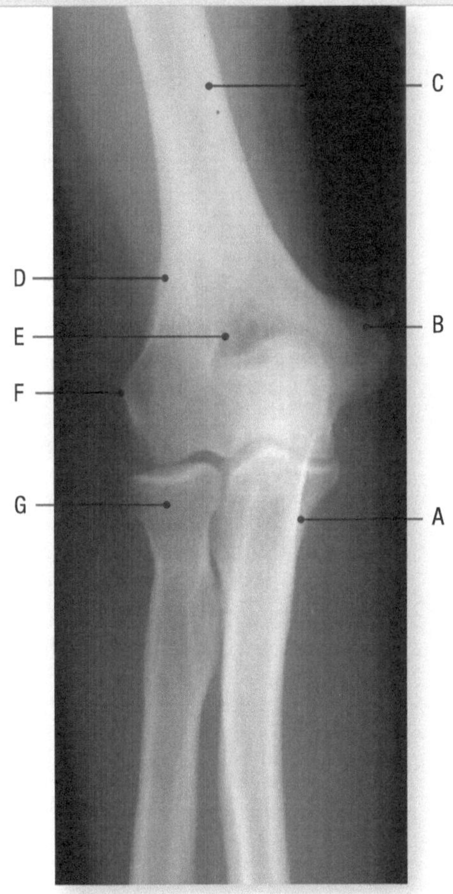


FIGURE 5.9.3 Adult elbow in flexion.

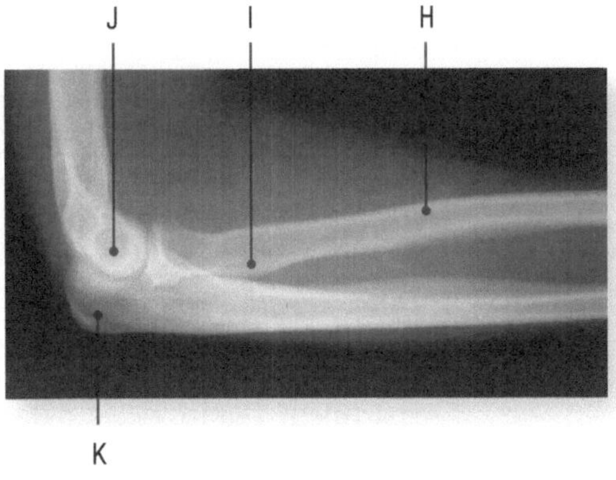

## CASE 5.10 Forearm Fracture with Acute Volar Compartment Syndrome

5.10 / **1.** *Based on the information presented in the case, determine the initial clinical diagnosis and the secondary clinical diagnosis based on the follow-up examination.*

The initial clinical diagnosis was a forearm fracture. However, the follow-up physical examination completed a couple of hours after the initial examination, presents with signs and symptoms associated with an acute volar compartment syndrome in combination with the forearm fracture.

5.10 / **2.** *Based on the clinical findings of the initial and secondary physical examinations, and your knowledge of the secondary clinical diagnosis, (a) what six signs and symptoms are common to the diagnosis? (b) In what order do they often present?*

a. The six signs and symptoms that should alert a clinician to the possibility of acute compartment syndrome are: pain, pressure, paresthesia, paresis, pallor, and pulselessness (in order of appearance).[62]

b. Pain over the involved compartment and/or throbbing pain, out of proportion to the injury and that is not relieved with analgesic medication, is normally the first sign to appear.[16] This occurs due to pressure or tension development in the soft tissue as a result of swelling and hemorrhaging within the compartment.[23] Next is paresthesia, which is subsequently followed by paresis. Daniels et al.[23] suggest that although paresthesia is an early indicator of compartment syndrome, it is not specific to this syndrome and is a sign of several other differential diagnoses. Pallor and pulselessness are the final two signs to appear as the condition worsens. In some situations such as when there is trauma to arteries of the forearm, pulselessness and pallor now may also be early signs of acute compartment syndrome. When all six signs and symptoms appear, the athlete will have experienced irreparable harm such as tissue necrosis and permanent loss of muscle function and nerve function from the ischemia.

5.10 / **3.** *Why did Tim seem so concerned about Derick experiencing pain with active and passive metacarpophalangeal and interphalangeal joint motion?*

The forearm contains three compartments: the volar, dorsal, and the mobile wad. The volar compartment is further divided into the superficial volar compartment, which contains the wrist flexors, and the deep compartment, which contains the flexor digitorum profundus, flexor pollicis longus, and pronator quadratus. Each of these compartments surrounds the muscular structures within its fascia that are responsible for wrist and finger movement. Trauma or some other precipitating factor causes interstitial swelling and pressure to increase within this closed myofascial compartment. This swelling and pressure lead to an eventual collapse of the vascular structures, compromising circulation (ischemia) to the muscles and nerves.[76] One of the most reliable symptoms of acute compartment syndrome is pain with passive movement or stretching of the involved tissue.[48,85] In this case, it is likely that the pain was worsened with passive extension of the finger from the flexed position and/or wrist extension. Active finger flexion and wrist flexion may also produce pain. As the condition progresses and ischemia worsens, muscle function will be gradually reduced and eventually lost.

5.10 / **4.** *If Derick presented with just paresthesia distal to the injury and minor throbbing over the injury site during the second assessment, how would you react? What could be occurring?*

Paresthesia distal to the injury and throbbing could simply be the result of the splint being applied too tight. Removing the splint and determining whether the athlete notes any changes or regains a normal neurovascular status would be the first step. If after a period of time these symptoms do not diminish, then the risk of further complications increases.

5.10 / **5.** *Overall, do you believe Tim adequately handled the situation and his interaction with Derick's parents? If not, what would you have done differently as the evaluating clinician?*

The answers to this question will vary among students. However, Tim may have overreacted and unnecessarily worried both Derick and his parents. If Tim's clinical diagnosis of acute volar compartment syndrome is wrong, then he has just damaged his reputation and unnecessarily scared both Derick and his parents. Calmly making the parents understand that the situation is critical and informing them that they need to have their son be seen immediately is probably adequate. Providing undue information, particularly when you are unsure of the outcome only serves to make matters worse.

## CASE 5.11 Pronator Teres Syndrome—Median Nerve

5.11 / **1.** *Based on the information presented in the case, determine the clinical diagnosis and the possible etiology.*

The clinical diagnosis is impingement of the median nerve resulting in pronator teres syndrome. Pronator teres syndrome was first described in 1951 and was believed to be the result of the entrapment of the median nerve between the two heads of the pronator teres.[78] Since Seyffarth's original description of pronator teres syndrome, four potential sites of compression or entrapment are now recognized. These sites include compression of the median nerve (1) under the ligament of Struthers in the distal humerus due to an anomalous bony spur on the medial epicondyle, (2) under the thickened lacertus fibrosis (bicipital aponeurosis), (3) under the tight fibrous arch of flexor digitorum muscle, and (4) the pronator teres muscle as result of muscle hypertrophy or an aberrant fibrous band.[45,68,77,79] For further explanation regarding the specific etiologies of pronator teres syndrome please refer to Lee and LaStayo's *Pronator Syndrome and Other Nerve Compressions that Mimic Carpal Tunnel Syndrome.*[45]

5.11 / **2.** *In your opinion, did Ron address all of the components of a thorough injury assessment? What if anything would you have added to the assessment?*

According to the injury assessment via HOPS (History, Observation, Palpation, Stress/Special Tests) and/or HIPS (History, Inspection, Palpation, Stress/Special Tests), it would appear that Ron omitted observing Harry for any deformities, open wounds, tenderness, or swelling. In the case of pronator teres syndrome an athlete may be observed for issues such as swelling, hypertrophy—particularly of the ulnar head of the pronator teres[77]—or functional use of the involved limb.

5.11 / **3.** *If Harry presented with pain in the proximal forearm or arm, loss of dexterity, and loss of the ability to pinch, would your clinical diagnosis be the same or different? Why and/or how did you come to this conclusion?*

If Harry presented with the above clinical signs and symptoms, a clinician would need to consider the possibility of anterior interosseous nerve compression syndrome. Unlike pronator teres syndrome, which can present with sensory deficits, entrapment or damage to the anterior interosseous results in motor deficits only. The anterior interosseous nerve is a motor branch arising from the median nerve running parallel to the interosseous membrane. The anterior interosseous nerve is responsible for innervating the flexor pollicis longus and the radial half of the flexor digitorum profundus.[21] Compression of the nerve at the tendinous origins of the deep head of the pronator teres or flexor digitorum[37] and/or trauma[86] causes flexion weakness of the interphalangeal joint of the thumb (flexor pollicis longus) and the distal interphalangeal joint of the index finger (flexor digitorum profundus), resulting in a positive pinch sign (Figures A5.11.1 and A5.11.2).

5.11 / **4.** *If you were the treating clinician, outline a conservative rehabilitation program.*

The answers to this question will vary among students. However, a conservative program will include:

- Identification of the cause and asking the patient to avoid these activities for a period of time. In this case weightlifting and the repetitive flexion-pronation motion of the elbow appear to be the cause. In severe cases a posterior splint may be warranted to avoid unwanted activity[77]; however, range of motion should be carried out each day while the splint is worn (approximately 2 weeks).[45] Remember to maintain cardiovascular function during this rest/immobilization period.

FIGURE A5.11.1

Negative pinch sign.

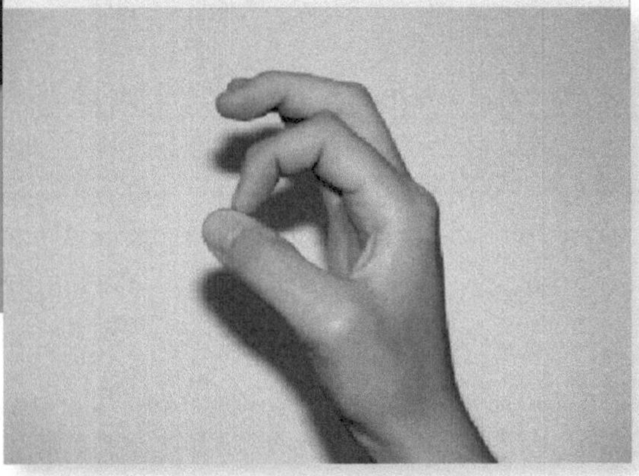

FIGURE A5.11.2

Positive pinch sign.

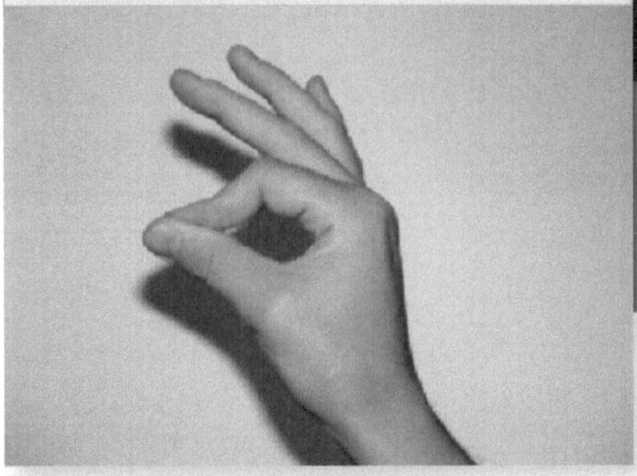

- A pharmacological course of oral steroid followed with non-steroidal anti-inflammatory medication.[6] A local cortisone injection may also be helpful both as a diagnostic and therapeutic tool.[68]
- Therapeutic modalities such as cryotherapy, ultrasound, electrical stimulation, and iontophoresis to control pain and facilitate tissue and nerve healing.
- Therapeutic exercises, including nerve gliding/mobilization to improve nerve function and movement and soft tissue mobilization to improve muscle relaxation and decrease muscle tension. If nerve gliding/mobilization appears to increase pain and neurological symptoms, discontinue at once. Also, consider using soft-tissue mobilization prior to any type of nerve gliding/mobilization.

5.11 / **5.** *As mentioned in the case, Ron suggests referral to another physician if conservative treatment does not work. What type of physician would you consider referring Harry to, and why?*

If conservative treatment fails, referring Ron to an orthopedic surgeon would typically be the first step. If possible, consider referring him to an orthopedic surgeon specializing in elbows.

5.11 / **6.** *Overall, do you believe Ron adequately evaluated Harry's condition? If not, what would you have done differently as the evaluating clinician, and why?*

The answers to this question will vary among students. The final diagnosis of pronator teres syndrome is often made with a good physical exam and diagnostic testing to rule out other conditions. The signs and symptoms and results of the physical examination presented in the case should be enough for an initial clinical diagnosis. One item Ron did seem to omit was any type of special test beyond the Tinel's sign. Lee and LaStayo[45] provide several objective tests that can be used by clinicians to assess for pronator teres syndrome. To determine the site of the entrapment, Lee and LaStayo recommend "creating maximal tension on the anatomical sites that can contribute to compression of the median nerve as it courses from the elbow to the wrist." The pronator compression test is another test used to assess for pronator teres syndrome. Pressure is placed on the pronator teres muscle bilaterally, with a positive finding being a reproduction of the sensory deficits into the thumb and index and middle finger within 30 seconds.[45] Gainor[33] found that of the ten patients with a diagnosis of pronator teres syndrome, all developed paresthesia in the hand within 30 seconds of compression over the median nerve. Eight of these patients also presented with a positive Tinel's sign.[33] Another study of 36 patients found the most common physical finding was a positive pronator compression test, followed by median nerve hypesthesia.[58] Lastly, Schultz, Houlgum, and Perrin[76] describe the pronator teres test, which also assesses for median nerve compression due to hypertrophy of the pronator teres.

## CASE 5.12 Cubital Tunnel Syndrome—Ulnar Nerve

5.12 / **1.** *Based on the information presented in the case, determine (a) the differential diagnoses and (b) the clinical diagnosis.*

a. Differential diagnoses: thoracic outlet syndrome, C8-T1 nerve root compression, medial brachial plexus cord compression, ulnar collateral sprain, and medial epicondylitis[11,71,77]

b. Clinical diagnosis: cubital tunnel syndrome, probably from compression or entrapment of the ulnar nerve

5.12 / **2.** *Celina asked several history questions to guide her physical examination. Based on the information presented in the case, do you believe she took an adequate history? If not, what questions would you have asked as the treating clinician?*

The answers to this question will vary among students. Overall, Celina appeared to generate an adequate history. Some additional information to assist in the physical examination might include the following:

- Determine whether or not the medial epicondyle had been exposed to constant resting pressure on a hard surface[13,80] or extreme periods of elbow flexion,[71] which causes the nerve to be compressed.
- Determine whether the patient has experienced any popping or snapping sensations.
- Ask about any changes in sleeping patterns that cause the patient to wake at night.[80]
- Although rare, abnormal strain on the ulnar nerve over the sulcus from sleeping with one or both arms in a flexed position can cause cubital tunnel syndrome.[10,31] Normal flexion of the elbow causes the ulnar nerve to elongate 4.7 to 8.0 mm, as well as the arcuate ligament, which decreases the ulnar nerve's canal volume 55 percent, thereby increasing the risk of ulnar nerve damage.[10]
- If Recruit Jones had still been a throwing athlete (a baseball player), the number of throws in one game or in a series of games is considered to correlate with the occurrence of cubital tunnel syndrome.[5] Also, identifying any changes in throwing mechanics would be necessary, because the strain placed on the proximal aspect of the cubital tunnel increases significantly with elbow flexion in the stance, wind-up, and middle cock-up phases of throwing.[5]

5.12 / **3.** *If Recruit Jones had reported a popping or clicking sound or sensation with elbow flexion, (a) how would this have affected your clinical diagnosis? (b) Would you have altered your evaluation?*

a. A patient reporting a popping or clicking sensation with elbow flexion and extension is typically experiencing an ulnar nerve subluxation or recurrent dislocation.[14] Recurrent dislocations may occur because of congenital or developmental laxity of the soft tissue responsible for holding the ulnar nerve in the cubital tunnel.[74] Previous injuries may also cause the nerve to become adhered in an irregular manner in the epicondylar groove.[74] Clinically, the subluxing ulnar nerve may feel thickened or doughy and can be manually displaced from the epicondylar groove. The clinical diagnosis of cubital tunnel syndrome or ulnar neuritis is still plausible; however, what may change is the etiology. Whether the ulnar neuritis is caused by compression, traction, or friction, the components of the physical assessment are similar.

b. The evaluation should then include a test for a subluxing ulnar nerve. Ask the patient to flex and extend the involved elbow while palpating the ulnar nerve as it dislocates anteriorly from the groove during flexion and returns into the cubital tunnel during extension.[14]

5.12 / **4.** *(a) What is the elbow flexion test, and (b) how is it performed? (c) If you were the evaluating clinician would you have performed this test? Why or why not? If not, (d) what other test might you have performed?*

a. The elbow flexion test is a provocative test used to diagnose ulnar nerve compression or entrapment in the cubital tunnel by putting the nerve on tension through full elbow flexion.

b. The test is normally performed with the patient standing or sitting with both elbows maximally flexed and the wrists extended. A positive finding occurs when the patient experiences tingling and paresthesia in the ulnar distribution of the forearm and hand. However, the testing position and length of time for the test (1–5 min) vary, as do the results. Buehler and Thayer[15] found that after 3 minutes of elbow flexion, pain, numbness (in the sensory distribution of the ulnar nerve), and tingling were found in 93 percent, 86 percent, and 86 percent of the patients, respectively, in subjects with confirmed cases of cubital tunnel syndrome. Studies of healthy subjects[67] found that in 20 elbows in 15 subjects (10%) flexion tests were positive with the wrist and shoulder placed in a neutral position, while 27 elbows in 20 persons (13%) tested positive with the wrist extended and shoulder abducted. Novack, Lee, Mackinnon, and Lay[56] evaluated the clinical usefulness of four provocative testing procedures by comparing 32 subjects with diagnostically assessed cases of cubital tunnel syndrome against 33 control subjects. They demonstrated that the sensitivity of the Tinel's sign was 0.70, and after 30 and 60 seconds of testing, the sensitivity of the elbow flexion test was 0.32 and 0.75 respectively. A pressure provocation at 30 and 60 seconds had a sensitivity of 0.55 and 0.89 respectively, and a combination pressure-flexion test was the highest at 0.98 for 60 seconds. All tests demonstrated a specificity of .95 or higher, with the flexion test having the highest at .99. Finally, Rosati et al.[73] evaluated the elbow flexion test in 216 subjects without compression of the ulnar nerve at the cubital tunnel. They found that the percentage of positive tests was greater at the 3-minute mark (16%) than the one-minute mark (3.6%).

c. Yes, as this is a commonly used test in diagnosing cubital tunnel syndrome. However, a couple of other tests may be utilized.

d. Two other special tests that could be performed include Wartenberg's sign and the Froment's sign. Wartenberg's sign assesses the patient's ability to bring his passively spread fingers together again. A positive finding is the inability to squeeze the little finger to the reminder of the hand.[51] The Froment's sign, first described by Jules Froment, results in reduced function and muscular weakness in pinch-grip strength. Patients are asked to hold a piece of paper between the thumb and index finger. When the clinician pulls the piece of paper away, the distal phalanx of the thumbs flexes (the flexor pollicis longus is compensatory) due to paralysis of the adductor pollicis muscle, which is innervated by the ulnar nerve, indicating ulnar nerve palsy.[51]

5.12 / **5.** *After completing the physical examination, Celina documented her findings and sent a copy of the report to Dr. Taylor's office. Please document your findings as if you were the treating clinician. If the case did not provide information you believe is pertinent to the clinical diagnosis, please add this information to your documentation.*

Answers will vary. Students should consider writing a SOAP note (see textbook Appendix B) using the ABCD format when writing the short- and long-term goals.

## CASE 5.13 Olecranon Bursitis

5.13 / **1.** *Based on the information presented in the case, identify what you believe was Bill's original clinical diagnosis and what the clinical diagnosis should have been.*

Bill's clinical diagnosis on the initial assessment was olecranon bursitis. Given the original information, Figure 5.13.1, and the information reported on Dr. Pedersen's follow-up physical examination, the clinical diagnosis should have been septic olecranon bursitis.

5.13 / **2.** *Why do you believe Dr. Pedersen asked Helen to prepare a 20mL syringe and a 22 gauge, 1-inch needle?*

Given the findings of her physical examination, Dr. Pedersen needed to aspirate the bursa to collect fluid for a culture. When aspirating for a culture, a sterile technique should be used.[19] If sepsis is not suspected but the fluid from the aspirated elbow is cloudy, a culture is warranted.

5.13 / **3.** *(a) Overall, do you believe Bill handled the situation correctly? If not, what would you have done differently as the evaluating clinician? (b) Should Bill have had more concern for Chris's condition?*

a. The answers to this question will vary among students because the situation presented in this case had many flaws. All students should agree that Bill failed to properly assess Chris and did not refer him to appropriate medical personnel. Bill failed to complete the injury assessment and missed several red flags, such as pain with palpation and movement, warmth and erythema, and the wound. Acute olecranon bursitis can be painful[19,65] and presents with a some loss of function from increased pressure,[76] but repetitive olecranon bursitis is normally painless.[19,20] For this reason, an athletic trainer must be diligent, consider all possibilities, and avoid making hasty clinical decisions. He must also be able to adequately document his findings.

b. Bill certainly needed to have much more concern for this condition than he did. Failure to refer Chris to the appropriate medical personnel for care increases the risk of septicemia. Septicemia is a systemic condition caused by a failure of the body's defense mechanisms to prevent the proliferation of gram-negative bacteria.

5.13 / **4.** *What professional standards, if any, did Bill fail to follow?*

To determine if Bill acted in a professional manner or if he failed to follow professional standards, students should examine the Board of Certification's *Standards of Professional Practice*[9] (see Appendix B in the textbook) as well as the States' Practice Act. According to Code 1: Patient Responsibility sections 1.2, 1.5, and 1.7 of the *Standards of Professional Practice:* "1.2 Protects the patient from harm, acts always in the patient's best interests, and is an advocate for the patient's welfare." In this case, Bill's actions were clearly not in the best interest of Chris. In fact, Bill's actions were negligent.

"1.5 Communicates clearly and truthfully with patients and other persons involved in the patient's program, including, but not limited to, appropriate discussion of assessment results, program plans, and progress." If Chris did present with warmth and erythema around the elbow, and on initial assessment Bill blatantly withheld this information from Dr. Pedersen, he would be in violation of this code.

"1.7 Exercises reasonable care, skill, and judgment in all professional work." There are four prerequisites that must be met in order to be found negligent in a civil case. One of these is breach of duty. Under this point, a plaintiff must demonstrate that an athletic trainer breached her duty to exercise reasonable care by failing to use reasonable care. The plaintiff must show that there is a connection between this failure in reasonable care and that this either caused the injury or worsened the condition. If Chris had in fact developed septicemia, required hospitalization, and incurred pain and suffering and medical bills, the likelihood of Bill being held accountable for his action or inaction is great.

Further evaluation of the *BOC Standards of Professional Practice* (provided in the Appendix of the textbook) may reveal violations of other practice codes. The *BOC Standards of Professional Practice* may also be found at http://www.bocatc.org/images/stories/multiple_references/standardsprofessionalpractice.pdf.

5.13 / **5.** *If you were Dr. Pedersen, how would you address this situation with Bill?*

The answers to this question will vary among students. However, all practicing athletic trainers and athletic training students need to understand that all credentialed athletic trainers are held accountable to these standards. In fact, the *BOC Standards of Professional Practice* states: "The BOC requires all athletic trainers and applicants to comply with the Code. The BOC may discipline, revoke or take other action with regard to the application or certification of an individual that does not adhere to the Code." Students should refer to the BOC's website and to their instructor for further information on disciplinary procedures that Dr. Pedersen can take and whether Dr. Pedersen should have reported Bill to the BOC.

## CASE 5.14 Lateral Epicondylitis

5.14 / **1.** *Based on the information presented in the case, determine (a) the differential diagnoses and (b) the clinical diagnosis.*

a. Differential diagnoses: radial head dislocation, radial collateral ligament sprain/instability, cervical lesions, arthritic disease, radial tunnel syndrome, posterior interosseous nerve syndrome, radiocapitellar chondromalacia[20,77]

b. Clinical diagnosis: lateral epicondylitis

5.14 / **2.** *In addition to the information Crystal gained from the history, identify three to four additional history questions she could have asked to help guide the physical examination and to help rule out the differential diagnoses.*

The following are some examples of additional history questions.[30,50]

- Is there any history of previous trauma; if so, what?
- Do you have any ache or morning stiffness?
- If the trauma is repetitive, describe the occupational or athlete exposure, such as load, repetitions, postures, and sporting equipment.
- Is this your dominant hand?
- Is there any change or difficulty in activities of daily living, such as tying shoes, turning a doorknob, or lifting heavy objects with the involved limb?
- Is there any numbness or tingling? (Lateral elbow pain can be caused by several neurological pathologies.)
- Is there any instability, giving way, locking, or catching when lifting heavy objects?
- Are there any prior or current neck, shoulder, or wrist injuries?

5.14 / **3.** *Why did Richard have significant discomfort with palpation of the lateral epicondyle?*

Lateral epicondylitis often is caused by overuse of the forearm common extensor muscles originating at the lateral epicondyle, especially when stabilizing the wrist in slight extension.[51] Muscles originating on the common extensor origin include the extensor carpi radialis brevis, extensor carpi radialis longus, extensor carpi ulnaris, extensor digitorum communis (middle finger slip), and the extensor digiti minimi. The extensor carpi radialis brevis is the tendon most often involved in cases of lateral epicondylitis, because it crosses both the elbow and the wrist and contracts eccentrically at both ends during certain movements.[61]

5.14 / **4.** *(a) Do you believe that Crystal thoroughly evaluated Richard's condition? If not, (b) what would you have done differently as the evaluating clinician?*

a. Crystal could have performed more tests to rule out neurological pathology. Such tests might include: Tinel's sign, pinch-grip test, upper-limb tension test, dermatome and peripheral nerve testing, brachial plexus compression test, and thoracic outlet syndrome test.[51]

b. She could have ruled out instability in the elbow by performing laxity tests on the radial collateral ligament and ulnar collateral ligament. Further ROM and strength testing of the shoulder and wrist may have revealed loss of ROM and/or additional muscular weakness that may be related to the condition. The testing could have also ruled out other joint involvement. The above would need to be addressed in rehabilitation.

Two other provocative maneuvers for soft tissue irritability could also have been used to assess for lateral epicondylitis: the Maudsley's test and the chair lift/pick-up test.

- The Maudsley's test (middle finger test) originally elicited pain in 36 patients with signs and symptoms of tennis elbow and was believed to indicate compression of the radial nerve by the contracting extensor carpi radialis brevis.[72] Recently, Fairbank and Corlett[28] challenged this notion and suggested that the Maudsley's test probably indicates pathology to the extensor digitorum communis (EDC) muscle rather than the extensor carpi radialis brevis, because the EDC is the major extensor of the middle finger. A review of 10 patients with a confirmed diagnosis of lateral epicondylitis upon clinical physical exam found a high prevalence of positive Maudsley's test (5 of 7 patients with VAS pain scores higher on middle finger extension and wrist extension reported tenderness over the most lateral aspect of the anterior surface of the lateral epicondyle where the EDC—middle finger originates), suggesting that the EDC plays a greater role in tennis elbow than once thought.
- The chair-lift test, or chair pick-up test, is a clinical assessment of elbow function and a provocative test in patients with lateral epicondylitis. It is part of "The Orthopedic Research Institute Tennis-Elbow Testing System,"[61] which is designed to simulate the load placed on the origin of the extensor tendons of the hand by forcefully gripping an object with the hand in palmar flexion, wrist ulnarly deviated, and forearm pronated. The "Paoloni, Appleyard, and Murrell System"[61] consists of a vertical handboard attached to a horizontal level arm, which is attached to a tensile cord and load cell used to collect force data. Subjects grasp a coronally aligned handboard with the thumb on the side of the handboard nearest their body and the other four digits on the side farthest from their body, ensuring pronation of forearm. With the elbow in 90° of flexion, subjects lift the handboard superiorly while maintaining the lever arm horizontal to the floor for 10 seconds (i.e., simulating lifting a chair from the floor by holding the top with the thumb and digits). Their results indicated that the chair pick-up test demonstrated high interrater reliability with intraclass correlation coefficient (ICC) for mean peak and total force, right and left arms (.86 to .93). A negative correlation between patient-rated activity pain and mean peak and total force (–.87 to 1.00) in patients with lateral epicondylitis was identified.

5.14 / **5.** *If you were the athletic trainer in this case, what would your next step be, knowing that Richard is on his way out to the first practice of the season?*

Answers will vary among students, but several possible answers might include:

- Address the pain and swelling to keep him at practice. Begin a round of over-the-counter anti-inflammatory medication, ultrasound treatments to the lateral epicondyle before practice, followed by stretching the forearm extensors, use of bracing during practice, and cryotherapy after practice.
- As pain and swelling decrease, implement strengthening exercises to prevent the injury from recurring.
- Follow up with the team physician in one week if the treatment fails to control or reduce symptoms.

## CASE 5.15 Medial Epicondylitis

5.15 / **1.** *Based on the information presented in the case, determine (a) the differential diagnoses and (b) the clinical diagnosis.*

a. Differential diagnoses: cervical radiculopathy, UCL ligament injury, flexor pronator strain, medial epicondyle avulsion, growth alteration of the medial epicondyle, osteochondrits of the capitulum or radial head, and apophysitis[91]

b. Clinical diagnosis: medial epicondylitis; however, given the age of the patient, little league elbow is possible. "Little league elbow" is a term used to describe a variety of pathologies that occur around the elbow in immature athletes[43]

5.15 / **2.** *Overall, do you believe that Anita completed a thorough history? What if anything would you have done differently?*

The answers will vary among students, but overall, the history obtained by Anita appeared to be sufficient. Some questions she may have considered would be:

- Any changes in pitching velocity and accuracy?
- What type of pitches do you throw (i.e., curve balls vs. fastballs)?
- Which phase of the throwing motion causes pain?[69]

5.15 / **3.** *In this case, the clinical diagnosis appears not to be an isolated injury but rather a symptom of a larger problem. Discuss what the larger problem is and how it may exist.*

The answers will vary among students. However, students should realize the need to focus their physical examination not only at the joint in question but to the joints above and below the injury site, especially in the case of an overuse throwing injury. Students should realize and appreciate the relationships of the elbow joint in the kinetic chain and its effect on other joints or vice versa. For example, scapular muscular weakness and lack of motor control can cause pain and dysfunction to the distal structures, which in turn causes changes in joint mechanics, which ultimately results in damage to the stressed tissue (i.e., the elbow in this case).

5.15 / **4.** *What are your thoughts regarding Jenny's pitch count? Is she within the pitching limits required by USA baseball?*

According to the publication, "Protecting Young Pitching Arms: The Little League Pitch Count Regulation Guide for Parents, Coaches and League Officials" (endorsed by the American Sports Medicine Institute), starting with the 2007 season, "pitchers in all divisions of Little League, from age 7 to 18, will have specific limits for each game, based on their age." Furthermore, "the number of pitches delivered in a game will determine the amount of rest the player must have before pitching again." In this, at the age of 14, Jenny is allowed 85 pitches. Her rest period as a pitcher age 16 and under must adhere to the following rest requirements:

- If a player pitches 61 or more pitches in a day, 3 calendar days of rest must be observed.
- If a player pitches 41 to 60 pitches in a day, 2 calendar days of rest must be observed.
- If a player pitches 21 to 40 pitches in a day, 1 calendar day of rest must be observed.
- If a player pitches 1 to 20 pitches in a day, no calendar day of rest need be observed.

A complete listing of the new Little League Pitching Rules can be found at LittleLeague.org (see www.littleleague.org/Assets/old_assets/media/Pitch_Count_Publication_2008.pdf).

5.15 / **5.** *Why do you believe Anita wanted to refer Jenny to a specialist? Would you have made a similar recommendation?*

Referral to a specialist such as an orthopedic surgeon for an immature athlete presenting with the above finding is warranted. Even with a good history and physical examination, further diagnostic testing, such as radiographs, is necessary to rule out osseous changes occurring from repetitive valgus forces applied to the elbow, which can result in submaximal injury, apophyseal fragmentation, acute avulsion of the medial epicondyle apophysitis, or other conditions, depending on the age and development of the athlete.[17,43,69]

## CASE 5.16 Condylar, Epicondylar, or Intercondylar Fracture

5.16 / **1.** *Based on the information presented in the case, determine (a) the differential diagnoses and (b) the clinical diagnosis.*

a. Differential diagnoses: dislocated elbow, distal supracondylar ridge fracture, distal humeral shaft fracture, olecranon fracture

b. Clinical diagnoses: condylar, epicondylar, or intercondylar fracture of the humerus

5.16 / **2.** *What is the common mechanism for this type of injury?*

The MOI for condylar fractures (medial) is a valgus force with the elbow extended,[31] which transmits forces up through the condyle and humerus.

5.16 / **3.** *If you were in Barry's situation, how would you have managed the situation?*

First, the area around Tuppu should be cleared to prevent harm to Tuppu or others while managing this injury. The coach or referee would need to move the players to another side of the field for the remainder of practice. Because a fracture is suspected, the clinician can: (1) use a SAM SPLINT to secure the area, making sure that the splint covers the elbow and wrist joints; (2) use an air splint, covering the elbow and inflating to secure the area; or (3) use a rapid form immobilizer to secure the area.

Once the area is secure, a sling and swath should be applied to the arm and secured to the athlete, allowing ease of transport and better security to the body to prevent other complications. Finally, an assessment of the distal neurovascular status is necessary before and after stabilization.

5.16 / **4.** *Suppose Barry removed the player from the field, splinted the injured area, and noticed the distal pulses were compromised. What should he then do?*

Most likely, Barry secured the splint too tightly. He would have to loosen the pressure and retake the pulse. If, after doing so, distal pulses are still absent, Barry would need to get medical attention rapidly. Trauma to the distal humerus increases the risk of damage to the brachial artery, can result in a diminished or absent radial pulse,[55] and increases the risk of a Volkmann's ischemic contracture.

5.16 / **5.** *Should Barry, who is the only athletic trainer on the field, call for emergency medical services and, if necessary, go with the athlete to the hospital?*

In this scenario, with a suspected fracture, the emergency action plan should be activated and followed. The emergency action plan should identity the individual responsible for calling the emergency medical services.[3] Barry would be responsible for maintaining the athlete's comfort as much as possible and immobilizing the fracture site. When emergency personnel arrive, the athlete should be transported to the hospital. Barry would need to stay at practice to care for the other athletes, and either a coach or fellow player should go with the injured athlete to the hospital.

5.16 / **6.** *Based on this type of injury, what are some complications that could result?*

The epiphyseal plate can be compromised in younger athletes,[47] and limited blood supply to the trochlea, ulnar nerve pathology from fractured bony segments, collateral ligament damage, and compromise to the brachial artery are all possible.

# REFERENCES


1. Altner P, Hartman J. Isolated fractures of the ulnar shaft in the adult. *Surg Clin North Am.* 1972;52:155–170.
2. American Red Cross. *Emergency Response.* Yardley, PA: Staywell; 2001.
3. Anderson JC, Courson R, Kleiner D, McLoda T. National Athletic Trainers' Association Position Statement: Emergency planning in athletics. *J Ath Training. 2002;37(1):99–104.*
4. Andrews JR, Wilk KE, Satterwhite YE, Tedder JL. *Physical examination of the thrower's elbow.* J Orthop Sports Phys Ther. 1993;17(6):296–304.
5. Aoki M, Takasaki H, Muraki T, Uchiyama E, Murakami G, Yamashita T. Strain on the ulnar nerve at the elbow and wrist during throwing motion. *J Bone Joint Surg, [Am].* 2005;87-A(11):2508–2514.
6. Azar FM, Andrews JR, Wilk KE, Groh D. Operative treatment of ulnar collateral ligament injuries of the elbow in athletes. *Am J Sports Med* [electronic version]. 2000;28:16–23. Available from: http://ajs.sagepub.com/cgi/content/abstract/28/1/16. Accessed June 19, 2007.
7. Bensahel H, Csukonyi Z, Badelon O, Badaoui S. Fractures of the medial condyle of the humerus in children. *J Ped Ortho.* 1986;6:430–433.
8. Berg EE. Elbow dislocation with arterial injury. *Orthop Nurs.* 2001;20(6):57–59.
9. Board of Certification. BOC Standards of Professional Practice [electronic version] 2006. Available from: http://www.bocatc.org/images/stories/multiple_references/standards professionalpractice.pdf. Accessed December 27, 2009.
10. Bozentka DJ. Cubital tunnel syndrome pathophysiology. *Clin Orthop.* 1998;351:90–94.
11. Bracker MD, Ralph LP. The numb arm and hand. *Am Fam Physician.* 1995;51(1):103–116.
12. Branch G, Wieting D. Biceps rupture. *eMedicine.* [electronic version]. 2008. Available from: http://emedicine.medscape.com/article/327119-overview. Accessed June 4, 2009.
13. Budd GM, Piccioni LH. Identifying and treating common problems in the elbow. *Am J Nurse Pract.* 2005;9(2):41.
14. Budoff JE, Nirschl RP. *Office examination of the elbow: how provocative tests can help clinch the diagnosis.* Consultant. 2001;41(7):1004–1005, 1009–1010, 1012–1013.
15. Buehler MJ, Thayer DT. The elbow flexion test: a clinical test for the cubital tunnel syndrome. *Clin Orthop.* 1988;Aug(233):213–216.
16. Burns KJ. Extremity and vascular trauma. In Sheehy SB, Blansfield JS, Danis DM, Gervasini AA, (eds.). *Manual of Clinical Trauma: The First Hour* (3rd ed.). St. Louis, MO: Mosby; 1999:292–293.
17. Cain EL, Dugas JR, Wolf RS, Andrews JR. Elbow injuries in throwing athletes: a current concepts review. *Am J Sports Med* [electronic version]. 2003;31:621–635. Available from: http://ajs.sagepub.com/cgi/content/abstract/31/4/621. Accessed July 7, 2007.
18. Callaway GH, Field LD, Deng XH, Torzilli PA, O'Brien SJ, Altchek DW, et al. Biomechanical evaluation of the medial collateral ligament of the elbow. *J Bone Joint Surg [Am].* 1997;79-A(8):1223–1231.
19. Cardone DA, Tallia AF. Diagnostic and therapeutic injection of the elbow region. *Am Fam Physician.* 2002; 66(11):2097–2100.
20. Chumbley EM, O'Connor FG, Nirschl RP. Evaluation of overuse elbow injuries. *Am Fam Physician* [electronic version]. 2000;61:691–700. Available from: http://www.aafp.org/afp/20000201/691.html. Accessed July 30, 2007.
21. Clarkson HM. *Musculoskeletal Assessment: Joint Range of Motion and Manual Muscle Strength.* Philadelphia, PA: Lippincott Williams & Wilkins; 2000.
22. Cohen MS, Bruno RJ. The collateral ligaments of the elbow: anatomy and clinical correlation. *Clin Orthop.* 2001;(383):123–130.
23. Daniels JM, Zook EG, Lynch JM. Hand and wrist injuries: part II. Emergent evaluation. *Am Fam Physician.* 2004;69:1949–1956.
24. Deschamp C. Prehospital management of pediatric pain. *Journal of Emergency Medical Services* [electronic version]. 2006. Available from: http://www.jems.com/news_and_articles/articles/Prehospital_Management_of_Pediatric_Pain.html. Accessed July 31, 2007.
25. Disabella VN. Elbow and forearm overuse injuries *eMedicine* [electronic version]. 2008. Available from: http://emedicine.medscape.com/article/96638-overview. Accessed December 27, 2009.
26. Docherty MA, Schwab, RA, John O. Can elbow extension be used as a test of clinically significant injury? *South Med J.* 2002;95(5):539–541.
27. Eygendaal D, Safran MR. Postero-medial elbow problems in the adult athlete. *Br J Sports Med* [electronic version]. 2006;40:430–434. Available from: http://bjsm.bmj.com/cgi/content/abstract/40/5/430. Accessed May 1, 2006.
28. Fairbank SR, Corelett RJ. The role of the extensor digitorum communis muscle in lateral epicondylitis. *J Hand Surg [BR].* 2002;27B(5):405–409.
29. Farrar EL, Lippert FG. Avulsion of the triceps tendon. *Clinical Orthopaedics.* 1981;161:242–247.
30. Field LD, Savoie FH. Common elbow injuries in sport. *Sports Med.* 1998;26(3):193–205.
31. Finsterer J. Ulnar neuropathy at the elbow due to unusual sleep position. *European Journal of Neurology.* 2000;7(1):115–117.
32. Fowles J, Kassab M. Displaced fractures of the medial humeral condyle in children. *J Bone Joint Surg [Am].* 1980;62A:1159–1163.
33. Gainor BJ. The pronator compression test revisited: a forgotten physical sign. *Orthop Rev.* 1990;19(10):888–892.
34. Hamilton W, Ramsey ML. Rupture of the distal tendon of the biceps brachii. *University of Pennsylvania Orthopaedic Journal.* 1999;12:21–26.
35. Hawksworth C, Freeland P. Inability to fully extend the injured elbow: an indicator of significant injury. *Arch Emerg Med.* 1991;8:252–256.
36. Hendricks S, Counselman FL. Managing common upper extremity fractures [electronic version]. *Emergency Medicine.* 2004;36:26–36. Available from: http://www.emedmag.com/html/pre/cov/covers/051504.asp. Accessed July 2, 2007.

37. Hill NA, Howard FM, Huffer B. The incomplete anterior interosseous syndrome. *J Hand Surg [Am]*. 1985;10:4–16.

38. Houshian S, Mehdi B, Larsen MS. The epidemiology of elbow fracture in children: analysis of 355 fractures, with special reference o supracondylar humerus fractures. *J Orthop Sci*. 2001;6:312–315.

39. Jensen SL, Deutch SR, Olsen BS, Sojbjerg JO, Sneppen O. Laxity of the elbow alter experimental excision of the radial head and division of the medial collateral ligament: efficacy of ligament repair and radial head prosthetic replacement: a cadaver study. *J Bone Joint Surg [BR]*. 2003;85-B(7):1006–1010.

40. Kacprowicz RF, Chumbley E. Ulnar collateral ligament injury. *eMedicine* [electronic version]. 2007. Available from: http://www.emedicine.com/sports/topic139.htm. Accessed June 4, 2009.

41. Kaminski TW, Power ME, Buckley B. Differential assessment of elbow injuries. *Ath Ther Today*. 2000;5(3):6–11.

42. Keany JE, McKeever D. Dislocation, elbow. *eMedicine* [electronic version]. 2009. Available from: http://emedicine.medscape.com/article/823277-overview. Accessed December 27, 2009.

43. Kocher MS, Waters PM, Micheli LJ. Upper extremity injuries in the paediatric athlete. *Sports Med*. 2000;30(2):117–135.

44. Langer P, Fadale P, Hulstyn M. Evolution of the treatment options of ulnar collateral ligament injuries of the elbow. *Br J Sports Med* [electronic version]. 2006;40:499–506. Accessed July, 31, 2007.

45. Lee MJ, LaStayo PC. Pronator syndrome and other nerve compressions that mimic carpal tunnel syndrome. *J Orthop Sports Phys Ther*. 2004;34(10):601–609.

46. Lee P, Hunter TB, Taljanovic M. Musculoskeletal colloquialisms: how did we come up with these names? *RadioGraphics* [electronic version]. 2004;24:1009–1027. Available from: http://radiographics.rsnajnls.org/. Accessed May 15, 2009.

47. Leet A, Young C, Hoffer M. Medial condylar fractures of the humerus in children. *Journal of Pediatric Orthopedics*. 2002;22(1):2–7.

48. Leigh W, Pai V. Beware: compartment syndrome of the hand. *N Z Med J* [electronic version]. 2005;118. Available from: http://www.nzma.org.nz/journal/118-1209/1300/.

49. Levangie PK, Norkin CC. *Joint Structure and Function: A Comprehensive Analysis*. Philadelphia, PA: F.A. Davis; 2001.

50. MacDermid JC, Michlovitz SL. Examination of the elbow: linking diagnosis, prognosis, and outcomes as a framework for maximizing therapy interventions. *J Hand Ther*. 2006;19(2):82–97.

51. Magee DJ. *Orthopedic Physical Assessment* (5th ed.). Philadelphia, PA: WB Saunders; 2007.

52. McKee MD, Schemitsch EH, Sala MJ, O'Driscoll SW. The pathoanatomy of lateral ligament disruption in complex elbow in stability. *Journal of Shoulder and Elbow Surgery*. 2003;12:391–396.

53. Moore K, Dalley A. *Clinically Oriented Anatomy* (5th ed.). Baltimore, MD: Lippincott Williams & Wilkins; 2005.

54. Nassab PF, Schickendantz MS. Evaluation and treatment of medial ulnar collateral ligament injuries in the throwing athlete. *Sports Medicine and Arthroscopy Review*. 2006;14:221–231.

55. Noaman HH. Microsurgical reconstruction of brachial artery injuries in displaced supracondylar fracture humerus in children. *Microsurgery*. 2006;26(7):498–505.

56. Novak CB, Lee GW, Mackinnon SE, Lay L. Provocative testing for cubital tunnel syndrome. *J Hand Surg. [AM]*. 1994;19-A(5):817–820.

57. O'Driscoll SWM, Lawton RL, Smith AM. The "Moving Valgus Stress Test" for medial collateral ligament tears of the elbow. *Am J Sports Med* [electronic version]. 2005;33:231–239. Available from: http://ajs.sagepub.com/cgi/content/abstract/33/2/231. Accessed June 18, 2007.

58. Olehnik WK, Manske PR, Szerzinski J. Median nerve compression in the proximal forearm. *J Hand Surg*. 1994;19(1):121–126.

59. Otsuka NY, Kasser JR. Supracondylar fractures of the humerus in children. *J Am Acad Orthop Surg*. 1997;5:19–26.

60. Paksima N, Panchal A. Elbow fracture-dislocations: the role of hinged external fixation. *Bull Hosp Jt Dis Orthop Inst*. 2004;62(1 & 2):33–39.

61. Paoloni JA, Appleyard RC, Murrell GAC. The Orthopaedic Research Institute-Tennis Elbow Testing System: a modified chair pick-up test—interrater and intrarater reliability testing and validity for monitoring lateral epicondylosis. *Journal of Shoulder and Elbow Surgery*. 2004;13(1):72–77.

62. Perron AD, Brady WJ, Keats TE. Orthopedic pitfalls in the ED: acute compartment syndrome. *Am J Emerg Med*. 2001;19(5):413–416.

63. Roche Pharmaceuticals. Toradol. 2007. Available from: http://www.rocheusa.com/products/toradol/. Accessed July 7, 2007.

64. Platt B. Supracondylar fractures of the humerus. *Emergency Nurse*. 2004;12(2):22–30.

65. Prentice WE. *Arnheim's Principles of Athletic Training: A Competency-Based Approach* (13th ed.). Boston, MA: McGraw Hill Publishing; 2009.

66. Rabee HM, Al-Salman MM, Iqbal K, Al-Khawashki H. Vascular compromise associated with supracondylar fractures in children. *Saudi Medical Journal*. 2001;22(9):790–792.

67. Rayan GM, Jensen C, Duke J. Elbow flexion test in the normal population. *J Hand Surg, [AM]*. 1992;17-A(1):86–89.

68. Rehak DC. Pronator syndrome. *Clin Sports Med. 2001;20(3):531–540.*

69. *Rettig AC. Managing elbow problems in throwing athletes.* Journal of Musculoskeletal Medicine. 2007;24:129–135.

70. Rettig AC, Sherrill C, Snead DS, Mendler JC, Mieling P. Nonoperative treatment of ulnar collateral ligament injuries in throwing athletes. *Am J Sports Med* [electronic version]. 2001;29:15–17. Available from: http://ajs.sagepub.com/cgi/content/abstract/29/1/15. Accessed June 18, 2007.

71. Robertson C, Saratsiotis J. A review of compressive ulnar neuropathy at the elbow. *J Manipulative Physiol Ther*. 2005;28(5) 345e:341–318.

72. Roles NC, Maudsley RH. Radial tunnel syndrome: Resistent tennis elbow as a nerve entrapement. *J Bone Joint Surg [Br]*. 1972;23-B:499–508.

73. Rosati M, Martignoni R, Spagnolli G, Nesti C, Lisanti M. Clinical validity of the elbow flexion test for the diagnosis

of ulnar nerve compression at the cubital tunnel. *Acta Orthopaedica Belgica.* 1998;64(4):366–370.

74. Safran MR, Bradley JP. Elbow injuries. In Fu FH, Stone DA (eds.), *Sports Injuries: Mechanisms, Prevention, Treatment* (2nd ed.). Philadelphia, PA: Lippincott Williams & Wilkins; 2001:1049–1084.
75. Schubert H. Radial head fracture. *Canadian Family Physician.* 2000;46:1759–1761.
76. Schultz SJ, Houglum PA, Perrin DH. *Examination of Musculoskeletal Injuries* (2nd ed.). Champaign, IL: Human Kinetics; 2005.
77. Sellards R, Kuebrich C. The elbow: diagnosis and treatment of common injuries. *Prim Care.* 2005;32(1):1–16.
78. Seyffarth H. Primary myoses in the M. pronator teres as cause of lesion of the N. medianus (the pronator syndrome). *Acta psychiatrica et neurologica Scandinavica. Supplementum.* 1951;74:251–4.
79. Shah KC, Rajshekhar V. Reliability of diagnosis of soft cervical disc prolapse using Spurling's test. *Br J Neurosurg.* 2004;18(5):480–483.
80. Shah MA, Sotereanos DG. Recognizing and managing compression neuropathies of the elbow. *Journal of Musculoskeletal Medicine. 1999;16(2):116.*
81. Singh H, Osbahr DC, Wickham MQ, Kirkendall DT, Speer KP. *Valgus laxity of the ulnar collateral ligament of the elbow in collegiate athletes.* Am J Sports Med [electronic version]. 2001;29:558–561. Available from: http://ajs.sagepub.com/cgi/content/abstract/29/5/558. Accessed June 18, 2007.
82. Singh RK, Pooley J. Complete rupture of the triceps brachii muscle. *Br J Sports Med* [electronic version]. 2002;36:467–469. Available from: http://bjsm.bmj.com/cgi/content/abstract/36/6/467. Accessed June 26, 2007.
83. Skaggs DL. Elbow fractures in children: diagnosis and management. *J Am Acad Orthop Surg.* 1997;5:303–312.
84. Sojbjerg JO, Ovesen J, Nielsen S. Experimental elbow instability after transection of the medial collateral ligament. *Clin Orthop.* 1987;218:186–190.
85. Starkey C, Ryan J. *Evaluation of Orthopedic and Athletic Injuries* (2nd ed.). Philadelphia, PA: F.A. Davis; 2002.
86. Stern MB. Anterior interosseous nerve entrapment (Kiloh-Nevin syndrome): report and follow-up study of three cases. *Clin Orthop.* 1984;187:223–227.
87. Stirmont TJ, An KN, Morrey BF. Elbow joint contact study: comparison of technique. *J Biomech.* 1985;18:329–336.
88. Temple A, Bache CE, Gibbons PJ. Fractures of the elbow: supracondylar fractures. *Trauma.* 2006;8(3):123–130.
89. Walsh JJ, Patterson LA. Medial humeral condyle fracture. *eMedicine* [electronic version]. 2008. Available from: http://emedicine.medscape.com/article/1231290-overview. Accessed December 27, 2009.
90. Wu J, Perron AD, Miller MD, Powell SM, Brady WJ. Orthopedic pitfalls in the ED: pediatric supracondylar humerus fractures. *Am J Emerg Med.* 2002;(6):544–550.
91. Young CC. Medial epicondylitis. *eMedicine* [electronic version]. 2008. Available from: http://emedicine.medscape.com/article/97217-overview. Accessed December 27, 2009.

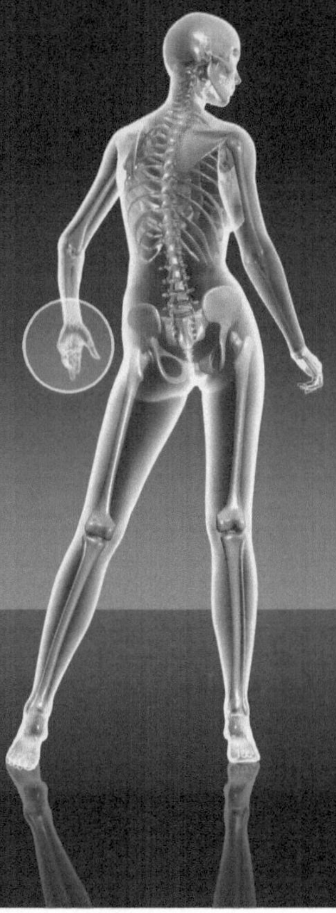

CHAPTER

# 6 Wrist, Hand, and Fingers

## QUICK REFERENCE

# ANSWERS TO CASE QUESTIONS

## CASE 6.1 Ulnocarpal and Ulnar Collateral Sprain

6.1 / **1.** *Based on the information presented in the case, determine (a) the differential diagnoses and (b) the clinical diagnosis.*

a. Differential diagnoses: ulna styloid fracture, carpal fracture, midcarpal instability, triangular fibrocartilage lesions, distal ulna joint arthritis, and wrist strain[51]
b. Clinical diagnosis: ulnocarpal/ulnar carpal sprain

6.1 / **2.** *Ray presented with tenderness along the palmar and medial wrist joint surface as shown in Figure 6.1.1. Identify the structures responsible for providing palmar and medial joint stability.*

Joint stability is provided by extrinsic and intrinsic ligaments of the wrist, which when damaged can lead to chronic wrist pain and carpal instability. The palmar (volar) extrinsic ligaments are the most important ligaments responsible for wrist stability (Table 6.2 in the Introduction); the intrinsic ligaments serve as a restraint to rotational movements. Medial joint stability is provided by the ulna collateral ligament. The UCL arises from ulna styloid process running distally to the medial aspect of the dorsal triquetrum and the pisiform palmarly. This ligament becomes taut during the end ranges of flexion and extension and is responsible for limiting radial deviation.[61,90]

6.1 / **3.** *As part of the physical examination, Genki performed a wrist glide that was positive. Which wrist glide do you think he used and how would you perform it?*

An posterior-anterior (PA) glide would be the position demonstrating the greatest amount of translation. The PA glide is used to examine wrist extension mobility. To perform the PA glide, the athlete should be placed in a seated position with the wrist and hand over the end of the table in a pronated position. The athletic trainer will need to stabilize the distal forearm while grasping the proximal carpal row. A downward force is then applied to the proximal carpal row.[87]

6.1 / **4.** *Genki decided that referral to the USTFA's orthopedic surgeon was warranted in this case. Do you believe this was an appropriate decision? Why or why not?*

The answers to this question will vary among students. Referring an athlete such as Ray to an orthopedic surgeon, particularly one specializing in the wrist and hand, would be an appropriate action given the information provided in the case. Injuries to the wrist and hand are often treated as minor or inconsequential injuries. In fact, trauma to the wrist is often diagnosed as a wrist sprain in the absence of gross injury. Injuries such as radial fractures and carpal fracture are sometimes misdiagnosed as wrist sprains and strains by ER physicians.[33,34] With this in mind, it would be best for Ray to be seen by a professional who can properly diagnosis and treat his injury.

6.1 / **5.** *Describe how to properly apply a volar splint.*

The answers to this question will vary among students, because volar splints can be applied many different ways. However, regardless of which method students choose, they need to check for signs of circulation, sensation, and movement before and after immobilization of the extremity; cover all open wounds with a sterile dressing; and apply cryotherapy in and around the area to decrease edema formation and to control pain.

To apply a volar splint using a SAM SPLINT (Figure A6.1.1):

FIGURE A6.1.1 C-curve SAM SPLINT.

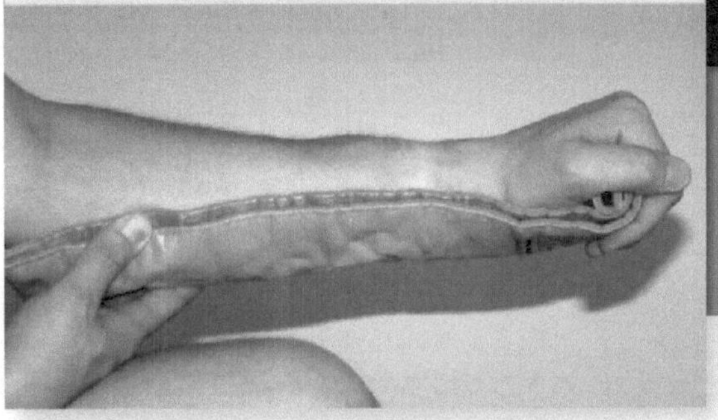

- Stabilize and support the extremity.
- Assess the distal neurovascular status.
- Roll the edge in order to allow the hand to assume a position of function, and create a C-curve.
- Using your arm as a model, mold the splint in the position of function.
- Apply the splint to the athlete from the proximal forearm to the distal palmar crease, and secure the splint using elastic wrap, cravat, or roller bandage.
- Place a gauze pad between the sling and swathe knots for comfort.
- Reassess the distal neurovascular status, and document findings.

To apply a rigid volar splint:

- Stabilize and support the extremity.
- Assess the distal neurovascular status.
- Place a padded rigid splint on the volar surface of the involved forearm.
- Place a roller bandage in the athlete's hand so the hand assumes a position of function.
- Secure the splint using elastic wrap, cravat, or roller bandage.
- When dealing with a trauma to the bone, be sure to immobilize the wrist to limit flexion and extension.
- Provide additional support by using a sling and swathe with the forearm in a slightly elevated position, if comfortable.
- Place a gauze pad between the sling and swathe knots for comfort.
- Reassess the distal neurovascular status, and document findings.

# CASE 6.2 Volar Plate Rupture

6.2 / **1.** *Based on the information presented in the case, determine (a) the differential diagnoses and (b) the clinical diagnosis.*

a. Differential diagnoses: dislocated PIPJ, subluxed PIPJ, volar plate avulsion, collateral ligament sprain, phalange fracture[17,85]

b. Clinical diagnosis: distal volar plate injury

6.2 / **2.** *Given the MOI, why did Nadal find increased laxity when she performed an anterio-posterior glide of the proximal interphalangeal joint?*

The volar plate lies on the volar aspect of phalange's PIPJ, forming the floor of the joint and separating the joint space from the flexor tendons. It is ligamentous at the proximal origin and cartilaginous at the distal insertion,[85] and that allows the flexor tendon to glide past the joint without catching.[17] According to Combs and Schultz, Houlgum, and Perrin,[17,87] the volar plate may be damaged two different ways. The volar plate can be detached from the proximal attachment, resulting in a pseudo-boutonniere deformity. Rupture from the distal attachment results in a swan-neck deformity; an avulsion from its distal bony attachment from the base of the middle phalanx results in a "chip fracture." An anterioposterior glide of the PIPJ therefore increases the stress applied to the volar plate, similar to the hypertension MOI in this case, resulting in an increase in joint laxity and/or pain.

6.2 / **3.** *Do you believe Nadal adequately evaluated Carter's condition? If not, what would you have done differently as the evaluating clinician?*

The answers to this question will vary among students. However, there is no report of Nadal palpating Carter's PIPJ. This could be clinically significant, because an injury to the volar plate often results in a dorsal dislocation or subluxation of the middle phalanx. Although an acute dislocation would have been observable, an athlete may instinctively reduce a PIPJ[17] dislocation by applying longitudinal traction (Figure A6.2.1), making it more difficult to recognize the extent of the injury and increasing the index of suspicion for PIPJ injuries.[65] Had Nadal palpated the PIPJ, she would have recognized that Carter was extremely tender on the volar surface of the PIPJ, indicting possible damage to the volar plate of the PIPJ.

FIGURE A6.2.1 Application of self-applied longitudinal traction.

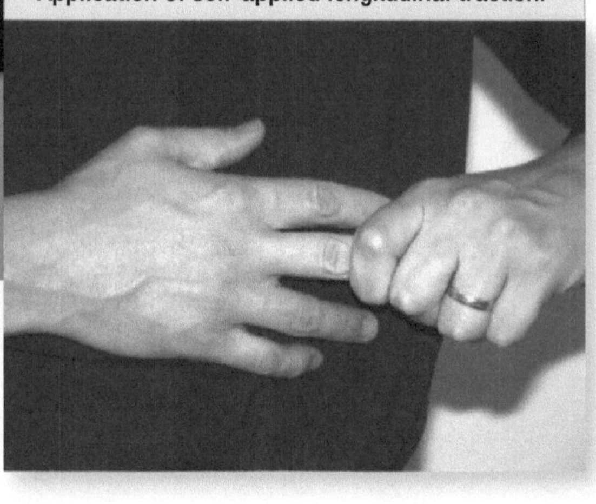

6.2 / **4.** *Based on the information presented in the case, identify the types of splints the orthopedic surgeon may have recommended for Carter.*

Patients suffering from volar plate injuries can be splinted in different ways. When an injury is stable, it is often treated symptomatically and can be splinted using an anatomical splint, normally for six weeks.[65] Unstable injuries, which are normally associated with joint fracture/avulsion and dislocation, are treated using a dorsal extension-block splint.[17,65] A dorsal blocking splint prevents full PIPJ extension during the first few weeks by initially blocking extension to 30° allowing full flexion.[13] The amount of extension is increased incrementally during the next three to four weeks, followed by approximately three months of anatomical splinting.[17] These splints can be bought commercially or fabricated using a thermoplastic and Velcro™.[13]

6.2 / **5.** *(a) Do you believe Nadal made the correct decision by referring Carter to the orthopedic surgeon? (b) If this had been an athlete, would you have treated him differently? Why, or why not?*

a. The answers to this question may vary among students. However, given the fact that Carter was hurt performing his assigned job duties, he may be entitled to workers' compensation benefits. Athletic trainers working in an industrial setting should become familiar with their individual state's laws, rules, and statutes governing workers' compensation. In the state of Utah, for example, an employer is required to file "Employer's First Report of Injury—Form 122" within seven days of the accident, injury, or occupational disease. The form is used for reporting accidents, injuries, or occupational diseases.[91] This form also serves as notice to OSHA. In conjunction with form 122, form 123, "Physician's Initial Report of Work Injury or Occupational Disease," must also be completed. This form is used by physicians and chiropractors to report their initial treatment of an injured employee.[91]

b. If this had been an athlete, the correct decision would still have been to refer the athlete to an orthopedic surgeon, particularly for radiographs. All too often, finger injuries are ignored because they are "just fingers." In this case, radiographs would be warranted because of the risk of chip fractures[17,65] and secondary damage occurring with a possible subluxation of the PIPJ.

## CASE 6.3 Gamekeeper's Thumb

6.3 / **1.** *Based on the information presented in the case, what is the differential diagnosis for both patients?*

Based on both scenarios, the differential diagnosis may include: Bennett's fracture, phalange fracture, de Quervain's tenosynovitis, bowler's thumb (perineural fibrosis of the subcutaneous ulnar digital nerve), tendonitis of the flexor pollicis brevis, tendonitis of the adductor pollicis, and tendonitis of the opponens pollicis.[27]

6.3 / **2.** *Based on the information presented in the cases, (a) what is the clinical diagnosis? (b) What is the common term used to describe the clinical diagnosis?*

a. Even though the MOIs for both scenarios were very different and involved different activities, the clinical diagnosis is ulnar collateral ligament sprain of the thumb.
b. The clinical diagnosis is commonly known as "gamekeeper's thumb." Gamekeeper's thumb is also known as "skier's" or "ski pole" thumb. Gamekeeper's thumb takes its name from the gamekeeper of the royal court who was likely to injure the UCL of the MCP joint when twisting or snapping the necks of fowl hunted for the king.[11] However, although the terms are often used interchangeably, "gamekeeper's thumb" tends to be more chronic in nature, whereas the term "skier's thumb" denotes more of an acute injury to the UCL.[35]

6.3 / **3.** *Even though Tom's and Valerie's accidents were very different, (a) why did they both end up with similar injuries? (b) Which of the scenarios shows the more common MOI?*

a. Tom tried to catch a football, which hit his thumb forcing it into hyperextension and abduction and injuring his ulnar collateral ligament. On the other hand, Valerie fell on her hand. Normally this wouldn't injure the UCL. However, a skier grasps the skipole in the webspace between the thumb and forefinger. When she lands on her hand, the pole jams back against her thumb, injuring the UCL. In both cases, the patient experienced sustained hyperabduction and radial deviation of the thumb's MCP joint.[70,72]
b. Tom's scenario demonstrates the more common MOI for a UCL sprain of the thumb.

6.3 / **4.** *What subjective factors gave Joel the impression that both injuries call for the same clinical diagnosis?*

The answers will vary among students. Both Tom and Valerie reported an MOI consistent with trauma to the UCL,[50,70,72] and both experienced pain and swelling along the ulnar aspect of the metacarpophalangeal joint. Patients will typically report pain at this point, because the proper collateral ligament arises from the metacarpal head and progresses volarly to insert onto the proximal phalanx. An accessory collateral ligament, which assists the proper collateral ligament (i.e., the ulnar collateral ligament), originates palmarly to the proper collateral ligament and inserts onto the thumb's sesamoid and volar plate.[61]

6.3 / **5.** *What objective factors gave Joel the impression that both injuries call for the same clinical diagnosis?*

The answers will vary among students, however, both patients presented with a fair amount of ecchymosis running from the MCP joint into the thenar eminence. This is consistent with trauma to the UCL.[65] Also, Tom was able to flex the MCP joint only 70°, compared with the typical 90° normally allotted for this joint.[4,16] A positive pinch test (as indicated by the inability of the patients to grip a card between thumb and forefinger) and a positive valgus stress test to the UCL of the thumb were both present in both cases. Tom's valgus stress test exhibited pain with increased movement (indicating moderate sprain); Valerie's UCL had 30° more laxity than her uninjured thumb (indicating a disruption of the ligament).

6.3 / **6.** *If you were in Joel's position, what directions for care would you provide Tom and Valerie at the end of their first visits?*

The answers will vary among students. An athletic trainer should consider referring the patients for evaluation by a physician, particularly in a situation where significant trauma such as an avulsion fracture is suspected. Any overlooked and untreated injury can lead to pain and instability. This would be followed by immobilizing both patients' thumbs in a gamekeeper's thumb splint or hand-based thumb spica cast with the IP joint left free for two to four weeks. They should be instructed to return in 10–14 days for re-evaluation. If the pinch mechanism is still weak, they would need to be referred to a hand specialist to determine if the UCL is healing properly or if surgery is indicated.

## CASE 6.4 Wrist Strain—Flexor Carpi Ulnaris Muscle

6.4 / **1.** *Based on the information presented in the case, determine the clinical diagnosis.*

The most likely clinical diagnosis would be a strained wrist, particularly to the flexor carpi ulnaris.

6.4 / **2.** *If Paige also presented with neurological symptoms, what could you conclude about the injury? What type of neurological symptoms may be present?*

If neurological symptoms were present, it could be a result of trauma (stretching) of the ulnar nerve. Remember from Chapter 5 that normal flexion of the elbow can cause the ulnar nerve to elongate 4.7 to 8.0 mm.[10] Simultaneous wrist extension may further elongate the nerve, predisposing it to injury. Damage to the ulnar nerve would result in decreased wrist flexion and decreased ulna deviation strength, because the ulnar nerve innervates the flexor carpi ulnaris. Changes to the peripheral sensory distribution of the ulnar nerve may be noted in the area of the palmar surface of the fourth and fifth metacarpals, the fifth phalange, and the medial half of the fourth phalange.

6.4 / **3.** *If you were the evaluating clinician, (a) how would you assess wrist flexion and extension muscle strength? (b) How could you isolate the clinical diagnosis?*

a. Wrist flexion and extension resistive range could be assessed with Paige in a sitting position with the wrist and hand over the edge of the table. To assess flexion, the clinician should stabilize the distal forearm while resistance is applied to the palmar surface of the supinated forearm (Figure A6.4.1). To assess extension, Earlene should stabilize the distal forearm while resistance is applied to the dorsal surface of the pronated forearm (Figure A6.4.2).

b. To isolate the flexor carpi ulnaris, a patient should be in a seated position with the wrist and hand over the edge of the table. The clinician places the patient's wrist into a flexed and ulnar deviated position. While stabilizing the distal forearm, resistance is applied over the hypothenar eminence attempting to move the wrist into extension and radial deviation.[16]

FIGURE A6.4.1 Resistive range of motion in wrist flexion.

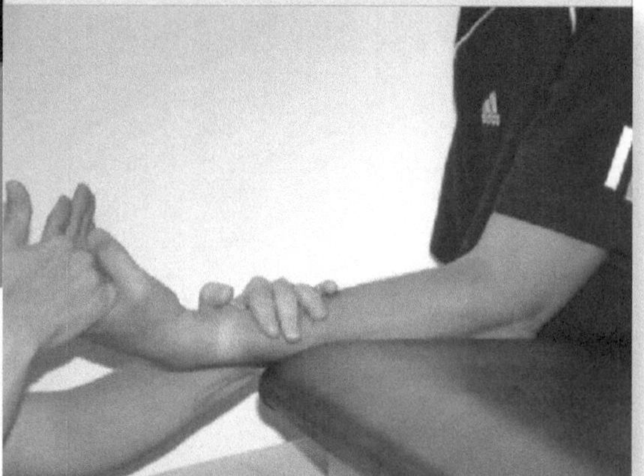

FIGURE A6.4.2 Resistive range of motion in wrist extension.

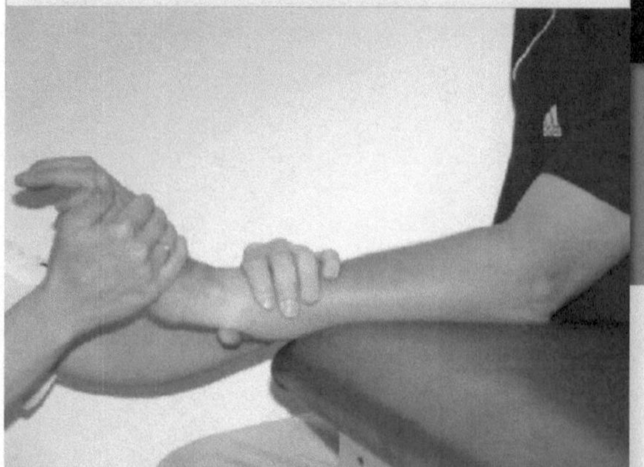

6.4 / **4.** *Overall, do you believe Earlene adequately evaluated Paige's condition, considering the provided information? If not, what would you have done differently as the evaluating clinician?*

The answers to this question will vary among students. Given the athlete's history and physical examination, Earlene appeared to complete a relatively thorough clinical evaluation.

6.4 / **5.** *As a clinician, discuss how you would explain to a patient or athlete the proper mechanics of performing the weight lifting technique known as a "clean"?*

The clean is a lifting technique in which an individual is asked to lift a barbell from the ground to chest height in a continuous smooth movement. This is accomplished by generating a significant amount of force over a short period of time, thereby increasing strength and power.

The clean can be broken down into seven different positions:

1. Starting position
2. First pull
3. Scoop
4. Second pull
5. Descent under the bar
6. The catch
7. Downward movement

A detailed video description of the clean can be found at www.nsca-lift.org/videos/Clean/defaultclean.shtml.

In this case, as Paige moved to the "catch" phase, she was maximally flexed at the elbow and extended at the wrist in order to rack the bar before moving to the finishing position. As she moved to the finishing position, she apparently felt a tearing sensation in her wrist. This could be caused by poor body position, loss of support base, improper technique, or other causes.

## CASE 6.5 Distal Phalange Fracture

6.5 / **1.** *Based on the information presented in the case, determine (a) the differential diagnoses and (b) the clinical diagnosis. What are the distinguishing characteristics of this injury?*

a. Differential diagnoses: phalange fracture, phalange dislocation, extensor digitorum rupture, and soft tissue injury[1]

b. Clinical diagnosis: distal phalange fracture

This is one of the most commonly fractured structures in the hand.[54] The injury is caused by crushing[9,17,64] MOI (e.g., fingers caught between two football helmets and being stepped-on). Distal phalange fractures may present with concomitant tendon injury[64] and/or may be open or closed, stable or unstable, displaced, and/or angulated.[103]

6.5 / **2.** *Amanda asked a few history questions to guide the physical examination. Based on the information presented in the case, do you believe Amanda took an adequate history? If not, what additional questions would you ask as the evaluating clinician?*

According to the clinical diagnosis, there may be several other questions Amanda could have asked, in addition to gathering information about the MOI. Questioning should focus on patient-related questions such as age, general health, occupation, previous injury, hand dominance, and type of equipment used.[20,70] Other questions to guide the physical examination include:

- How much and what kind of force was involved?
- Were there any unusual sounds or sensations?
- What type of physical activities are you involved in?[20,45]

6.5 / **3.** *Figure 6.5.1 in the textbook demonstrates Andy's fingers at rest. What is the name of this finger position, and why is it a cause of concern for an athletic trainer observing this position?*

Figure 6.5.1 demonstrates a flexion cascade. A flexion cascade can be used to detect subtle deformities (i.e., angulation, rotation, and displacement) of the fingers and should be compared with the fingers on the uninvolved side. When no deformity, particularly rotation, is present, all the tips of the fingers will be on the same plane pointing to the region of the scaphoid at the base of the palm.[17,51] If the fingertips do not lie in the same plane, the patient should be immediately referred for proper medical care to prevent any permanent deformity that may affect hand function.

6.5 / **4.** *Compression and percussion tests are often performed when evaluating the clinical diagnosis, and they were used in this case. Do you believe these are reliable tests? Is there another test that Amanda could have performed?*

a. Compression and percussion tests are commonly used to elicit pain that is indicative of a possible simple fracture.[43,62] These clinical tests are particularly useful to athletic trainers when making return-to-play decisions when diagnostic tests such as radiographs are not readily available.[43] They are commonly described in many traditional athletic training texts[44,87,90] and are widely utilized, but their reliability has yet to be validated.

b. Researchers have utilized tuning forks at 128 Hz and auscultation with a stethoscope to detect fractures in adults (i.e., femoral neck),[6] children (i.e., femoral neck, shaft, and tibia),[59] and the presence of stress fractures.[4] Moore[62] compared the use of a 128

Hz tuning fork and stethoscope with the use of compression and percussion testing (compared to the gold standard, radiographs) to assess possible fractures. He found that the tuning fork and stethoscope was an effective and valid diagnostic tool for evaluating possible fractures, yielding a success rate of 89.2 percent when compared to radiographs. Percussion and compression fracture testing methods yielded only a rate of 67.6 percent and 64.9 percent respectively. Calculation of sensitivity, specificity, and positive and negative likelihood ratios are located in Table A6.5.1.

6.5 / **5.** *If you were the evaluating clinician in this case, what if anything would you have done differently or elaborated on?*

The answers to this question will vary among students. Students should recognize the need to perform a more thorough observation of the hand and fingers. Any observation of the hand should include an adequate assessment of the attitude of the hand and fingers, including cuts, abrasions, ecchymosis, swelling, and color of the skin.[17,39] The next step is to observe the general appearance of the nails. Trauma to the fingertips, particularly in the presence of a crush injury, as in this case, may lead to the development of subungual hematoma or nail-bed lacerations.[17,103] In fact, the throbbing pain reported by Andy could have been the result of a subungual hematoma, a painful condition in which bleeding develops beneath the nail, causing the hematoma to become trapped between the rigid structures of the nail on top and the distal phalanx below.[103]

**TABLE A6.5.1** Calculation of sensitivity, specificity, and positive and negative likelihood ratios.

| MEASURE | COMPRESSION VS. RADIOGRAPHS | PERCUSSION VS. RADIOGRAPHS | TUNING FORK AND STETHOSCOPE VS. RADIOGRAPHS |
|---|---|---|---|
| Sensitivity | .47 | .50 | .78 |
| Specificity | .80 | .78 | .95 |
| Positive likelihood ratio | 2.35 | 2.27 | 15.6 |
| Negative likelihood ratio | .66 | .64 | .23 |

## CASE 6.6 Proximal Interphalangeal Joint Dislocation

**6.6 / 1.** *Based on the information presented in the case, (a) what is the likely clinical diagnosis? (b) What is the likelihood of perceiving the injury visually as presented in Figure 6.6.1 after the injury has occurred?*

a. The clinical diagnosis in this case is a probable dislocated proximal interphalangeal joint or a possible fracture-dislocation of the joint.

b. Trauma to the hand and fingers in particular are often treated as inconsequential injuries, with the mentality, "it is just a finger." In fact, many athletes and/or teammates will instinctively reduce the finger using longitudinal traction (refer back to Figure A6.2.1) on the field,[90,106] which may explain the decreased likelihood of direct visual perception of the injury after the injury has occurred.

**6.6 / 2.** *(a) Given the MOI, what would you have expected to observe? (b) Is this a common MOI?*

a. Based on the MOI, a deformity of the PIPJ should have been observed. This may provide some indication as to the extent of the trauma.

b. Hyperextension, the mechanism noted in this case, is the most common MOI.[17,50,81] It would typically result in a dorsal dislocation of the PIPJ where the proximal middle phalanx moves dorsally in relation to the distal proximal phalanx,[42,50,81,106] resulting in a rupture of the volar plate from its distal attachment[81] or in a fracture-dislocation of the PIPJ.[42]

A hyperflexion force or a varus or valgus force coupled with a volar thrust to the middle phalanx can result in a volar PIPJ dislocation.[42,50,75] In this case, the athlete will present with a volar displacement of the proximal portion middle phalanx relative to the distal portion proximal phalanx and having a rotational component (all of the fingernails should all lie in the same plane) resulting from damage to the collateral ligament central slip. An angulated PIPJ, radially or ulnarlly, indicates damage to one or both of the collateral ligaments and volar plate and is commonly referred to as a lateral PIPJ dislocation.

**6.6 / 3.** *If you were the evaluating clinician in this case and you arrived before Dr. Smith, what if anything would you have done differently during the initial evaluation?*

The answers to this question will vary among students. Students should recognize the need to perform a more complete physical examination, observing for joint effusion and edema and rotation of phalanges, palpating for joint tenderness over the volar plate, assessing joint function (if applicable), and checking the neurovascular status of the phalanges. If a fracture-dislocation is suspected, immediate referral to a physician is necessary.

**6.6 / 4.** *Do you believe the actions of Dr. Smith were appropriate? If Paul sustained secondary damage as a result of Dr. Smith's actions, could Dr. Smith be held liable for his actions?*

Clearly, while Dr. Smith may have had good intentions, he most likely acted outside his scope of medical practice. In Utah for example, the Chiropractic Physician Practice Act, 58-73 (May 5, 2008) states: " 'Practice of chiropractic' means a practice of a branch of the healing arts: (a) the purpose of which is to restore or maintain human health, in which patient care or first aid, hygienic, nutritional, or rehabilitative procedures are administered; (b) which places emphasis upon specific vertebral adjustment, manipulation, and treatment of the articulation and adjacent tissues of the spinal column, musculoskeletal structures of the body, and nervous system."

Fingers are not adjacent tissues to the vertebral column. This means that if Dr. Smith had treated Paul in the state of Utah he may have violated the state practice act. However, Dr. Smith was not in Utah and would be likely to maintain that he was acting as a "Good Samaritan" and that because he was not being paid for his service and acted in good faith, his actions were not negligent.

Now, the argument would focus around the question of whether the care rendered by Dr. Smith is considered "standard of care." That is, would another prudent and reasonable individual with similar training and knowledge in this situation provide the same level of care? Given the MOI and the findings of a complete physical examination, a trained physician or athletic trainer would have strongly suspected a possible fracture-dislocation of the PIPJ and should have taken the appropriate steps to rule out such an injury. Therefore, it could be argued that Dr. Smith did not provide appropriate care and may be liable.

6.6 / **5.** *What steps could be taken to minimize the risk of outside interference with an injured athlete occurring at your university or college?*

The answers to this question will vary among students, depending on their level. A key step is to ensure that there is adequate medical coverage during high-profile athletic events such as the one cited in this case. This concept should extend beyond special events and be applied to the normal day-to-day operations of any athletic training facility. In 2003 (revised in 2007), the NATA[67] published *Recommendations and Guidelines for Appropriate Medical Coverage of Intercollegiate Athletics* (available at http://www.nata.org/statements/support/amciarecsandguides.pdf) as a resource to address specific applications of staffing issues in an athletic training program to ensure adequate health care coverage.[67] Additionally, the NCAA provides information on emergency care coverage in the *2009–2010 Sports Medicine Handbook*[68] and also addresses the need for "the presence of a person qualified and delegated to render emergency care to a stricken participant." They also state, "Players or non-medical personnel should not touch, move or roll an injured player." Athletic training programs may also institute a policy whereby anyone not officially authorized by the athletic training staff is not permitted to touch or move an injured student-athlete.

6.6 / **6.** *In this case, an on-field event occurred that unfortunately does occasionally occur in the athletic training profession. Putting yourself in the role of Bayden, discuss how you would have wanted the athletic director to assist in handling this situation. In reality, has this or something like this ever occurred to any of your clinical instructors?*

Answers to these questions will vary greatly among students. In fact, this question is best answered as a group discussion, because there is not necessarily only one correct answer. Certainly, the actions of the Dr. Smith were at best inappropriate and could have been handled much differently.

## CASE 6.7 Lunate Dislocation

6.7 / **1.** *(a) Based on the information presented in the case, what is the most likely clinical diagnosis? (b) What is the typical MOI?*

a. The most likely clinical diagnosis is a dislocation of the lunate.

b. Perilunate and lunate dislocations are likely to occur in high-energy impact sports or falls from a significant height.[12,31,66] Injury results when the athlete experiences excessive radiocarpal hyperextension (normally greater than 100°) and ulnar deviation, in combination with axial loading and a pronated forearm.[31,66,78,81] The final position of the wrist when contact is made will determine the specific perilunar or radiocarpal injury.

6.7 / **2.** *Do you believe the medical team adequately evaluated the condition? If not, what would you have done differently as the evaluating clinician?*

The answers to this question will vary among students. It would appear that the medical team provided adequate care, given the information presented in the case. Discussion addressing the need for spinal stabilization and helmet removal would be appropriate in this case scenario.

6.7 / **3.** *(a) What is a Murphy's sign and a fat carpus sign? (b) How is the Murphy's sign performed?*

FIGURE A6.7.1 Murphy's sign.

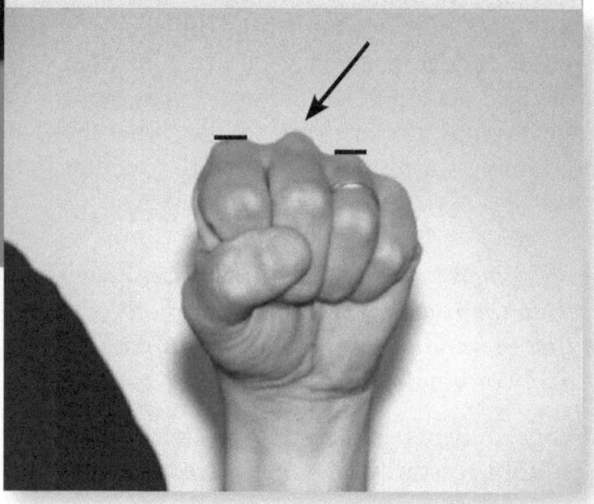

Normally the third MCPJ should be higher than the second and fourth MCPJ.

a. A Murphy's sign is a test used to assess for a possible dislocation of the lunate. A fat carpus sign is viewed on a lateral radiograph when the lunate is volar to the radius and indicates a dislocated lunate.[68]

b. To perform a Murphy's sign begin with the athlete in a seated or standing position. The athlete is instructed to make a fist (Figure A6.7.1). The examiner observes the position of the third metacarpal. If the third metacarpal is level with the second and fourth metacarpals, then either a volar or dorsal displacement of the lunate is indicated.[44] This test is described in some text books as a clinical sign,[29,44,90] but a review of literature examining the origins of Murphy's sign could not be located. One should not confuse the Murphy's sign used to diagnoses lunate dislocation with that of the Murphy's sign used to diagnoses cholecystitis (i.e., inflammation of the gallbladder).

6.7 / **4.** *Karen assessed Kal's neurological status and found numbness and tingling in the lateral palm and into the second and third fingers. What is/are the possible cause(s) of this?*

Median nerve injury is commonly associated with lunate dislocations[19,22,58,66,81] because the volarly displaced lunate compresses the median nerve, which runs through the carpal tunnel.

6.7 / **5.** *If you were a collegiate or high school athletic trainer and an athlete presented with wrist pain and swelling over the proximal carpal row, decreased grip strength, and decreased ROM (i.e., ulnar deviation) with no apparent history of injury, (a) what clinical diagnosis would you suspect? (b) What would be the MOI?*

a. The most likely clinical diagnosis would be Kienböck's syndrome or disease.

b. Kienböck's, a degenerative condition of the lunate, was first described by Kienböck in 1910 in Europe.[30] It develops as a result of repeated trauma to the lunate in patients with anatomical predispositions.[56] Repetitive low impact stress compromises the vascular supply to the lunate,[79,80] resulting in avascular necrosis of the lunate. In fact, patients with Kienböck's disease are believed to have only a single palmar artery, rather than the normal double artery, supplying the lunate bone.[56] The disease is diagnosed with imaging studies, and treatment depends on the stage and severity of disease process and the amount of carpal collapse.[80]

## CASE 6.8 Scaphoid Fracture

6.8 / **1.** *Based on the information presented in the case, determine (a) the differential diagnoses and (b) the clinical diagnosis.*

a. Differential diagnoses: distal radius and/or ulna fracture, metacarpal fracture, carpal fracture (trapezium and scaphoid in particular), and wrist sprain

b. Clinical diagnosis: scaphoid fracture

6.8 / **2.** *If Ian was comparing Tim's wrist bilaterally, the swelling around the radial distal and proximal carpal rows would obscure which anatomical landmark?*

Immediate swelling would obliterate the anatomical snuff box, which is demarcated by the extensor pollicis longus (medial border), abductor pollicis longus and extensor pollicis brevis (lateral), and scaphoid (floor).[39]

In situations where an athlete presents with diffuse swelling on the dorsolateral side of the wrist, other types of wrist injuries should be suspected.[40] In fact, the clinical signs of a scaphoid fracture have been shown to have a high sensitivity but a low specificity.[24,28,32,102] Research has found that anatomical snuff-box tenderness is reported to be 90 to 100 percent sensitive; however specificity is only 29 to 40 percent.[28,32]

6.8 / **3.** *The MOI in this case was not typical for the clinical diagnosis. Based on the clinical diagnosis, identify the most common MOI and explain the etiology.*

Scaphoid fractures typically occur when a victim falls on an outstretched hand with the wrist extended at least 90° and radially deviated 10°, or during hyperextension[2,57,104] as the bone is compressed against the dorsal lip of the radius and the second row of carpal bones.[40] A hyperextension mechanism of injury in conjunction with tenderness in the anatomical snuff box is suggestive of a possible scaphoid fracture.[57]

6.8 / **4.** *(a) Did Ian make the correct decision in removing Tim from the game? (b) Which, if any other, special test would you have performed?*

a. Based on the information presented in the case, it would appear that Ian made a conservative but appropriate decision in removing Tim from physical activity. It is recommended that athletes presenting with pain to the floor of the anatomical snuff box be suspected of a possible scaphoid fracture, because tenderness in this area is considered a possible clinical indicator of such an injury.

b. Ian could have also performed a scaphoid compression test by applying a compression force through the first phalange longitudinally. The range of sensitivity of this test is reportedly 71 to 100 percent, but the specificity of the test has a much greater range, 22 to 80 percent,[15,24,32] suggesting that the compression test alone may not be a good indicator of a scaphoid fracture. Other pathologies mimicking a fractured scaphoid include traumatic de Quervain's disease, a fractured trapezium and radial styloid, and osteoarthritis of the carpometacarpal joint.[15,99] Grover[32] also found significant swelling of the wrist joint in the presence of a scaphoid fracture, suggesting that marked swelling about the wrist in the presence of positive scaphoid compression tenderness provides clinical suspicion of a possible scaphoid fracture. This would then prompt the need for radiographs. In fact, once radiographs are requested by a physician, she is "obliged to treat the injury as a scaphoid fracture even if the films reveal no immediate fracture."[99]

6.8 / **5.** *What type of initial care should Ian provide before Tim sees the orthopedic surgeon?*

Initial care in this case would consist of protection, rest, ice, compression and elevation (PRICE). The area should be splinted with a volar splint or a thumb spica splint made from a SAM SPLINT® or Orthoplast® (or similar splinting material). Remember to assess the athlete's circulation, sensation, and movement before and after the removal of the splint.

6.8 / **6.** *Based on the case report describe how Ian could have performed a grip strength test while assessing Tim on the sidelines.*

Sideline assessment of grip strength in this case would require Ian to ask Tim to grab at least two of his fingers and squeeze as hard as possible. Although this is a subjective finding, any significant deficit in grip strength would be noted. During an off-field or clinical assessment, a hand dynamometer would provide a clinician with objective data regarding deficits in grip strength. However, given the circumstances of the case, this was not feasible.

6.8 / **7.** *What are the special risks of this fracture, and how should this affect any approach to a wrist fracture/sprain?*

Among the carpal bones, the scaphoid is the most commonly fractured bone (60% to 79%)[2,32,89] and is at increased risk of developing avascular necrosis (death or decay of tissue due to local ischemia) because of the bone's poor vascular supply.[80] Thus, it is usually wise to treat all suspected wrist fractures or sprains as clinical fractures until a scaphoid fracture can be ruled out.[40,80]

## CASE 6.9 Colles' Fracture with TFCC Damage

6.9 / **1.** *Based on the information presented in the case, do you agree with Inga's clinical diagnosis? If not, what do you believe is the correct clinical diagnosis in this particular situation?*

The most likely clinical diagnosis is a Colles' fracture. A wrist sprain is a possible differential diagnosis, but Inga's rushed evaluation missed several key signs and symptoms of a Colles' fracture, with possible secondary triangular fibrocartilage complex damage.

6.9 / **2.** *Because of Inga's indifference to Cory, she missed several key signs. If you were the evaluating athletic trainer, what if any other signs would you have assessed during the general observation component of the physical examination that may have helped you determine the clinical diagnosis?*

Some of the key signs missed in this case include the classic dorsal angular deformity known as a "silverfork" or "dinnerfork" deformity.[29,93] However, radial deformity may not be present in all cases, and not all distal radial fractures are true Colles' fractures.[75,93] Other signs of a radial fracture beside ecchymosis and swelling include (1) dorsal displacement of the radius, (2) radial angulation (outward displacement), (3) radial displacement, (4) loss of radial styloid height, and (5) supination of the distal fragments.[7,52]

6.9 / **3.** *Based on the clinical diagnosis, which component of the physical examination do you believe Inga forgot to complete, if any? What is the clinical significance of omitting this part of the examination?*

It would appear that Inga failed to assess Cory's neurovascular status and test for possible fractures. Inga would have been wise to assess the circulatory and sensory function by assessing the radial artery and the radial, ulnar, and median nerves for evidence of damage as a result of the trauma. Trauma to the distal radius increases the likelihood of neurovascular damage. The neurovascular status should also be checked both before and immediately after joint immobilization.

6.9 / **4.** *Identify the structures comprising the proximal and distal carpal rows. Identify which carpal bones align with each of the five metacarpals.*

The proximal carpal row from lateral to medial is comprised of the following:

- Scaphoid, which is palpable with ulnar deviation and comprises the floor of the anatomical snuff box
- Lunate, which is proximal to the capitate and distal to Lister's tubercle and covered by the extensor carpi radialis brevis
- Triquetrum, which with radial deviation allows the carpal to move out from underneath the ulnar styloid process
- Pisiform, which is located on the anterolateral surface of the triquetrum and is formed within the flexor carpi ulnaris tendon

The distal carpal row is comprised of the following:

- Trapezium, which articulates with the first metacarpal
- Trapezoid, which articulates with the second metacarpal
- Capitate, the largest of all carpal bones, which articulates with the third metacarpal and is located within a depression when the wrist is in neutral position

- Hamate and hook of the hamate, which lie in a direct line between the pisiform and the web space of the thumb and index finger. The fourth and fifth metacarpals articulate with the hamate.

6.9 / **5.** *During the examination, Inga assessed the stability of the radial and ulnar collateral ligaments. If you were the evaluating athletic trainer, would you perform these exams? Why, or why not?*

Based on the MOI, Inga should not have performed these exams. If Inga had taken the time to complete a thorough observation and taken into account the increased pain with PROM, she should have recognized the potential for a distal radius fracture. In this case, Inga should not have performed ligamentous testing until a physician confirmed the presence or absence of a distal radius fracture. Following this confirmation, stress testing of the distal radioulnar and radiocarpal joints may be warranted to assess for damage to structures such as the radial collateral ligament, ulnar collateral ligament, palmar radiocarpal ligaments, dorsal radiocarpal ligaments, and triangular fibrocartilage complex.

# CASE 6.10 Bennett's Fracture

6.10 / **1.** *Based on the information presented in the case, determine the clinical diagnosis and describe the injury.*

The clinical diagnosis in this case would be a Bennett's fracture. Bennett's fracture is an intra-articular fracture-dislocation of the thumb's carpometacarpal joint, with the fracture occurring at the base of first metacarpal (a small fragment of the first metacarpal continues, to articulate with the trapezium) and with a dorsal dislocation or subluxation of the first metacarpal[14,38] (Figure A6.10.1). The fracture was first described in 1882 by Dr. Edward Bennett.[8]

FIGURE A6.10.1 Example of a Bennett's fracture.

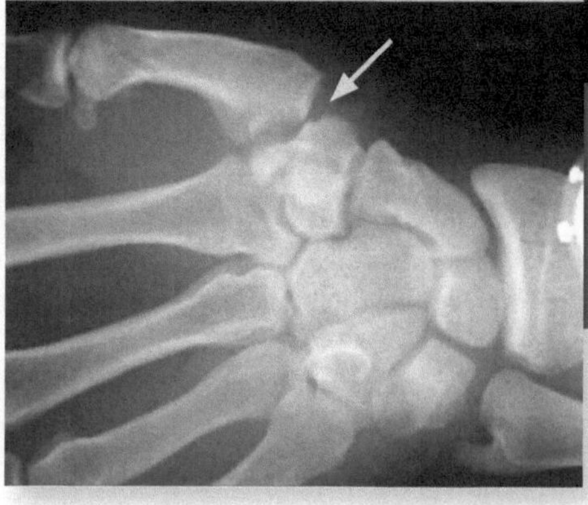

*Source:* www.learningradiology.com, with permission.

6.10 / **2.** *The MOI in this case appeared to be an excessive adduction force applied to Art's partially flexed thumb. What other possible MOI exists for this clinical diagnosis?*

Bennett's fractures typically occur when an axial force is applied to a partially flexed thumb, such as when punching with a closed fist.[28,75,87]

6.10 / **3.** *In this case, Marion believed she observed a laterally displaced first metacarpal shaft. Based on the clinical diagnosis, what would cause the first metacarpal shaft to be laterally displaced?*

Dorsal, radial, and proximal displacement of the first metacarpal may occur because of the unopposed pull of the abductor pollicis longus,[2,38,87] which inserts into the base of the first metacarpal bone.

6.10 / **4.** *Obviously, this case presented with an on-field event that cut short Marion's evaluation of Art's thumb. Identify what, if any, further evaluation would be required in this case.*

The answers to this question will vary among students. However, an athletic trainer may continue to assess for joint crepitus and false joint motion. Considering the pain and instability with PROM, stress testing is probably not warranted. A neurological evaluation should be completed. Radiographs, including a true lateral view of the thumb and a CT scan, would be necessary in making an accurate diagnosis of a Bennett's fracture.[81]

6.10 / **5.** *In this case, an on-field event occurred that unfortunately does occur occasionally in the athletic training profession. Putting yourself in the role of the athletic training student in this case, discuss how you would have responded during and after the coach's outburst. In reality, has this or something like this ever occurred to you? Was the coach right or wrong?*

Answers to this question will vary greatly among students. In fact, this question is best answered as a group discussion, because there is not necessarily only one correct answer. Certainly, the actions of the coach were at best inappropriate and could have been handled much differently.

## CASE 6.11 Boxer's Fracture

6.11 / **1.** *Based on the information presented in the case, determine the clinical diagnosis and identify the layman's term(s) for the diagnosis.*

The clinical diagnosis in this case is a fracture of the fifth metacarpal, also known as a "boxer's fracture." Some physicians may use the term "brawler's fracture" rather than boxer's fracture. Professional and amateur boxers are skilled in the proper punching techniques and are less likely to sustain a fracture of the fifth metacarpal, because they understand the proper mechanics of throwing a punch.[37]

6.11 / **2.** *What are the common MOIs associated with this injury?*

One of the most common MOIs for boxer's fracture involves punching an immovable or firm object with some force behind it with a closed fist.[2,3,28] Although boxer's fractures usually occur when the hand is closed into a fist, they can also occur when the hand is not clenched and strikes a hard object. In urban areas, ER physicians routinely see boxer's fracture.[3] Those diagnosed with boxer's fractures are predominately men (92% compared with 58% for all other injuries).[3] Another MOI involving axial forces or compressive forces is being stepped on by another individual's foot.[75]

6.11 / **3.** *What special test could have helped Kristi confirm the clinical diagnosis, and how is it performed?*

Sometimes no deformities may occur when an individual has a boxer's fracture, so it can be difficult to diagnose the injury. Kristi could have assessed for metacarpal fractures by using a compressive or axial force. The compression test or metacarpal fracture test is performed by having the patient relax his fingers so that the MCPJ is resting at 90°. A compressive force is then applied to the head of the metacarpal. If the patient reports pain with the force applied to the metacarpal, then an athletic trainer should suspect a possible fracture.

6.11 / **4.** *What could Kristi have done to prevent this incident from occurring?*

According to the BOC's *Role Delineation Study 5th Edition,* one of the domains of professional responsibility is to ensure a safe environment and risk management. Kristi or a safety team member designated by the facility should inspect the factory plant at regular intervals for safety hazards such as exposed pipes like the one Matt tripped on. These risks should be documented and disposed of immediately to decrease employee risk and reduce lost production time and workman compensation claims.

## CASE 6.12 de Quervain's Syndrome

6.12 / **1.** *Based on the information presented in the case, (a) determine the clinical diagnosis and (b) discuss the possible etiology.*

a. The clinical diagnosis is a stenosing tenosynovitis of the first dorsal compartment, often known as de Quervain's syndrome and sometimes referred to as Hoffman's disease.[75] It was first described by Fritz de Quervain in 1895.[46,47]

b. de Quervain's syndrome is caused by repetitive extension of the thumb and/or using the thumb to pinch or twist something while simultaneously moving the wrist (forceful grasping coupled with ulnar deviation), affecting the abductor pollicis longus and extensor pollicis brevis.[47,81,84,86] It is a common tendinitis about the wrist in athletes, particularly racquet sports[81] but has been reported in rowers[86] and piano players[46,47] and as an occupational musculoskeletal disorder in office workers.[71,100] Other factors involved in the development of de Quervain's syndrome are muscle fatigue, poor training technique,[86] and increased computer usage and postural deviations.[71,100]

6.12 / **2.** *In your opinion did Ryan address all the components of a thorough injury assessment? What, if anything, would you have added to the assessment?*

According to injury assessment by either HOPS (history, observation, palpation, stress/special tests) or HIPS (history, inspection, palpation, stress/special tests), it would appear that Ryan completed an adequate evaluation. When evaluating a wrist and hand, a thorough history is necessary, which includes the patient's vocational and recreational activities; the quality, radiation, severity, and timing of the injury; and the palliative and aggravating factors affecting the pathology.[26] During palpation, an athletic trainer may also want to consider assessing for crepitus in tunnel 1.

6.12 / **3.** *Ryan's assessment of Sally's thumb reveals palpable tenderness in tunnel 1. Identify the structures located in tunnel 1. Identify the remaining tunnels and the anatomical structures that lie within them.*

When palpating the wrist, Hoppenfeld recommends breaking the wrist down into specific clinical zones to assist the clinical evaluation.[39] Furthermore, located within some of these zones are tunnels or dorsal passageways for the tendons of the wrist and finger musculature. Hoppenfeld's specific clinical wrist zones and tunnels[39] are outlined in the following list.

- Wrist zone I: **tunnel 1**—abductor pollicis longus and extensor pollicis brevis
- Wrist zone II: (1) **tunnel 2**—extensor carpi radialis brevis and longus; (2) **tunnel 3**—extensor pollicis longus; (3) **tunnel 4**—extensor digitorum communis and extensor indicis (independent movement)
- Wrist zone III (ulnar styloid process): (1) **tunnel 5**—extensor digiti minimi; (2) **tunnel 6**—extensor carpi ulnaris

6.12 / **4.** *If you were the evaluating clinician, how would you have performed the Finklestein test?*

The Finklestein test is a provocative test used to diagnose de Quervain's syndrome. The test was first described by Finklestein in 1930 where he states "on grasping the patient's thumb and quickly abducting the hand ulnarward, pain over the styloid tip is excruciating."[25] However, Leao[48] stated that the test described by Finklestein was translated from a paper by Eichhoff in 1927 who described an experiment to confirm the theory that repetitive tendon stretching (ulnar deviation) could be the cause of syndrome.[23,25] Eichhoff's experiment reportedly required a patient to grasp the thumb with the other fingers while moving the hand into ulnar abduction which would cause an intense pain over the radial styloid.[23,48] This would appear to be the test that is commonly used and described today by most authors. Elliot[23] points out the need to perform the test correctly in order to diagnose de Quervain's with accuracy.

Today, the test is normally performed with the patient in a standing or sitting position. The athletic trainer passively ulnar deviates the wrist, with the patient's thumb flexed and adducted in the palm (Figure A6.12.1). A positive finding occurs when the patient experiences a reproduction of pain and tenderness over the abductor pollicis longus and extensor pollicis brevis over the radial styloid.

FIGURE A6.12.1 Finklestein's test.

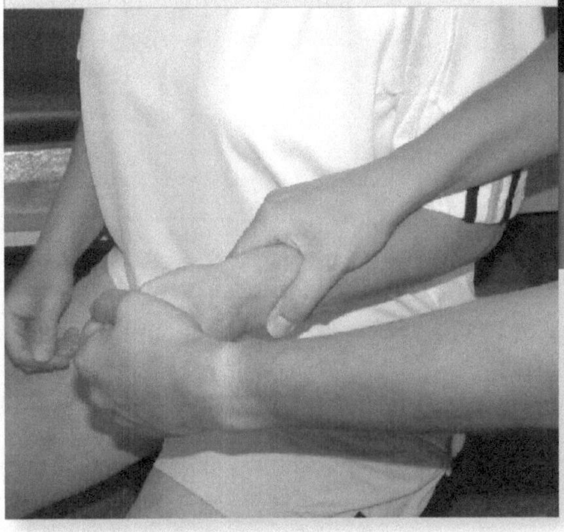

6.12 / **5.** *Outline a conservative rehabilitation program as if you were the treating clinician.*

The answers to this question will vary among students. However, a conservative program should include an identification of the cause and a recommendation that the patient avoid these activities for a period of time. In this case, limiting piano playing and squash may be indicated because use will continue to stimulate inflammation of the tendons. Limitation of thumb usage may require a splint that extends over the wrist to immobilize the affected tendons[84] and will often be accompanied by NSAIDs.[41,81,84] In cases involving athletes, remember to maintain cardiovascular function during this rest/immobilization period if play will be limited. Cryotherapy will also be indicated.

Some physicians will opt for steroid injection into the first dorsal compartment. The reported cure rates for a single injection range from 45 to 100 percent, as cited in Rettig[81] and in Jirarattanaphochai.[41] A supplemental oral administration of an NSAID (i.e., nimesulide) does not improve the effectiveness of a single injection of a steroid (i.e., triamcinolone acetonide) when treating de Quervain's syndrome.[41]

## CASE 6.13 Carpal Tunnel Syndrome

6.13 / **1.** *Based on the information presented in the case, determine (a) the differential diagnoses and (b) the clinical diagnosis.*

a. Differential diagnoses: cervical disc pathology, cervical myofascial pain, cervical spondylosis, lateral epicondylitis, diabetic neuropathy, thoracic outlet syndrome, multiple sclerosis, brachial plexus pathology[5]

b. Clinical diagnosis: carpal tunnel syndrome

6.13 / **2.** *Lt. Brown asked several history questions to guide her physical examination. Based on the information presented in the case, do you believe she took an adequate history? If not, what questions would you have asked as the evaluating clinician?*

The answers to this question will vary among students. Overall, Lt. Brown appeared to generate an adequate history, though there are some specific questions that she failed to identify based on the clinical diagnosis.

Determining hand dominance would be indicated. Based on the case, there was a 15 percent deficit in grip strength; however, without knowing hand dominance, how is a clinician able to determine whether or not this is significant? A positive grip strength test would suggest a 10-percent-or-more deficit on the injured non-dominant hand but a 5-percent-or-more deficit on the injured dominant hand.[90]

Occupation is another factor necessary in determining the clinical diagnosis. Because she works in logistics, it can be assumed that Sgt. Rabb spends a great deal of time working with computers. A systematic review found that the risk of carpal tunnel syndrome increased with use of a computer, especially with mouse use of more than 20 hours per week.[100] Computer usage has been reported as a possible etiology by other authors. However, a study examining work-related upper extremity disorders suggests that the prevalence of carpal tunnel syndrome as a work-related disorder is often overstated and is overshadowed by other physical findings.[71] In fact, Pascerelli found that only 8 percent of the individuals examined had carpal tunnel syndrome. More recently, it has been suggested that carpal tunnel syndrome has both work-related and personal risk factors,[105] which is why a complete medical history is also necessary to identify other causes of carpal tunnel such as metabolic disorders, infections, inflammatory conditions, aberrant anatomy, gender, and BMI.[60,92,96,101]

A patient should be asked about her sleep pattern and whether or not she is sleeping with the wrist flexed. It should also be determined whether the symptoms worsen during the day or at night.[4,18]

6.13 / **3.** *What is a flick sign, and is it an effective tool for detecting the clinical diagnosis?*

Individuals experiencing carpal tunnel syndrome often complain of pain that is worse at night and that usually awakens them from sleep. When the patient awakens, she often attempts to relieve the symptoms by flicking the hand. That is, she shakes her wrist as if she were trying to shake down a thermometer.[105] However, the usefulness of this test as a diagnostic tool is limited.[26] Hansen, Micklesen, and Robinson determined the flick sign's sensitivity and false-positive to be 37 and 26 percent, respectively. The positive predictive value for the flick sign was 74 percent, but the negative predictive value was 37 percent. However, they did determine that the flick sign detected more subjects with carpal tunnel than the Tinel's sign.[36]

6.13 / **4.** *Overall, do you believe Lt. Brown adequately evaluated Sgt. Rabb's condition? If not, what would you have done differently as the evaluating clinician and why?*

The answers to this question will vary among students. The final diagnosis of carpal tunnel syndrome is often made with a good history and physical examination. Location of the symptoms, hypoalgesia, and decreased thumb strength are suggested to be highly predictive findings in the diagnosis of carpal tunnel syndrome[19] There were, however, several items that were either omitted or performed incorrectly, including:

- Failure to assess joint strength, particularly of thumb abduction, flexion, opposition, and the lateral two lumbricals. These structures are innervated by the median nerve or branches from the median nerve (lumbricals).
- Inaccurate performance of Phalen's maneuver (as in textbook Figure 6.13.2). Phalen's maneuver is a traditional clinical test for diagnosing carpal tunnel syndrome, but Lt. Brown failed to execute the test correctly. Phalen's maneuver requires maximal flexion of the wrist for 60 seconds; however, the flexed elbows need to be brought below the horizontal plane passing through the wrists (Figure A6.13.1). A study reviewed clinical tests commonly used to diagnose carpal tunnel syndrome and found that the sensitivity of the test ranged from 40 to 87 percent, while the specificity ranged from 59 to 80 percent.[97] Phalen himself reported a sensitivity of 79 and 80 percent.[73,74] A more recent examination of 142 subjects suggests that Phalen's maneuver has a sensitivity of 34 percent. The positive predictive value was 73 percent, and the negative predictive value was 35 percent.
- Lt. Brown also failed to perform a Tinel's sign. A Tinel's sign is positive when repetitive tapping over the carpal tunnel elicits symptoms in the distribution of the median nerve (Figure A6.13.2).[44] However, a review of the clinical tests used to diagnose carpal tunnel syndrome found that the sensitivity of the test ranged from 44 to 60 percent, while the specificity ranged from 67 to 94 percent.[97] A more recent examination of 142 subjects suggests that the Tinel's sign has a sensitivity of 27 percent and a false-positive result of 8 percent. The positive predictive value was 87 percent, and the negative predictive value was 39 percent.

6.13 / **5.** *As mentioned in the case, Lt. Brown documented her findings and sent a copy of the report to Dr. Packer's office. Please document your findings as if you were the treating clinician. If the case did not provide information you believe is pertinent to the clinical diagnosis, please add this information to your documentation.*

Answers will vary. Students should consider writing a SOAP note (see textbook Appendix B) using the ABCD format when writing the short- and long-term goals.

FIGURE A6.13.1 Correct Phalen's maneuver.

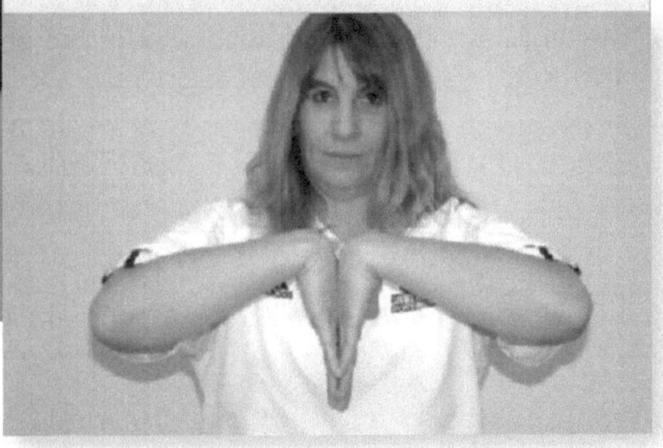

FIGURE A6.13.2 Tinel's sign.

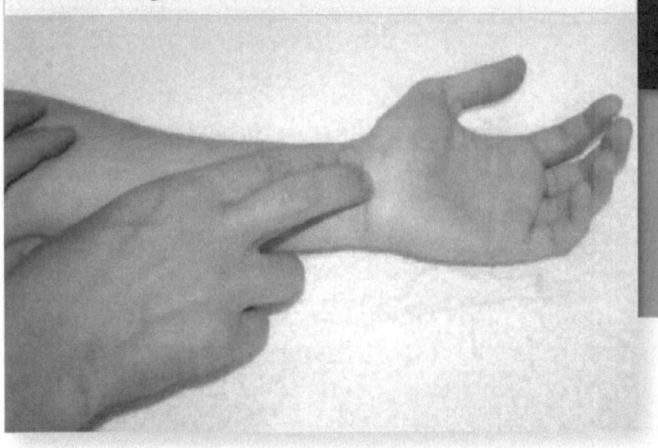

## CASE 6.14 Handlebar Palsy

6.14 / **1.** *Based on the information presented in the case, determine (a) the differential diagnoses and (b) the clinical diagnosis. (c) Identify the common term used to describe the clinical diagnosis.*

a. Differential diagnoses: carpal fracture, traumatic peripheral nerve injury, intracarpal instability, flexor muscle strain
b. Clinical diagnosis: ulnar neuropathy
c. "Handlebar palsy" or "cycle palsy"

6.14 / **2.** *Sienna assessed AROM and performed muscle testing of the fingers but failed to assess PROM. If you were the evaluating clinician, how would you assess passive flexion and extension ROM and what would you expect to find clinically?*

FIGURE A6.14.1 Passive finger ROM.

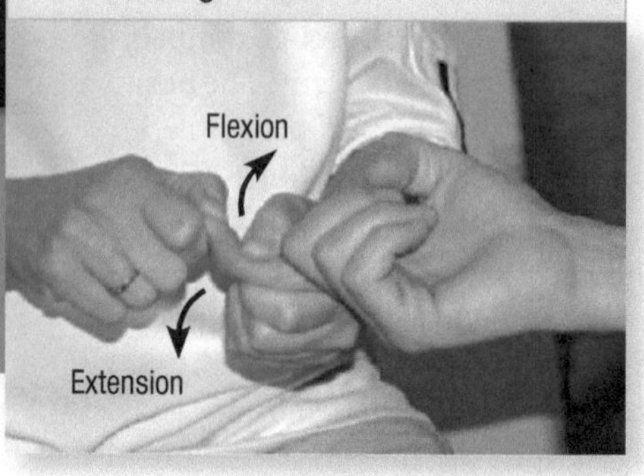


Finger flexion and extension passive range could be assessed with Jack in a supine or sitting position with the forearm resting on the table and the wrist in a neutral position, finger relaxed. Sienna should stabilize the metacarpal being assessed proximally, while grasping the distal phalange. Slight traction is applied through the distal hand while moving the finger through flexion and extension (Figure A6.14.1), applying overpressure at the end range of each motion.[16]

In this case, the PROM may be unremarkable; however, if there is severe atrophy and the athlete assumes a flexed position of the fourth and fifth phalangeal DIPJ and PIPJ, a firm pathological end-feel may be noted with DIP, PIP, and MCP extension.

6.14 / **3.** *(a) Identify the bony and soft tissue structures Sienna should have palpated as part of her evaluation specific to the wrist and hand. (b) Identify the neurological and vascular structures at greatest risk based on the clinical diagnosis. (c) Identify the anatomical landmarks in textbook Figure 6.14.3.*

a. The exact anatomical structures palpated will depend on the extent of the athlete's pain and apprehension. Given the information presented in the case, Sherrie would have been wise to palpate the carpal bones, particularly the pisiform and hook of the hamate, metacarpals, palmar muscles (thenar and hypothenar eminence).
b. The ulnar nerve as it passes through the Tunnel of Guyon is at greatest risk for ulnar nerve compression, entrapment, or palsy.[77] The median nerve is also at risk of trauma if the wrist is hyperextended for prolonged periods of time while cycling.[94] The ulnar artery, which also passes through the Tunnel of Guyon is also at risk for trauma. Prolonged pressure applied over the hypothenar eminence increases the risk of ulnar artery thrombosis.[63]
c. Answers to textbook Figure 6.14.3 (see the photo repeated on p. 147) are as follows: A = radius, B = scaphoid, C= trapezium, D = first metacarpal, E = third metacarpal, F = proximal phalange, G = capitate, H = triquetrum (pisiform is also in this area), I = lunate, J = ulna

6.14 / **4.** *Sienna performed the special test that was shown in textbook Figure 6.14.2. (a) What is the name of this test and what does it assess? (b) Describe how to perform this test.*

a. Froment's sign, named for Jules Froment, assesses for injury and/or paralysis to the ulnar nerve, presenting with decreased pinch grip strength.[83]

b. To perform a Froment's sign, begin with the patient in a seated or standing position. The patient is asked to grasp a piece of paper between the thumb and index finger. The clinician then attempts to pull away the piece of paper. A positive test occurs if the distal phalanx of the thumb flexes, as a result of paralysis of the adductor pollicis muscle (innervated by deep branch of the ulnar nerve), rather than remaining pulp to pulp with the index finger.

FIGURE A6.14.2

A/P view, adult wrist, and hand.

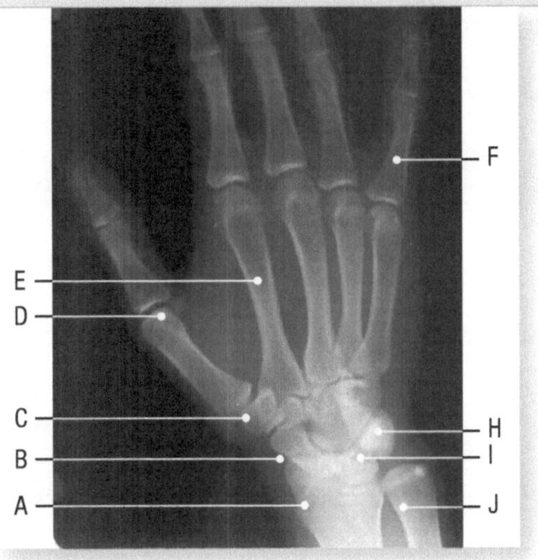


6.14 / **5.** *After completing the physical examination, Sienna discussed Jack's treatment options and prevention strategies. If you were the evaluating athletic trainer, what types of prevention strategies would you recommend?*

The answers to this question will vary among students; however, some prevention strategies may include the following:[21,76,77,95]

- Reduced road mileage
- Modification of the hand grip (moving the weight from the center of the palms to the outside edge of his palms) and changing hand grip frequently
- Padded gloves to absorb the shocks and jolts from the road
- Adjustment of the bike so that the cyclist sits in a more upright position, thereby decreasing the weight and pressure on the hands and wrists
- Use of aerobars to allow the cyclist to rest his forearms on pads

## CASE 6.15 Boutonniere Deformity

6.15 / **1.** *Based on the information presented in the case, determine (a) the differential diagnoses and (b) the clinical diagnosis.*

a. Differential diagnoses: dislocated PIPJ, volar plate rupture (proximal attachment), laceration of the central extensor tendon slip, rheumatoid arthritis[53]

b. Clinical diagnosis: boutonniere deformity

6.15 / **2.** *What is the common MOI associated with this injury?*

The typical MOI is a longitudinal force applied to the tip of the distal phalange, such as being stuck with a ball. This mechanism results in either forced flexion of the PIPJ or volar displacement, causing disruption of the central slip of the extensor tendon, which normally inserts into the dorsal base of the middle phalanx. However, dorsal crush injuries and lacerations of the extensor tendon[17] may also result in a boutonniere deformity or central slip injury.

6.15 / **3.** *David asked only a couple of history questions to guide the physical examination. Based on the information presented in the case, do you believe David took an adequate history? If not, what additional questions would you ask as the evaluating clinician?*

The answers to this question will vary among students. However, according to the clinical diagnosis there may be several other questions David could have asked. Examples are:

- Where did the ball strike the finger (e.g., did the ball strike the tip of the distal phalange)?
- What type and how much force was involved?
- Were there any strange sounds or sensations?
- What was your initial response (e.g., did Mike grab the finger and possibly reduce it)?
- Is there any history of finger injury?

6.15 / **4.** *Based on the information presented in the case, do you believe David cared for the injury appropriately?*

David applied the incorrect type of the splint to Mike's finger, as was shown in textbook Figure 6.15.2. Figure 6.17.1 on p. 151 demonstrates the splinting procedure for a mallet finger. In this case, because the PIPJ can be passively extended (i.e., demonstrates an extension lag) it should be immobilized using a static extension splint to hold the PIPJ in full extension to keep the ends of the tendon from separating as it heals. All this assumes that the injury is going to be treated nonoperatively.[14,17,75] The static splint should allow the DIPJ to move freely, and active and passive ROM should be performed daily to keep the lateral bands from moving volarly. The length of time required for use of the splint will depend on the extent of the trauma. However, a complete rupture of the central slip will normally require six to eight weeks of full-time splinting[17,72,75] and three weeks of night splinting. Once the splint is removed, it will be necessary to continue buddy taping the finger until full ROM is achieved and also during physical activity.

If the patient presents with a PIPJ flexion contracture or tightness of the oblique retinacular ligament (ORL), additional splinting strategies may need to be implemented. Mike should speak to his physician or a certified hand therapist to determine the most appropriate splint application for these situations.

6.15 / **5.** *Clearly Mike did not seem concerned about the status of his injury. If a recreational athlete asked you, "What further damage could I do at this point?" how would you respond?*

The answers to this question will vary among students. The patient should be informed that several types of injuries are possible to the finger after getting it "jammed." If a boutonniere deformity is suspected, the damage to the central slip causes the lateral bands of the extensor tendon to retract and displace volarly to the axis of the PIPJ, creating a flexor force on the joint and thereby resulting in hyperextension of the DIPJ.[72] Hyperextension of the DIPJ causes the oblique retinacular ligament to become taut, limiting joint ROM. An athletic trainer may also suggest to the patient that an additional trauma or usage of the finger could cause more swelling in and around the PIPJ and that, as the swelling worsens, the deformity is accentuated, resulting in a worsening of the condition.

## CASE 6.16 Jersey Finger

6.16 / **1.** *Based on the information presented in the case, determine the clinical diagnosis.*

The injury is a jersey finger, also known as disruption of the flexor digitorum profundus (FDP) from the insertion on the distal phalanx.[17,72,75] It is called "jersey finger" because this injury frequently occurs when a football tackler wraps a finger around an opponent's clothing (i.e., his jersey) while the opposing player pulls away,[49,88] causing forced hyperextension of the DIPJ while the finger is actively flexing.

6.16 / **2.** *What test(s) could a clinician add to Danni's evaluation to assist in determining the clinical diagnosis? How would you perform the test(s)?*

Trauma to the DIPJ can cause significant pain and swelling to the joint. The DIPJ should be tested in isolation to determine the extent of damage.[49] To isolate the FDP, an athletic trainer should stand in front of the patient and hold his fingers in extension except for the joint being tested. The athletic trainer then isolates the DIPJ and instructs the subject to flex. A positive finding would be the patient's inability to flex the DIPJ.

An athletic trainer could also perform a flexor tendon avulsion test by asking the patient to make a fist. A positive finding would be the patient's inability to flex the DIPJ.[44,49]

6.16 / **3.** *(a) How would performing a PROM test assist in determining the clinical diagnosis? (b) If you were the evaluating clinician how would you perform PROM testing on the DIPJ and PIPJ?*

a. A way to assess the integrity of the FDP is to passively move the wrist through flexion and extension, which results in extension and flexion of the digits, respectively. This test uses the tenodesis (stabilizing a joint by anchoring the tendons that move that joint) effect of the antagonistic tendons.[69]

b. To assess PROM of the DIPJ, the athletic trainer should grasp and stabilize the middle phalanx while moving the DIPJ through flexion and extension PROM. To assess PROM of the PIPJ, stabilize just proximal to the PIPJ and move the PIPJ through flexion and extension.

6.16 / **4.** *Which finger is the most susceptible to this injury?*

Leddy and Packer[49] found that 75 percent of FDP ruptures they examined involved the ring finger. In an examination of tendon avulsion injuries of the distal phalanx, Tuttle suggests that trauma to the ring finger flexors is a multi-factorial event[98] and cites three hypotheses: (1) the ring finger has the least independent motion of all the fingers; (2) the insertion of the ring finger FDP is weaker than that of the long finger; and (3) the ring fingertip becomes 5 mm more prominent and absorbs more force than the other fingers during grip.

6.16 / **5.** *Why is it necessary for a clinician to recognize this injury and refer the athlete as early as possible?*

Early recognition and proper management reduce the likelihood of complications such as poor tendon gliding, contractures, and repair failures from factors such as poor blood flow, prolonged retraction of the ruptured tendon, and development of adhesions between the FDP and FDS tendons.[49,88]

# CASE 6.17 Mallet Finger

6.17 / **1.** *Based on the information presented in the case, determine (a) the differential diagnoses and (b) the clinical diagnosis. (c) What is the colloquial term for this injury?*

a. Differential diagnoses: DIPJ fracture, DIPJ dislocation, DIJP sprain, DIPJ avulsion fracture

b. Clinical diagnosis: injury to the terminal slip of the extensor tendon

c. "Mallet finger" or basketball, baseball, or dropped finger[17,55,76]

6.17 / **2.** *Tyler asked several history questions to guide the physical examination. Based on the information presented in the case, what one question do you believe he should have asked to guide the physical examination?*

Based on the information provided, Tyler should have asked Madison about her ability to actively extend the DIPJ. Trauma to the terminal slip of the extensor tendon leaves patients unable to actively extend the joint, often referred to as a DIP extensor lag.

6.17 / **3.** *According to the case report, no special tests were performed—only PROM and muscle testing. Describe how Tyler might have assessed Madison's inability to extend her finger.*

Tyler in all likelihood should have performed an extensor avulsion test. This is done by stabilizing the PIPJ and instructing the patient to actively extend her DIPJ. If there is a rupture of the terminal slip of the extensor tendon, the patient will be unable to actively extend the DIPJ.[87]

6.17 / **4.** *A component of Tyler's care was to splint Madison's finger. Based on the information provided in the case, describe the splinting procedure proper to this clinical diagnosis.*

FIGURE A6.17.1 Mallet finger splint.

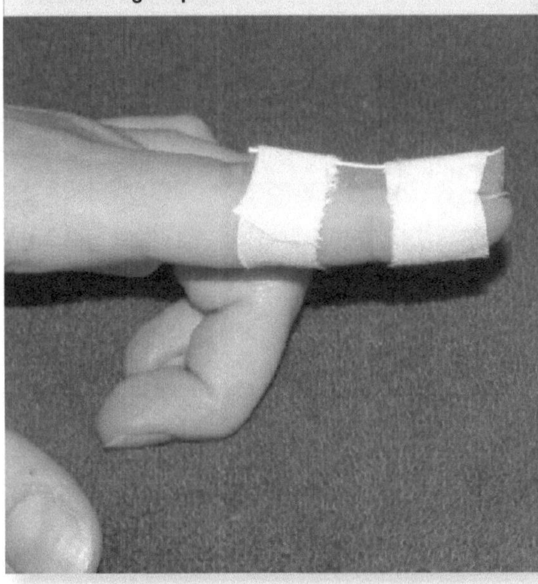

Several commercial splints are available to clinicians, or they can make their own (Figure A6.17.1). The Stack splint (Promedics, Blackburn, England) is a commonly used splint for mallet finger, but it does not always provide a proper fit and can lead to poor patient compliance.[55,82] Custom-made thermoplastic splints are often used in athletic training, and a prospective study assessing the results of such splints found the splints to be easy to make and fit and suitable for all finger shapes and sizes. They improved the deformity in 30 of 34 cases, with no cases of skin irritation.[82] However, the physician's diagnosis will typically determine exactly how the splint is applied. When a tendon-only rupture is suspected, the splint should be designed so that the DIPJ is in slight hyperextension (5°–10°).[13,17] Care should be taken to avoid excessive hyperextension, which can compromise circulation to the skin covering the dorsal aspect of the finger and cause eventual sloughing of the skin.[15] When the tendon injury involves a fracture, the DIPJ is kept at neutral. In either case, the splint should not interfere with PIPJ motion. The patient is instructed to wear the splint 24 hours per day for 6 weeks and then another 2 to 6 weeks at night.[13,17,82] The DIPJ must be maintained in extension, even when the patient is showering and changing the splint, and this should be clearly understood by the patient during the initial fitting of the splint. Any flexion movement of the DIPJ will result in a re-setting of the treatment time from the day of movement.

6.17 / **5.** *Would radiographic studies be useful in this case? Why, or why not?*

Yes, radiographs would prove useful. These would obliviously need to be ordered by Madison's referring physician, but radiographs help to rule of out concomitant fractures or other joint pathology,[14,17,38] such as an avulsion fracture, and would also determine the size of any bony fragments. A physician will typically order AP and true lateral radiographs.

# REFERENCES


1. Alke J, Schraga ED. Fracture, hand. *eMedicine* [electronic version]. 2009. Available from: http://emedicine.medscape.com/article/825271-overview. Accessed December 25, 2009.
2. Altizer L. Hand and wrist fractures: first part of a 2-part series. *Orthop Nurs.* 2003;22(2):131–138.
3. Altizer L. Boxer's fracture. *Orthop Nurs.* 2006;25:271–273.
4. Anderson JM. Carpal tunnel syndrome: common, treatable, but not necessarily work-related. *J Controversial Med Claims.* 2007;14(4):1–10.
5. Ashworth NL. Carpal tunnel syndrome *eMedicine* [electronic version]. 2006. Available from: http://www.emedicine.com/pmr/TOPIC21.HTM. Accessed January 15, 2008.
6. Bache JB, Cross AB. "The Barford Test" a useful diagnostic sign in fracture of the femoral neck. *Practitioner.* 1984; 228:305–307.
7. Bailey MM, Michalski J. Close-tip on Colles' fracture. *Nursing.* 1992;22(10):47–47.
8. Bennett EH. *Fractures of the Metacarpal Bones.* Dublin Journal of Medical Science. 1882;73:72–75.
9. Bowen JE, Malanga GA, Napolitano E, Tzeng A. Phalangeal fractures *eMedicine* [electronic version]. 2006. Available from: http://www.emedicine.com/sports/TOPIC101.HTM. Accessed January 3, 2008.
10. Bozentka DJ. Cubital tunnel syndrome pathophysiology. *Clin Orthop Relat Res.* 1998;351:90–94.
11. Campbell CS. Gamekeeper's thumb. *J Bone Joint Surg Br.* 1955;37-B(1):148–149.
12. Campbell RD, Lance EM, Yeoh CB. Lunate and perilunar dislocations. *J Bone Joint Surg Br.* 1964;46-B(1):55–72.
13. Chan DY. Management of simple finger injuries: the splinting regime. *Hand Surg.* 2002;7(2):223.
14. Chan O, Hughes T. Hand. *BMJ* [electronic version]. 2005; 330:1073–1075. Available from: http://bmj.com/cgi/content/full/330/7499/1073. Accessed January 17, 2008.
15. Chen S. The scaphoid compression test. *J Hand Surg Br.* 1989;14-B:323–325.
16. Clarkson H. *Joint Range of Motion and Function Assessment: A Research-Based Practical Guide* (3rd ed.). Baltimore, MD: Lippincott Williams and Wilkins; 2006.
17. Combs JA. It's not "Just A Finger". *J Athl Train.* 2000; 35(2):168–178.
18. Corrington KA, Fields K, Nasbelsky J. What is the best diagnostic approach to paresthesias of the hand? *J Fam Pract.* 2002;51(12):1078–1078.
19. D'Arcy CA, McGee S. The rational clinical examination. Does this patient have carpal tunnel syndrome? *JAMA.* 2000;283(23):3110–3117.
20. de Alwis W. Fingertip injuries. *Emerg Med Australas.* 2006;18(3):229–237.
21. Dettori NJ, Norvell DC. Non-traumatic bicycle injuries: a review of the literature. *Sports Med.* 2006;36(1):7–18.
22. Dimitriou CG, Chalidis B, Pournaras J. Bilateral volar lunate dislocation. *J Hand Surg Eur Vol.* 2007;32(4):447–449.
23. Elliott BG. Finkelstein's test: a descriptive error that can produce a false positive. *J Hand Surg.* 1992;17B:481–482.
24. Esberger DA. What value the scaphoid compression test? *J Hand Surg Br.* 1994;19-B(6):748–749.
25. Finklestein H. Stenosing tendovaginitis at the radial styloid process. *J Bone Joint Surg Am.* 1930;12-A:509–540.
26. Forman TA, Forman SK, Rose NE. A clinical approach to diagnosing wrist pain. *Am Fam Physician.* 2005;72(9): 1753–1758.
27. Foye PM, Raanan J, Stitik TP, Nadler SF. (2009). Skier's thumb. *eMedicine* [electronic version]. Available from: http://emedicine.medscape.com/article/98460-overview.
28. Freeland P. Scaphoid tubercle tenderness: a better indicator of scaphoid fractures? *Arch Emerg Med.* 1989;6(1):46–50.
29. Gallaspy JB, May JD. *Signs and Symptoms of Athletic Injuries.* St. Louis, MO: Mosby; 1996.
30. Gerwin M. The history of Kienbock's disease. *Hand Clin.* 1993;9(3):385–390.
31. Goldberg SH, Strauch RE, Rosenwasser MP. Scapholunate and lunotriquetral instability in the athlete: diagnosis and management. *Oper Techniques Sports Med.* 2006;14: 108–121.
32. Grover R. Clinical assessment of scaphoid injuries and the detection of fractures. *J Hand Surg Br.* 1996;21-B(3): 431–343.
33. Guly HR. Diagnostic error in an accident and emergency department. *Emerg Med J.* 2001;18:263–271.
34. Guly HR. Injuries initially misdiagnosed as sprained wrist (beware the sprained wrist). *Emerg Med J.* 2002;19(1):41–42.
35. Hannibal M, Rogers D. Gamekeeper's thumb *eMedicine* [electronic version]. 2007. Available from: http://emedicine.medscape.com/article/97679-overview. Accessed December 26, 2009.
36. Hansen PA, Micklesen P, Robinson LR. Clinical utility of the Flick Maneuver in diagnosing carpal tunnel syndrome. *Am J Phys Med Rehabil.* 2004;83(5):363–369.
37. Hernandez M, Ufberg JW. Boxer's fracture. *eMedicine Health.* 2005. Available from: http://www.emedicinehealth.com/boxers_fracture/article_em.htm. Accessed January 28, 2008.
38. Hodgkinson DW, Kurdy N, Nicholson DA, Driscoll PA. ABC of emergency radiology. *Hand.* 1994;308:401–405.
39. Hoppenfeld S. *Physical Examination of the Spine and Extremities.* Norwalk, CT: Appleton-Century-Croft; 1976.
40. Hunter D. Diagnosis and management of scaphoid fractures: a literature review. *Emerg Nurs.* 2005;13(7):22–26.
41. Jirarattanaphochai K, Saengnipanthkul S, Vipulakorn K, Jianmongkol S, Chatuparisute P, Jung S. Treatment of de Quervain disease with Triamcinolone injection with or without Nimesulide. *J Bone Joint Surg Am.* 2004;86-A(12):2700–2706.
42. Kang R, Stern P. Fracture dislocation of the proximal interphalangeal joint. *J Am Soc Surg Hand.* 2002;2(2):47–59.

43. Kazemi M. Tuning fork test utilization in detection of fractures: a review of the literature. *J Can Chiropractic Assoc.* 1999;43(2):120–124.
44. Konin JG, Wiksten D, Isear JA, Brader H. *Special Tests for Orthopedic Examination* (3rd ed.). Thorofare, NJ: Slack; 2006.
45. Kubiak EN, Klugman JA, Bosco JA. Hand injuries in rock climbers. *Bull NYU Hosp Jt Dis.* 2006;64(3–4);172–177.
46. Lackey E, Sutton R. Facts about de Quervain's tenosynovitis. *Gen Pract.* 2003a:79–79.
47. Lackey E, Sutton R. Investigating carpal tunnel syndrome. *Gen Pract.* 2003b:69–69.
48. Leao L. de Quervain's disease. *J Bone Joint Surg Am.* 1958;40-A:1063–1070.
49. Leddy J, Packer J. Avulsion of the profundus tendon insertion in athletes. *J Hand Surg Br Am.* 1977;2-A(1):66–69.
50. Leggit JC, Meko CJ. Acute finger injuries: part II: fractures, dislocations, and thumb injuries. *Am Fam Physician.* 2006;73(5):821–834.
51. Lichtman DM, Joshi A. Ulnar-sided wrist pain. *eMedicine* [electronic version]. 2009. Available from: http://emedicine.medscape.com/article/1245322-overview#Differential Diagnosis. Accessed December 29, 2009.
52. Lidstrom A. Fractures of the distal end of the radius. A clinical and statistical study of end results. *Acta Orthop Scand.* 1959;Suppl, 41:1–118.
53. Likes R, Ghidella S. Boutonniere deformity. *eMedicine* [electronic version]. 2008. Available from: http://www.emedicine.com/orthoped/topic24.htm. Accessed May 21, 2008.
54. Lubanah J, Hood J. Fractures of the distal interphalangeal joint. *Clin Orthop Relat Res.* 1996;327(6):12–20.
55. Maitra A, Dorani B. The conservative treatment of mallet finger with a simple splint: a case report. *Arch Emerg Med.* 1993;10:244–258.
56. McLennan M. Radiology rounds: Kienb^ck's disease (osteonecrosis of the lunate). *Can Fam Physician.* 1998;44:1607,1616–1608.
57. McNally C, Gillespie M. Scaphoid fractures. *Emerg Nurs.* 2004;12(1):21–25.
58. Melsom DS, Leslie IJ. Carpal dislocations. *Curr Orthop.* 2007;21(4):288–297.
59. Misurya RK, Khare A, Mallick A, Sural A, Vishwakarma GK. Use of tuning fork in diagnostic auscultation of fractures. *Injury.* 1987;18:63–64.
60. Moghtaderi A, Izadi S, Sharafadinzadeh N. An evaluation of gender, body mass index, wrist circumference and wrist ratio as independent risk factors for carpal tunnel syndrome. *Acta Neurol Scand.* 2005;112(6):375–379.
61. Moore K, Dalley A. *Clinically Oriented Anatomy* (5th ed.). Baltimore, MD: Lippincott Williams & Wilkins; 2005.
62. Moore MB. The use of a tuning fork and stethoscope versus clinical fracture testing in assessing possible fractures. Virginia Polytechnic Institute and State University, Blacksburg, VA; 2005.
63. Moore R, Levin S. Vascular disorder of the upper extremity. *University of Pennsylvania Orthopaedic Journal.* 1998; 11(Spring):52–58. Available from: http://www.uphs.upenn.edu/ortho/oj/1998/oj11sp98p52.html. Accessed January 17, 2008.
64. Moran DS, Mendal L. Current opinion. Core temperature measurement: methods and current insights. *Sports Med.* 2002;32(14):879–885.
65. Morgan WJ, Slowman LS. Acute hand and wrist injuries in athletes: evaluation and management. *J Am Acad Orthop Surg.* 2001;9(6):389–400.
66. Murray PM. Dislocations of the wrist: carpal instability complex. *J Am Soc Surg Hand.* 2003;3(2):88–99.
67. National Athletic Trainers' Association. Recommendations and guidelines for appropriate medical coverage of intercollegiate athletics. 2007. Available from: National Athletic Trainers' Association: http://www.nata.org/statements/support/amciarecsandguides.pdf. Accessed December 26, 2009.
68. National Collegiate Athletic Association. *2009–10 NCAA Sports Medicine Handbook.* Indianapolis, IN: National Collegiate Athletic Association; 2009.
69. Neumeister M, Wilhelmi B, Bueno R. Flexor tendon lacerations *eMedicine* [electronic version]. 2007. Available from: http://www.emedicine.com/orthoped/TOPIC94.HTM. Accessed May 23, 2008.
70. Osterman AL, Moskow L, Low DW. Soft-tissue injuries of the hand and wrist in racquet sports. *Clin Sports Med.* 1988;7(2):329–348.
71. Pascarelli EF, Yu-Pin H. Understanding work-related upper extremity disorders: clinical findings in 485 computer users, musicians, and others. *J Occup Rehabil.* 2001;11(1): 1–21.
72. Peterson JL, Bancroft LW. Injuries of the fingers and thumb in the athlete. *Clin Sports Med.* 2006;25(3):527–542.
73. Phalen GS. The carpal tunnel syndrome. Seventeen years' experience in diagnosis and treatment of six hundred fifty-four hands. *J Bone Joint Surg Am.* 1966;48-A(2):211–228.
74. Phalen GS. The carpal tunnel syndrome: clinical evaluation of 598 hands. *Clin Orthop Relat Res.* 1972;83:29–40.
75. Prentice WE. *Arnheim's Principles of Athletic Training: A Competency-Based Approach* (13th ed.). Boston, MA: McGraw Hill Publishing; 2009.
76. Rehak DC. Pronator syndrome. *Clin Sports Med.* 2001;20(3):531–540.
77. Rehak DC. Cyclist's hands: overcoming overuse injuries. *Hughston Health Alert* [electronic version]. 2003;Summer. Available from: http://www.hughston.com/hha/a_15_3_2.htm.
78. Rettig AC. Elbow, forearm and wrist injuries in the athlete. *Sports Med.* 1998;25(2):15–130.
79. Rettig AC. Athletic injuries of the wrist and hand: part I: traumatic injuries of the wrist. *Am J Sports Med.* 2003a;31(6):1038–1048.
80. Rettig AC. Tests and treatments of hand, wrist, and elbow overuse syndromes: 20 clinical pearls: sorting through disorders that commonly occur in the upper extremity . . . third in a special series of articles. *J Musculoskel Med.* 2003b;20(3):136.
81. Rettig AC. Athletic injuries of the wrist and hand: part II: overuse injuries of the wrist and traumatic injuries to the hand. *Am J Sports Med.* 2004;32, 262–273.

82. Richards S, Kumar G, Booth S, Naqui S, Murali S. A model for the conservative management of mallet finger. *J Hand Surg.* 2004;29(1):61–62.

83. Richardson C, Fabre G. Froment's sign. *J Audiovisual Media Med.* 2003;26(1):34.

84. Robb-Nicholson C. de Quervain's tenosynovitis. *Harv Women's Health Watch.* 2004;12(2):8.

85. Robinson M. Jammed fingers *eMedicine* [electronic version]. 2007. Available from: http://emedicine.medscape.com/article/98081-overview. Accessed May 19, 2009.

86. Rumball JS, Lebrun CM, Di Ciacca SR, Orlando K. Rowing injuries. *Sports Med.* 2005;35(6):537–555.

87. Schultz SJ, Houglum PA, Perrin DH. *Examination of Musculoskeletal Injuries* (2nd ed.). Champaign, IL: Human Kinetics; 2005.

88. Shippert B. A "Complex Jersey Finger": case report and literature review. *Clin J Sport Med.* 2007;17(4):319–320.

89. Simpson D, McQueen MM. Acute sporting injuries to the hand and wrist in the general population. *Scott Med J.* 2006;51(2):25–26.

90. Starkey C, Ryan J. *Evaluation of Orthopedic and Athletic Injuries* (2nd ed.). Philadelphia, PA: F.A. Davis; 2002.

91. State of Utah Labor Commission. Labor Commission, Industrial Accidents. Available from: http://www.rules.utah.gov/publicat/bulletin/2005/20050601/27900.htm. Accessed May 20, 2008, May 19, 2009.

92. Stevens JC, Beard CM, O'Fallon WM, Kurland LT. Conditions associated with carpal tunnel syndrome. *Mayo Clin Proc.* 1992;67:541–548.

93. Summers A. Recognizing and treating Colles' type fractures in emergency care setting. *Emerg Nurs.* 2005;13(6):26–33.

94. Thompson MJ, Rivara FP. Bicycle-related injuries. *Am Fam Physician.* 2001;63(10):2007–2014.

95. Toth C, McNeil S, Feasby T. Peripheral nervous system injuries in sport and recreation: a systematic review. *Sports Med.* 2005;35(8):717–738.

96. Treaster DE, Burr D. Gender differences in prevalence of upper extremity musculoskeletal disorders. *Ergon.* 2004;47(5):495–526.

97. Tuck NR Jr, Simper D, Schliesser J, Cramer GD. Evaluation of diagnostic procedures for carpal tunnel syndrome. *J Neuromusculoskeletal Syst.* 2000;8(1):1–9.

98. Tuttle H, Olvey S, Stern P. Tendon avulsion injuries of the distal phalanx. *Clin Orthop Relat Res.* 2006;445:157–168.

99. Unwin A, Jones K. *Emergency Orthopaedics and Trauma.* Oxford: Butterworth Heinemann; 1995.

100. Village J, Rempel D, Teschke K. Musculoskeletal disorders of the upper extremity associated with computer work: a systematic review. *Occup Ergon.* 2005;5(4):205–218.

101. von Schroede HP, Botte MJ. Carpal tunnel syndrome. *Hand Clin.* 1996;12(4):643–655.

102. Waizenegger M, Barton NJ, Davis TR, Wastie ML. Clinical signs in scaphoid fractures. *J Hand Surg.* 1994; 19-B(6):743–747.

103. Wang QC, Johnson BA. Fingertips injuries. *Am Fam Physician.* 2001;63(10):1961–1966.

104. Weber ER, Chao EY. An experimental approach to the mechanism of scaphoid waist fractures. *J Hand Surg.* 1978;3(2):142–148.

105. Werner RA. Evaluation of work-related carpal tunnel syndrome. *J Occup Rehabil.* 2006;16(2):207–222.

106. Williams J, Tomaino M. Hand and wrist injuries. In Fu F, Stone D, eds. *Sports Injuries: Mechanism, Prevention, Treatment* (2nd ed.). Baltimore, MD: Lippincott Williams & Wilkins. 2001:1085–1101.

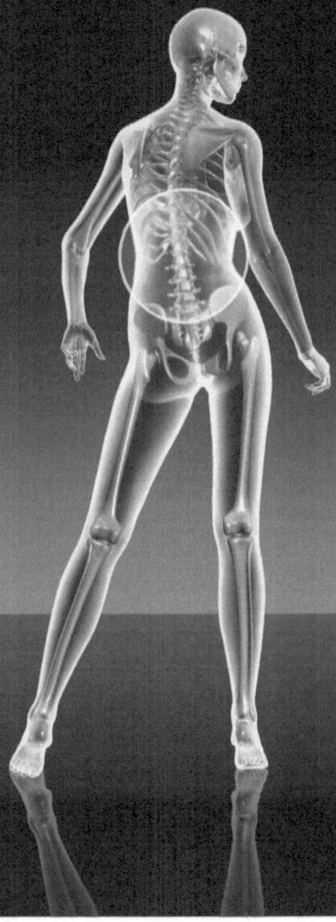

CHAPTER 7

# Thoracic and Lumbar Spine

## QUICK REFERENCE

CASE 7.1
**Lumbar Strain**

CASE 7.2
**Lumbar Intervertebral Disc Pathology**

CASE 7.3
**Lumbar Facet Syndrome**

CASE 7.4
**Spondylolisthesis**

CASE 7.5
**Lumbar Spinal Stenosis**

CASE 7.6
**Thoracic Strain**

CASE 7.7
**Thoracic Spine Fracture**

CASE 7.8
**Sciatica**

# ANSWERS TO CASE QUESTIONS

## CASE 7.1 Lumbar Strain

7.1 / **1.** *Based on the information presented in the case, determine (a) the differential diagnoses and (b) the clinical diagnosis.*

a. Differential diagnoses: lumbosacral disc injuries, lumbosacral discogenic pain syndrome, lumbosacral facet syndrome, lumbosacral radiculopathy, lumbosacral acute bony trauma, lumbosacral spondylolysis and spondylolisthesis, sacroiliac joint injury[35,50]

b. Clinical diagnosis: lumbar strain

7.1 / **2.** *Based on Coach Post's age and clinical presentation, do you believe Caroline's history was appropriate? If not, what would you have done differently as the evaluating clinician?*

The answers to this question will vary among students. Given his low-back injury, questioning further into Coach Post's related medical history is warranted to rule out serious systemic diseases and potential surgical emergencies. This is accomplished by asking specific red-flag questions, such as those shown earlier in textbook Table 7.1 in the anatomical review.[3,27,35] Two of the red-flag questions specific to Coach Post are shown in Table A7.1.1. Historical red-flag questions should center on the patient's risk of cancer, spinal infection, fracture, ankylosing spondylitis, and cauda equina syndrome.

Coach Post's age would raise a concern because being over 50 is considered a red flag[35] for both cancer and fracture and would warrant further medical evaluation.

7.1 / **3.** *If Coach Post also presented with neurological symptoms such as sensory changes over the anterior middle-thigh, over the patella, and the medial lower-leg to the great-toe, along with weakness in ankle dorsiflexion, (a) what could you conclude about the injury? (b) What deep-tendon reflex should be assessed with this clinical presentation?*

a. If sensory change over the anterior middle thigh, patella, and the medial lower leg to great toe were present, along with weakness in ankle dorsiflexion, this would suggest compression of the L4 nerve root, probably as a result of intervertebral disc injury (herniation).[27]

b. Assessment of the L4 or quadriceps deep-tendon reflex would be indicated in this case and would be decreased. The presence of dermatome, myotome, and deep-tendon reflex deficits requires referral to a physician for further diagnostic testing.[2]

**TABLE A7.1.1** Acute lumbar pain red-flag questions specific to Coach Post.

| RED FLAGS | QUESTIONS |
|---|---|
| Cancer | Ask about the patient's age (>50 or <20 years), history of cancer or strong suspicion of cancer, unexplained weight loss, progressive motor or sensory deficits, unrelenting night pain, failure to improve after 6 weeks of conservative therapy |
| Fracture | Ask about the patient's age, significant trauma, history of osteoporosis, chronic oral steroid use, and substance abuse |

7.1 / **4.** *Based on the clinical presentation, Caroline rated Coach Post's thoracolumbar extension strength as 3/5. Describe the test position required to make this determination.*

A muscle strength grade of 3/5 indicates that Coach Post is able to lift the head and sternum so that the xiphoid process is off the table with the hands held behind the back. Figure A7.1.1 shows the test position for this determination. Note, resistance does not need to be applied to the upper back as you are testing against gravity only.

FIGURE A7.1.1 Erector spinae muscle testing against gravity.

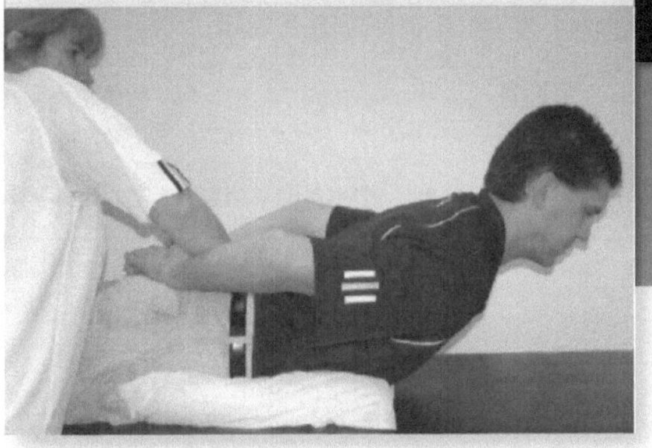

7.1 / **5.** *If you were the treating clinician, besides providing basic conservative therapy (i.e., cryotherapy, OTC anti-inflammatory medicine, muscle strengthening), what information should be included as part of Coach Post's rehabilitation plan?*

For all patients, regardless of the type of injury sustained, patient education (oral information or booklet information) is a vital component of the patient's recovery and prevention of further injury.[3,28,35,61] Patient education should be evidence-based and focus on the:

- Injury sustained
- MOI and aggravating factors to avoid
- Expected time course for improvement
- Modification in home, work, and recreational activities to reduce pain, speed recovery, and prevent chronic injury[9,28,35]

Patient educational booklets developed to provide evidence-based information and medical advice consistent with current clinical guidelines have been shown to have a positive effect on patients' beliefs and clinical outcomes.[9] Similarly, Undermann[61] found that half of chronic low-back-pain patients who read the educational book *Treat Your Own Back* had improvements in their pain immediately and at 9-month and 18-month follow-ups.

## CASE 7.2 Lumbar Intervertebral Disc Pathology

7.2 / **1.** *Based on the information presented in the case, determine (a) the differential diagnoses and (b) the clinical diagnosis.*

a. Differential diagnoses: lumbosacral disc injuries, lumbosacral discogenic pain syndrome, lumbosacral facet syndrome, lumbosacral radiculopathy, lumbosacral acute bony trauma, lumbosacral spondylolysis and spondylolisthesis, sacroiliac joint injury[33,35,50]

b. Clinical diagnosis: posterior disc herniation

7.2 / **2.** *The injury in this case is typically seen in the adult population, often as a result of twisting of the trunk while carrying or lifting weight. For adolescent athletes, (a) what is the likelihood of this injury? (b) What would be the MOI?*

a. As mentioned in the chapter introduction, ruptures of the lumbar intervertebral disc in the general population are very common, however, a herniated nucleus pulposus in children and adolescents appears to account for less than 2 to 6 percent of all reported cases of lumbar disc herniations,[31,46] though the actual incidence rate is not known.[46]

b. The MOI in children and adolescents appears to be slightly different from the MOI in adults. Typically, patients in the younger age group have a history of mechanical stress applied to the lumbar spine, normally as a result of a specific traumatic event or sports injury.[32,34,46]

7.2 / **3.** *During the physical examination, Kendrick notes that Eric is constantly shifting in his chair. As the evaluating clinician, what conclusion can you draw regarding this behavior?*

The direction of listing and rotation demonstrated by a patient is determined by the direction of disc herniation and may cause the body to bend toward or away from the side of involvement in order to alleviate symptoms. Because most disc herniations extrude posterolaterally, as a consequence of the relatively weak posterior longitudinal ligament,[20,21] pain is worse in positions such as sitting (flexion) that produce increased pressure on the annular fibers.[33] Increases in intradiscal pressure were reported to be higher in patients assuming a seated position or a seated position with flexion than in patients standing upright or assuming a recumbent position.[45] In fact, a more recent in vivo study found that the intradiscal pressure while sitting relaxed without a backrest was 90 percent of the pressure while standing; walking led to intradiscal pressure peaks of up to 130 percent, and flexion of the upper part of the body while standing demonstrated an intradiscal pressure at 216 percent when there is 36° of flexion between the thoracolumbar junction and the sacrum.[54] It is this increased disc pressure that probably exacerbated Eric's symptoms during sitting.

7.2 / **4.** *(a) What is the difference between lumbar and thoracolumbar motion? (b) How would you as the evaluating clinician assess lumbar motion? (c) Thoracolumbar motion?*

a. Lumbar motion, particularly flexion and extension, is isolated movement of the five lumbar vertebrae. Thoracolumbar flexion and extension involve combined movements of the lumbar and thoracic spine.

b. Lumbar flexion is assessed using a tape measure with the patient in a standing position. The starting point is S2 and 10 cm above the spinous process of S2 (mark the position). The patient is instructed to flex to the limit of motion, and the difference between the two points is recorded. Extension is measured in the prone position from the table to the suprasternal notch.

Lumbar flexion can also be measured with single and dual inclinometers. To measure lumbar ROM using a single inclinometer, place the inclinometer on the level of L1, and zero the instrument. The patient then flexes, and the measurement is taken. The patient then returns to the upright position. The inclinometer is placed on the sacrum, and the instrument is zeroed. The patient is then asked to flex again. The sacral measurement is subtracted from the L1 measurement to determine the lumbar flexion ROM. The same technique is used for extension ROM. To measure lumbar ROM using two inclinometers, place the inclinometer on the level of L1 and the sacrum, and zero both instruments. The patient then flexes the spine. The sacral reading is then subtracted from the L1 reading, giving the clinician the measurement of the lumbar flexion. The same method is performed for extension and lateral flexion, except that the inclinometer is placed on the T12 level for lateral flexion.

c. Thoracolumbar motion is assessed with the patient in a standing position and the clinician using a tape measure. In this case S2 is still the beginning position; however, the C7 spinous process is now the landmark. The patient flexes and extends the thoracolumbar spine while the clinician notes the differences between the starting and ending motions. Normal ROM is approximately 10 cm in flexion and 2.5 cm in extension.

An alternative method is to use single or dual inclinometers if available. Using a single inclinometer, follow the same technique as previously discussed with lumbar flexion ROM. This time, however, place the inclinometer on C7 and zero the instrument. The patient then performs the motion, and the measurement is taken. The inclinometer is then placed on the sacrum, the instrument is zeroed, and the patient performs the motion. The measurement is recorded. The sacral measurement is subtracted from the C7 measurement to determine thoracolumbar ROM. When using dual inclinometers, place an inclinometer on the level of C7 and the other on the sacrum. The inclinometers are then zeroed, and the patient is asked to flex or extend. The sacral inclinometer measurement is subtracted from the C7 measurement.

7.2 / **5.** *As part of the physical examination, Kendrick performed a neurological examination. Complete Table 7.2.1, which shows the sensory and motor deficits associated with nerve root involvement at each of the lumbar and sacral levels identified in the chart.*

A completed version of Table 7.2.1 is provided in Table A7.2.1.

7.2 / **6.** *(a) Why is Eric's pain worse in the morning and improved after exercise? (b) If you were treating Eric, what activities would you have him perform during his exercise phase to reduce his discomfort?*

a. Patients with disc herniations will typically experience an increase in pain upon wakening in the morning. This occurs because the nucleus pulposus is a semi-gelatinous substance composed mainly of water. During the day, constant movement, disc compression, and dehydration cause the disc to lose fluid, thereby decreasing the size of the disc. This results in less pressure on the nerve root. Periods of rest and inactivity cause the disc to rehydrate, allowing the nuclear material to increase pressure on the nerve roots again.

b. Many physicians recommend McKenzie exercises during rehabilitation to centralize the nucleus pulposus.[21] A recent systematic review suggests that McKenzie therapy results in more of a short-term decrease (<3 months) in pain and disability for LBP patients than other standard treatments, such as nonsteroidal anti-inflammatory medication,

**TABLE A7.2.1 Sensory and motor deficits in association with nerve root involvement at individual lumbar and sacral levels.[57]**

| DISC LEVEL | LOCATION OF DERMATOME SYMPTOMS | MOTOR DEFICITS |
|---|---|---|
| L1 | Back, over greater trochanter and groin | Hip flexion |
| L2 | Back, wrapping around to anterior superior thigh and medial thigh above knee | Hip flexion and adductors, diminished patellar tendon reflex |
| L3 | Back, upper gluteal, anterior thigh, medial knee, and lower leg | Knee extension, diminished patellar tendon reflex |
| L4 | Medial gluteals, lateral thigh and knee, anterior medial lower leg, dorsomedial aspect of foot and big toe | Ankle dorsiflexion and inversion (anterior tibialis), diminished patellar tendon reflex |
| L5 | Lateral knee and upper lateral lower leg, dorsum of foot | Great toe extension |
| S1 | Buttock, posterolateral thigh, lateral side and plantar surface of the foot | Ankle plantarflexion and eversion, diminished or absent Achilles reflex |
| S2 | Buttock, posteromedial thigh, posterior, medial heel | Knee flexion and great toe flexion |

back massage with back care advice, strength training with supervision, and spinal mobilization.[10,14] The long-term effects of McKenzie rehabilitation programs are unclear, and no studies have attempted to examine this question.[10]

# CASE 7.3 Lumbar Facet Syndrome

7.3 / **1.** *Based on the information presented in the case, determine (a) the differential diagnoses and (b) the clinical diagnosis.*

a. Differential diagnoses: nerve root impingement, intervertebral disc herniation, osteophytes, spinal stenosis, lumbar sprain, and lumbar strain[58]

b. Clinical diagnosis: facet joint syndrome at L4 to L5, sometimes referred to as spondylitis (inflammation of the vertebrae)

7.3 / **2.** *Steve asked several history questions to guide his physical examination. Based on the information presented in the case, do you believe he acquired an adequate history? If not, what questions would you have asked as the evaluating clinician?*

The answers to this question will vary among students. Overall, Steve appeared to generate an adequate history. Some specific questions assisting in the examination may include:

- Questions focusing on lumbar spine red flags (refer to textbook Table 7.1)
- Questions regarding neurologic history and social or psychological distress that may amplify the patient's pain are warranted[19]
- Questions focusing on determining referred pain patterns. For example pain emanating into the flank, hip, and upper lateral thigh would suggest an upper facet pathology; pain from the lower facet joints is likely to penetrate deeper into the thigh, usually laterally and/or posteriorly[16]

7.3 / **3.** *Textbook Figure 7.3.2 is an image of a DTR. What is a DTR? How would you as the evaluating clinician assess the DTR in Figure 7.3.2?*

a. The abbreviation "DTR" stands for deep tendon reflex. It is a form of reflex testing in which the motor pathway of a nerve produces an observable pattern of reaction when a sensory afferent neuron is stimulated. It can be elicited at almost any tendon and is used to assess for lower motor neuron lesions (LMNL). A lower motor neuron lesion indicates injury to the nerve structures in the anterior horn of the spinal cord and in the spinal and peripheral nerves, resulting in unilateral symptoms. In the case of the DTR, the involved muscles associated with the peripheral nerve or nerve root have diminished or absent spinal reflexes.

b. To assess the patella (L4) DTR, the patient is placed in a short sitting position with legs hanging over the edge of the table. This places the tendon on stretch while the clinician strikes the patella tendon using the flat end of the reflex hammer to elicit a response. If there is difficulty eliciting a response, attempt a Jendrassik maneuver by squeezing the feet together when assessing the upper extremity and clasping and pulling the hands apart when assessing the lower extremity to increase activity of the spinal cord. This maneuver helps to accentuate minimal reflex activity.

7.3 / **4.** *Steve suggested to Justin that he seek further medical assistance from an orthopedic surgeon and explained how the clinical diagnosis may be confirmed. How does injecting the area with an anesthetic and noting the changes in the symptoms assist in making the clinical diagnosis?*

Physicians commonly inject the facet joint as a diagnostic tool, and this is generally accepted in clinical practice as the most reliable means of diagnosing which facet joints are pain generators.[16,55] Using either a local anesthetic or by anesthetizing the medial branches of the dorsal rami that innervate the target joint, physicians can determine if the facet joint is the source of pain. If the pain is not relieved, the injected joint cannot be considered the source of pain. The actual source of pain may be another facet joint or some other structure[41,55] or pathology.

7.3 / **5.** *After completing the physical examination, Steve documented his findings electronically and sent a copy of the report to Justin's orthopedic surgeon. Using your athletic training room's computer tracking software, document your findings electronically as if you were the treating clinician. If the case did not provide information you believe is pertinent to the clinical diagnosis, please add this information to your documentation. If you do not have access to injury-tracking software, consider downloading a trial version from CSMI Solutions (Sportsware) by going to www.csmisolutions.com/cmt/publish/service_software_dl.shtml and following the on-screen directions.*

Answers will vary. Students should consider writing a SOAP note (see textbook Appendix B) using the ABCD format when writing the short- and long-term goals.

## CASE 7.4 Spondylolisthesis

7.4 / **1.** *Based on the information presented in the case, determine (a) the differential diagnoses and (b) the clinical diagnosis.*

a. Differential diagnoses: lumbar disk pathology, lumbosacral discogenic pain syndrome, lumbosacral facet syndrome, lumbosacral acute bony injury, lumbosacral sprain and/or strain, spondylolysis (defect in the pars interarticularis), sacroiliac joint injury[49]

b. Clinical diagnosis: spondylolisthesis (forward displacement of a vertebral body in relation to the body immediately below it)

7.4 / **2.** *Overall, do you believe Tim took an adequate history? What if anything would you as the evaluating clinician have done differently?*

The answers to this question will vary among students. Overall, Tim performed an adequate history assessment. There are several other specific questions Tim may have asked to further guide the physical examination. These include, but are not limited to:[29,30,37,44,56]

- Do you remember any episodes of acute injury to the low back?
- Do you have any pain that radiates to the buttocks or posterior thigh?
- Do you have any disturbance in bowel or bladder function?
- Have you experienced a sudden growth spurt?
- Has there been a sudden increase in training, such as in intensity, frequency, or activity (particularly repetitive lumbosacral extension activities)?
- Have you added any new skills to your routine that you have not yet mastered?
- Other questions identifying risk factors, such as family history, menstrual irregularities, decreased bone mass, poor nutrition/disordered eating patterns, osteopenia, rate of weight loss, and psychological stresses, all of which play a significant role in the development of spondylolisthetic conditions.

7.4 / **3.** *(a) Based on the clinical diagnosis, what else may have Tim noted during his palpation of Rochelle, particularly if the injury had a significant progression? (b) Is this a reliable clinical indicator of the clinical diagnosis?*

a. Depending on the degree of the spondylolisthesis Rochelle may have demonstrated a palpable step-off deformity[29,48] or step sign[44] of the lumbar spine and protective lumbosacral paravertebral muscle spasms.

b. Bryk and Rosenkranz[8] describe the spinous process step sign (as seen on radiographs) as a step-off deformity that runs along the posterior margins of the spinous processes at the interspace superior to the involved vertebra as identified on radiographs. The anecdotal correlation of the radiological step sign with a palpable step-off deformity during the physical examination has become commonplace and taught as a method to detect the presence of spondylolisthesis.[17] In fact, in Collaer's[17] examination of the diagnostic utility of static lumbar spinous palpation as a means of detecting isthmic (a narrow passage connecting two larger cavities) spondylolisthesis in patients with LBD, the researcher found that validity testing revealed a sensitivity of 60 percent (95% CI, 14.7–94.7) and a specificity of 87.2 percent (95% CI, 72.6–95.7) (Table A7.4.1). They also found poor-to-fair inter-rater detection of spondylolisthesis, suggesting that palpation of the static spinous process by itself is not a definitive method for the detection of spondylolisthesis, and question its use as a single diagnostic indicator.

**TABLE A7.4.1 Static palpation of step-off deformities compared with radiographs.**

| | SPONDYLOLISTHESIS PRESENT RADIOGRAPH POSITIVE | SPONDYLOLISTHESIS ABSENT RADIOGRAPH NEGATIVE |
|---|---|---|
| Positive Palpation | 3 True positives | 5 False positives |
| Negative Palpation | 2 False negatives | 34 True negatives |

Note: Sensitivity = # of True Positives / # of True Positives + # of False Negatives

Specificity = # of True Negatives / # of True Negatives + # of False Positives

Positive Likelihood Ratio = sensitivity / 1– specificity

Negative Likelihood Ratio = 1– sensitivity / specificity

7.4 / **4.** *(a) What is the name of the special test performed in textbook Figure 7.4.2? (b) What is considered a positive finding?*

a. The special test performed in textbook Figure 7.4.2 is commonly referred to as a Stork test, Stork stand, one-leg standing with lumbar extension, or single-leg hyperextension.[12,21]

b. The test assesses for possible damage to the pars interarticularis region of the involved spinal region[36] and is typically performed while the patient stands on one leg with the sole of the non-weight-bearing foot resting on the medial aspect of the knee of the weight-bearing limb. The patient balances on one leg while simultaneously performing a lumbar extension movement. A complaint of pain is normally noted in the lumbar spine or sacroiliac area. If the lesion is to the pars interarticularis unilaterally, pain will typically be evoked on the opposite side to the leg being lifted; a bilateral fracture results in pain when either leg is lifted.

   A recent study evaluating whether the one-legged hyperextension test or Stork stand can assist in the clinical detection of active spondylolysis found that the one-legged hyperextension test is not useful in detecting active spondylolysis. It was furthermore recommended that it should not be relied on to exclude the diagnosis.[42] Remember that spondylolysis is often but not always the precursor to the development of spondylolisthesis. When compared to the gold standard, MRI is inferior to bone scintigraphy (with SPECT)/computed tomography. Bone scintigraphy (with SPECT), followed by limited computed tomography (when a bone scintigraphy is positive) should remain the first-line investigation of active athletes with LBP.[42]

7.4 / **5.** *Based on textbook Figure 7.4.3 how would the clinical diagnosis be graded?*

The diagnosis of spondylolisthesis is often made with lateral lumbar plain films and can be graded according to the amount of displacement of the involved vertebrae.[17,29,64] In Meyerding's five-category classification of spondylolisthesis, a clinician would observe the percentage of slippage by taking a lateral view of the lumbosacral junction and measuring the slip as a percentage of the length of the superior border of the sacrum.

- First degree with <25 percent slippage
- Second degree with 25–50 percent slippage
- Third degree with 50–75 percent slippage
- Fourth degree with 75–100 percent slippage
- Fifth degree with >100 percent slippage

Textbook Figure 7.4.3 demonstrates a forward slippage that is equal to about 1/4 to 1/2 of the anteroposterior diameter of S1. So this is a Grade 1 to Grade 2 spondylolisthesis.

# CASE 7.5 Lumbar Spinal Stenosis

7.5 / **1.** *Based on the above case scenario, what do you suspect is wrong with Doris's spinal column?*

The differential diagnoses are degenerative joint disease, nerve root impingement, centrally herniated discs, degenerative spondylolisthesis, SI dysfunction, facet syndrome, piriformis syndrome, epidural abscess, and trauma/fractures.[1,25]

The clinical diagnosis is lumbar spinal stenosis presenting with neurogenic claudication. Neurogenic claudication is limping or lameness accompanied by pain and paresthesia in the back, buttocks, and legs that is relieved by the stooping commonly seen in patients with lumbar spinal stenosis.[25]

7.5 / **2.** *Many times, this condition can be found in other regions of the spine and may cause other signs and symptoms. If other problems were to occur, what are some of the complications that you as the evaluating clinician may need to observe or determine as part of the history?*

The following is a list of potential complications and/or medical issues resulting in other potential signs and symptoms.[13,26] Students may provide additional answers.

- Position-related radiculopathy occurring when patients experience a reproduction in pain and paresthesia based on their position
- Loss of balance or gait unsteadiness as a result of muscular atrophy and weakness
- Chronic cauda equina syndrome, which develops from gradually progressing lumbar spinal stenosis. This normally results in bladder dysfunction and perineal (the area between the thighs extending from the coccyx to the pubis and lying below the pelvic diaphragm) pain presenting as loss of bladder/bowel function (partial or sometimes complete urinary /fecal incontinence). When working with older patients in whom this condition is more common and these symptoms are present, referral to the appropriate medical personnel is necessary.
- Infections occurring not as a direct cause but when sensations to the extremities are comprised because of the stenosis. Any external wound that is not noticed or treated appropriately may become infected.

7.5 / **3.** *Based on the clinical diagnosis, what are some of the most common diagnostic tests used when diagnosing this condition?*

The following are four of the most common tests and their recommended purposes.

- Radiographs are recommended to evaluate bone continuity, fractures, tumors, or other defects suspected with lumbar spinal stenosis and should include anteroposterior (AP) and lateral radiographs of the lumbosacral spine.[13]
- Magnetic resonance imaging is recommended to evaluate the intervertebral disk, neural elements, and soft-tissue elements of the spinal canal.[13,47] This has been shown to be as accurate as CT myelography and diagnostically superior to either myelography or CT alone[6] and has demonstrated moderate-to-substantial intra- and inter-reader reliability.[40] Results have also found that axial loading increases the severity of lumbar canal stenosis, and the effect of axial loading is greatest at the L4–L5 and L5–S1 levels.[63]
- Computerized tomography scans use a radiation beam to produce cross-sectional images to evaluate the canal dimensions (shape and size) and configuration and

identify disk abnormalities and herniation, facet degeneration and hypertrophy, ligamentous hypertrophy and redundancy, and spondylosis.[13] A CT myelogram is radiography of the spinal cord and nerve roots using an injected dye into the spinal column, which provides a contrast medium to produce an image of the spinal cord and nerves, disks, and even tumors or bone spurs. These are not the first diagnostic tests recommended.

- Bone scans use a radioactive solution injected into a vein that attaches itself to bone. The radioactive materials are detected by a gamma camera producing images of the bone and pathologies of the bone.

7.5 / **4.** *If you were the treating clinician, what types of conservative therapy would you consider for this clinical diagnosis to help alleviate pain and discomfort?*

The answers will vary among students; however, conservative care is normally recommended when treating mild cases of spinal stenosis. In severe cases, decompressive surgery is often warranted to remove the bone and ligaments around the stenosis only after conservative treatment has failed to resolve the symptom.[59,65] Conservative treatment may consist of bed rest, activity modification, physical therapy (i.e., to maintain strength and flexibility and to correct biomechanical deficits), braces and corsets (to reduce loads across the spine), traction, electrotherapy, spinal manipulation, narcotic analgesics, and/or epidural steroids.[3,59,65] Examination of treatments of lumbar spinal stenosis found that conservative care such as local anesthetic block reduces symptoms and increases walking distance but only on a short-term basis (one month). Epidural steroids offer no additional benefit. An 8- to 10-year follow-up examination comparing patients treated surgically with nonsurgically treated patients revealed that patients with lumbar spinal stenosis demonstrated similar LBP relief, predominant symptom improvement, and satisfaction with the current state with either treatment, but leg pain relief and back-related functionality were greater in those initially receiving surgical treatment.[4]

7.5 / **5.** *As the evaluating clinician, if Doris asked about her options and wanted you to elaborate on the three most common surgical techniques, how would you respond?*

Because of the relationship established between many clinicians and patients, clinicians must often explain and/or elaborate on information provided by the physician. In this case, the clinicians should begin by describing the two main goals of surgical intervention. These are decompression of the affected neural elements throughout their entire course from the central canal to their exit through the neural foramina and maintenance of spinal stability or restoration of stability in cases of preoperative degenerative instability.[13,65] Three common procedures follow.

- Laminotomy: only the portion of the lamina is removed that may help relieve pressure or be used to gain access to a disk or to bone spurs to decrease any nerve pressure.
- Spinal fusion: two or more vertebral bodies are fused or connected together by bony pieces from other parts of the body such as the pelvis. Sometimes, screws, rods, or wires can be used.
- Laminectomy: complete removal of the entire lamina of the vertebrae to allow more room for the spinal nerves to expand and also to allow access to spurs or disks.

## CASE 7.6 Thoracic Strain

7.6 / **1.** *Based on the information presented in the case, (a) what is the likely clinical diagnosis? (b) What is the normal MOI?*

a. The most likely clinical diagnosis is a thoracic strain, possibly to the iliocostalis thoracis, longissimus thoracis, spinalis thoracis, and semispinalis thoracis.

b. Isolated muscular strains to the thoracic spine normally result from a single episode of mechanical overload with an eccentric muscular contraction or from the violent stretching of the tissue into flexion, extension, rotation, and/or a combination of movements.[57] In this case, the injury was a result of violent stretching of the intrinsic muscles acting on the thoracic spinal column.

7.6 / **2.** *In this case, Sig was initially evaluated and treated by Gene during a medical time-out. However, Sig was forced to retire from the match because he could not receive any additional care. Why?*

The National Collegiate Athletic Association (NCAA) follows the rules governed by United States Tennis Association (USTA) rules and modifications adopted by the NCAA DI Tennis Committee and the Intercollegiate Tennis Association (ITA). According to USTA Regulation III.E, when an obvious injury occurs, a coach may assist and touch the player until an athletic trainer arrives to diagnose and treat the injury. However, once the athletic trainer reaches the player, he has a maximum of five minutes for diagnosis and treatment. Also, any player suffering from a treatable medical condition (e.g., asthma) may be allowed one medical time-out of 3 minutes for the treatment of that medical condition. Once this time-out is used, any medical conditions must be handled by the athlete during the changeover. This is the reason why Gene was allowed on the court only once. Considering that the immediate on-field actions could affect the playing status of a player, it is imperative for all athletic trainers to understand the rules governing the sports they are assigned to cover.[62]

7.6 / **3.** *(a) Identify the posterior extrinsic muscles acting on the spinal column that Maria should have palpated as part of her evaluation. (b) Identify the different layers of the intrinsic muscles acting on the posterior spine. (c) Identify the muscles that make up the erector spinae muscle group, and describe the technique used to identify this muscle group.*

a. Given the information presented in the case, Maria would have been wise to palpate the following extrinsic muscles acting on the spine:
   - latissimus dorsi
   - upper, middle, and lower trapezius
   - levator scapulae
   - rhomboids major and minor
   - serratus anterior (deep extrinsic muscles)
   - deltoid, supraspinous, infraspinatus, teres minor, and teres major

   These muscles attach to the upper limb of the axial skeleton and primarily function to control humeral and scapular motions.

b. The intrinsic muscles acting on the posterior column are divided into three layers: superficial, intermediate, and deep. The superficial layer consists of the splenius muscles (capitis and cervicis) and is responsible for laterally flexing and rotating the head and neck to the same side (unilaterally) and extending the head and neck (bilaterally). The intermediate layer is also known as the erector spinae muscle group and will be reviewed below. The deep layer consists of several short muscles (semispinalis, multifidus, and rotatores) known as the transversospinal muscles because the fibers run from the transverse processes to the spinous superior to them. Acting unilaterally and/or bilaterally, the transversospinal muscles act in extension of the cervical and thoracic spine (semispinalis thoracis and cervicis), rotation towards the contralateral side (multifidus, rotators, and semispinalis thoracis), and extension of the head (semispinalis capitis).[60]

c. The erector spinae muscle group consists of three pairs of vertical columns of muscle. The columns from lateral to medial include the iliocostalis (lateral column), the longissimus (intermediate column), and the spinalis (medial column). The iliocostalis is divided into three sections, including the iliocostalis lumborum (acts on the lumbar spine), iliocostalis thoracis (acts on the thoracic spine), and iliocostalis cervicis (acts on the cervical spine). The longissimus is divided into the longissimus thoracis (acts on the thoracic spine), the longissimus cervicis (acts on the cervical spine), and longissimus capitis (acts on the head). Finally the spinalis is divided into the spinalis thoracis (acts on the thoracic spine), spinalis cervicis (acts on the cervical spine), and spinalis capitis (acts on the head). Acting bilaterally, the three columns of the erector spinae function to extend the head and part or all of the vertebral column. Unilaterally, the erector spinae laterally flexes the head or the vertebral column. The erector spinae muscle group also acts eccentrically to control trunk flexion.

7.6 / **4.** *The tennis coach in this case was obviously unhappy when he confronted Gene in the athletic director's office the morning after the match. What was he upset about? How could this situation be prevented?*

In this case, the athletic training student violated laws regarding patient confidentially.[51,52] If this had been a certified athletic trainer, not only would she have violated federal and state laws regarding privacy, she would also have violated the BOC Standards of Professional Practice regarding patient privacy (see textbook Appendix B). In this case, the athletic training student was confronted by an individual who was apparently a news reporter and struck up a seemingly innocent conversation. However, the act of sharing patient information is not only against the law but also destroys the much needed trust between a patient and clinician. Although many individuals in the collegiate or high school athletic training setting may require access to a patient's records, every attempt must be made to limit how that information is disclosed and to whom.

## CASE 7.7 Thoracic Spine Fracture

7.7 / **1.** *Based on the information presented in the case, determine (a) the differential diagnoses and (b) the clinical diagnosis.*

a. Differential diagnoses: transverse process fracture, spinous process fracture, pneumothorax, rib fracture, dislocated rib

b. Clinical diagnosis: thoracic spine fracture[38]

7.7 / **2.** *Why do you think that the condition did not manifest itself acutely after the incident?*

The thoracic spine is protected by the rib cage. The relative shape (kyphosis shape) and biomechanical aspects of the thoracic spine make it very stable, decreasing the incidence of fractures to this area.[22] Most patients who suffer a thoracic spine fracture do not report neurological symptoms, making diagnosis of the injury difficult. In addition, many cases present with only slight pain and stiffness, with the major symptoms of point tenderness only at the specific level of the spine where the trauma occurred.[18,22,39]

7.7 / **3.** *The literature lists catastrophic injuries to pole vaulters as rare. Please describe the common MOIs that athletic trainers must nevertheless be aware of, and closely prepared for, when supervising pole vaulters.*

The most common mechanism reported occurs when a pole vaulter lands on the edge of the landing pad with his head striking the ground surface. The second most common mechanism occurs when the vaulter releases the pole prematurely or lands in the pole's planting box. The third most common mechanism occurs when an athlete does not land on the padding at all.[7]

7.7 / **4.** *Based on the case, if the pole vaulter was suspected of having a catastrophic injury, what management steps should Lauren and Samantha follow in order to spineboard the athlete?*

The answers to this question should *not* vary from student to student. They must include the following steps. For further information, please discuss this case with your staff athletic trainer to determine how he may handle this situation.

- Determine the level of responsiveness.
- Immediately activate EMS.
- Assess for and manage for compromise to the airway, to breathing, and to circulation. Manage any external bleeding.
- Provide in-line stabilization and apply a cervical collar. Maintain head stabilization throughout the spineboarding process until the head and neck are securely attached to board. Prepare to spineboard, and make sure you have additional trained assistance.
  a. Place spine board adjacent to athlete.
  b. Place arms of athlete at side.
  c. Have other rescuers at shoulders, waist/thigh, and lower legs of athlete.
  d. Assign another rescuer to move spine board into position.
  e. Rescuer at head will provide all commands.
  f. Athlete should be rolled toward rescuers. A 6-plus person lift may be used in some situations when enough rescuers are present.

g. When the athlete is perpendicular to the ground, the spine board is placed next to the body at an angle. When a 6-person lift is used, the spine board is slid under the body into the proper position.

h. Slowly return spine board and athlete into supine position and fasten athlete to the spine board.

i. Secure body first (chest, abdomen, legs), followed by head and neck, filling any voids as necessary.

j. Perform ongoing assessment. Please refer to your school's Emergency Action Plan for the procedures used in your athletic training program.

## CASE 7.8 Sciatica

7.8 / **1.** *Based on the information presented in the case, determine (a) the differential diagnoses and (b) the clinical diagnosis.*

a. Differential diagnoses: lumbar disk herniation, sacroiliac joint dysfunction, hamstring syndrome, ischial tuberosity overgrowth[43]

b. Clinical diagnosis: sciatica, secondary to piriformis syndrome

7.8 / **2.** *Hannah assessed several body areas during the physical examination. Based on the information presented in the case, do you believe it was necessary for her to perform all of these tests?*

The answers to this question may vary among students. However, students should recognize the following:

- Numerous injuries and conditions can cause inflammation of the sciatic nerve or sciatica.[60] Sciatica occurs secondary to an injury or condition. As a result, a complete evaluation must be conducted to determine the causative injury/condition.
- As listed in the differential diagnoses, lumbar disc and sacroiliac joint pathology are more common causes of sciatic nerve inflammation than the piriformis syndrome presented in this case. Therefore, a complete evaluation of these areas should be conducted to rule out these injuries/conditions, which may require further diagnostic testing.
- Based on a confirmed causative injury/condition of sciatica as in the case, an appropriate treatment and rehabilitation protocol can be developed for piriformis syndrome.

7.8 / **3.** *Which findings in the history and physical examination possibly led Hannah and the team orthopedist to the clinical diagnosis above?*

Although the condition is uncommon, sciatica caused by piriformis syndrome has been described in the literature.[24,53] Several proposed characteristics of this condition can be found in the case above and include:

- Mechanism of injury: overtraining (i.e., conclusion of competitive season, triathlon training, history of stress fracture)
- Signs and symptoms: pain and numbness in posterior hip and buttocks (i.e., gluteus maximus and piriformis) with radiating symptoms into the posterior thigh
- Leg length discrepancy
- Weakness with active hip abduction
- Positive special tests: Freiberg sign, Lasegue's test, Pace sign, and resisted external rotation
- Unremarkable thoracic and lumbar spine evaluation, neurological tests, and radiographs

7.8 / **4.** *Describe the anatomical factors in the development of the clinical diagnosis.*

The piriformis and sciatic nerve exit the pelvis through the sciatic notch, along with other structures. Commonly, the sciatic nerve exits the notch below the piriformis. However, anatomical variations of the sciatic nerve and piriformis have been described, such as passing of the nerve through the piriformis and separate trunks of the nerve passing above and below to the piriformis.[5] Regardless of the anatomical relationship, inflammation of the piriformis can cause subsequent compression and inflammation of the sciatic nerve.

7.8 / **5.** *If you were Hannah, and Jim asked, "What is the plan for treatment and rehabilitation of my condition," what would be your response?*

The answers to this question may vary among students. Treatment and rehabilitation should focus on reduction of inflammation and pain and improvement of flexibility and muscular strength. Oral anti-inflammatory medication may prove useful. A pain-free flexibility and strengthening program for the lumbar, hip, pelvis, and lower extremities will address ROM and strength deficits. Core strength and stability should also be included.[11] Modifications of training and of the routine of prolonged sitting will assist with the reduction of inflammation and pain. Referral to the team's orthopedist for further evaluation and treatment is warranted if symptoms persist.

# REFERENCES


1. Alverez JA, Hardy RH. Lumbar spinal stenosis: a common cause of back and leg pain. *Am Fam Physician* [electronic version]. 1998;59:1825–1834, 1839–1840. Available from: http://www.aafp.org/afp/980415ap/alvarez.html.
2. Anderson M, Parr G, Hall S. *Foundations of Athletic Training: Prevention, Assessment, and Management* (4th ed.). Baltimore, MD: Lippincott Williams & Wilkins; 2008.
3. Atlas S, Deyo R, Keller R, et al. The Maine Lumbar Spine Study, part III, 1-year outcomes of surgical and nonsurgical management of lumbar spinal stenosis. *Spine.* 1996;21:1787–1794.
4. Atlas S, Keller R, Wu Y, Deyo R, Singer D. Long-term outcomes of surgical and nonsurgical management of lumbar spinal stenosis: 8 to 10 year results from the Maine lumbar spine study. *Spine.* 2005;30(8):936–943.
5. Beaton L, Anson B. The relation of the sciatic nerve and of its subdivisions to the piriformis muscle. *Anat Rec.* 1937;70:1–5.
6. Bischoff R, Rodriguez R, Gupta K, Righi A, Dalton J, Whitecloud T. A comparison of computed tomography-myelography, magnetic resonance imaging, and myelography in the diagnosis of herniated nucleus pulposus and spinal stenosis. *J Spinal Disord.* 1993;6(4):289–295.
7. Boden BP, Osbahr DC. High-risk stress fractures: evaluation and treatment. *J Am Acad of Ortho Surg.* 2000;8(6):344–353.
8. Bryk D, Rosenkranz W. True spondylolisthesis and pseudospondylolisthesis: the spinous process sign. *Can Asso Radiologists J.* 1969;20:53–56.
9. Burton A, Waddell G, Tillotson K, Summerton N. Information and advice to patients with back pain can have a positive effect: a randomized controlled trial of a novel educational booklet in primary care. *Spine.* 1999;24(2484–2491).
10. Busanich B, Verscheure S. Does McKenzie therapy improve outcomes for back pain? *J Athl Train.* 2006;41(1):117–119.
11. Byrd J. Piriformis syndrome. *Oper Tech Sports Med.* 2005; 13:71–79.
12. Cassas K, Cassettari-Wayhs. Childhood and adolescent sports-related overuse injuries. *Am Fam Physician.* 2006; 73:1014–1022.
13. Chen AL, Spivak JM. Degenerative lumbar spinal stenosis. *Physician and Sportsmed.* 2003;31(8):25–34.
14. Clare H, Adams R, Maher C. A systematic review of efficacy of McKenzie therapy for spinal pain. *Aust J Physiother.* 2004;50:209–216.
15. Clarkson H. *Musculoskeletal Assessment: Joint Range of Motion and Manual Muscle Strength.* Philadelphia, PA: Lippincott Williams & Wilkins; 2000.
16. Cohen MS, Bruno RJ. The collateral ligaments of the elbow: anatomy and clinical correlation. *Clin Orthop Relat Res.* 2001;(383):123–130.
17. Collaer JW, McKeough M, Boissonnault WC. Lumbar isthmic spondylolisthesis detection with palpation: interrater reliability and concurrent criterion-related validity. *J Man & Manipulative Ther.* 2006;14(1):22–29.
18. Deluca S. Thoracic spine fractures. *Am Fam Physician.* 1990;42(2):419–421.
19. Deyo R, Rainville J, Kent D. What can the history and physical examination tell us about low back pain? *JAMA.* 1992;268(6):760–765.
20. Ebraheim NA, Hassan A, Lee M, Xu R. Functional anatomy of the lumbar spine. *Semin Pain Med.* 2004;2(3):131–137.
21. Eddy D, Congeni J, Loud K. A review of spine injuries and return to play. *Clin J Sports Med.* 2005;15:453–458.
22. Elattrache N, Fadale P, Fu F. Thoracic spine fracture in a football player: a case report. *Am J Sports Med.* 1983;21(1):157–160.
23. Elveru R, Rochstein J, Lamb R, Riddle D. Methods for taking subtalar joint measurements: a clinical report. *Phys Ther.* 1988;68:678–682.
24. Furman MB, Puttiliz KM, Pannullo R, Simon J. Spinal stenosis and neurogenic claudication. *eMedicine* [electronic version]. 2009. Available from: http://eMedicine.medscape.com/article/310528-overview. Accessed June 9, 2009.
25. Freiberg A. Sciatic pain and its relief by operations on the muscle and fascia. *Arch Surg.* 1937;34:337–350.
26. Goh KJ, Khalifa W, Anslow P, Cadoux-Hudson T, Donaghy M. The clinical syndrome associated with lumbar spinal stenosis. *Eur Neurol.* 2004;52(4):242–249.
27. Heck JF, Sparano JM. A classification system for the assessment of lumbar pain in athletes. *J Athl Train.* 2000;35(2):204–211.
28. Henrotin Y, Cedraschi C, Duplan B, Bazin T, Duquesnoy B. Information and low back pain management: a systematic review. *Spine.* 2006;31:E326–E334.
29. Herman MJ, Pizzutillo PD. Spondylolysis and spondylolisthesis in the child and adolescent: a new classification. *Clin Orthop Relat Res.* 2005;434:46–54.
30. Herring S, Bergfeld J, Boyajian-O'Neill L, et al. Female athlete issues for the team physician: a consensus statement. *Med Sci Sports Exerc.* 2003;35(10):1875–1793.
31. Hoffman H. Childhood and adolescent lumbar pain: differential diagnosis and management. *Clin Neurosurg.* 1980;27:553–576.
32. Hood-White R, Lowdon JD. Herniated nucleus pulposus with radiculopathy in an adolescent: successful nonoperative treatment. *South Med J.* 2002;95(8):932–933.
33. Humphreys SC, Eck JC. Clinical evaluation and treatment options for herniated lumbar disc. *Am Fam Physician.* 1999;59(3):575–582.
34. Kazemi M. Adolescent lumbar disc herniation in a Tae Kwon Do martial artist: a case report. *J Can Chiropractic Assoc.* 1999;43(4):236.
35. Kinkade S. Evaluation and treatment of acute low back pain. *Am Fam Physician.* 2007;75:1181–1188, 1190–1182.
36. Konin JG, Wiksten D, Isear JA, Brader H. Special tests for orthopedic examination (3rd ed.). Thorofare, NJ: Slack; 2006.
37. Konz R, Goel V, Grobler, L, et al. The pathomechanism of spondylolytic spondylolisthesis in immature primate lumbar spines: in vitro and finite element assessments. *Spine.* 2001;26(4):E38–E49.

38. Leahy M, Rahm M. Thoracic spine fractures and dislocations. *eMedicine* [electronic version]. 2009. Available from: http://emedicine.medscape.com/article/1267029-overview. Accessed December 26, 2009.
39. Lischyna N, Karim R. Thoracic spine compression fractures following a snowboarding accident: a case study. *J Can Chiropractic Assoc.* 2003;47(2):110–115.
40. Lurie J, Tosteson A, Tosteson T, et al. Reliability of readings of magnetic resonance imaging features of lumbar spinal stenosis. *Spine.* 2008;55(14):1605–1610.
41. Manchikanti L, Boswell M, Singh V, Pampati V, Damron K, Beyer C. Prevalence of facet joint pain in chronic spinal pain of cervical, thoracic, and lumbar regions. *BMC Musculoskeletal Disorders* [electronic version]. 2004. Available from: http://www.biomedcentral.com/1471-2474/5/15. Accessed September 28, 2009.
42. Masci L, Pike J, Malara F, Phillips B, Bennell K, Brukner P. Use of the one-legged hyperextension test and magnetic resonance imaging in the diagnosis of active spondylolysis. *Br J Sports Med.* 2006;40(11):940–946.
43. Mayrand N, Fortin J, Descarreaux M, Normand M. Diagnosis and management of posttraumatic piriformis syndrome: a case study. *J Manipulative Physiol Ther.* 2006;29:486–491.
44. Motley G, Nyland J, Jacobs J, Caborn D. The pars interarticularis stress reaction, spondylolysis, and spondylolisthesis progression. *J Athl Train.* 1998;33(34):351–358.
45. Nachemson A. Disc pressure measurements. *Spine.* 1981;6:93–97.
46. Ozgen S, Konya D, Toktas OZ, Dagcinar A, Ozek MM. Lumbar disc herniation in adolescence. *Pediatr Neurosurg.* 2007;43(2):77–81.
47. Panagiotis ZE, Athanasios K, Panagiotis D, Minos T, Charis M, Elias L. Functional outcome of surgical treatment for multilevel lumbar spinal stenosis. *Acta Orthop.* 2006;77(4):670–676.
48. Patel DP, Shivdasani V, Baker RJ. Management of sport-related concussion in young athletes. *Sports Med.* 2005;35(8):671–684.
49. Perrin A, Shiple B. Lumbosacral spondylolisthesis. *eMedicine* [electronic version]. 2008. Available from: http://www.emedicine.com/sports/TOPIC70.HTM. Accessed June 26, 2010.
50. Radebold A. Lumbosacral spine sprain/strain injuries. *eMedicine* [electronic version]. 2007. Available from: http://www.emedicine.com/sports/topic69.htm. Accessed August 10, 2008.
51. Rankin J, Ingersoll C. *Athletic Training Management.* Dubuque, IA: McGraw-Hill College Publishing; 2006.
52. Ray R. *Management Strategies in Athletic Training* (3rd ed.). Champaign, IL: Human Kinetics; 2005.
53. Robinson D. Piriformis syndrome in relation to sciatic pain. *Am J Surg.* 1947;73:355–358.
54. Rohlmann A, Claes L, Bergmann G, Graichen F, Neef P, Wilke HJ. Comparison of intradiscal pressures and spinal fixator loads for different body positions and exercises. *Ergon.* 2001;44(8):781–794.
55. Saal J. General principles of diagnostic testing as related to painful lumbar spine disorders. *Spine.* 2002;27(22):2538–2545.
56. Sadiq S, Meir A, Hughes SPF. Surgical management of spondylolisthesis overview of literature. *Neurol India.* 2005;53(4):506–511.
57. Schultz SJ, Houglum PA, Perrin DH. *Examination of Musculoskeletal Injuries* (2nd ed.). Champaign, IL: Human Kinetics; 2005.
58. Shin CH, Slipman, CW. Lumbar facet arthropathy. *eMedicine* [electronic version]. 2009. Available from: http://emedicine.medscape.com/article/310069-overview. Accessed December 26, 2009.
59. Snyder DL, Doggett D, Turkelson C. Treatment of degenerative lumbar spinal stenosis. *Am Fam Physician.* 2004;70(3):517.
60. Starkey C, Ryan J. *Evaluation of Orthopedic and Athletic Injuries* (2nd ed.). Philadelphia, PA: F.A. Davis; 2002.
61. Udermann B, Spratt K, Donelson R, Mayer J, Graves J, Tillotson J. Can a patient educational book change behavior and reduce pain in chronic low back pain patients? *Spine J.* 2004;4(4):425–435.
62. United States Tennis Association. The Rules of Tennis. 2009. Available from: http://www.usta.com/AboutUs/~/media/USTA/Document percent20Assets/2007/02/09/doc_13_16051.ashx. Accessed May 25, 2009.
63. Wang Y, Jeng C, Wu C, et al. Dynamic effects of axial loading on the lumbar spine during magnetic resonance imaging in patients with suspected spinal stenosis. *J Formos Med Assoc.* 2008;107(4):334–339.
64. Wicker A. Spondylolysis and spondylolisthesis in sports. *Int SportMed J.* 2008;9(2):74–78.
65. Yuan PS, Albert TJ. Nonsurgical and surgical management of lumbar spinal stenosis. *J Bone Joint Surg Am.* 2004;86-A(10):2320–2330.

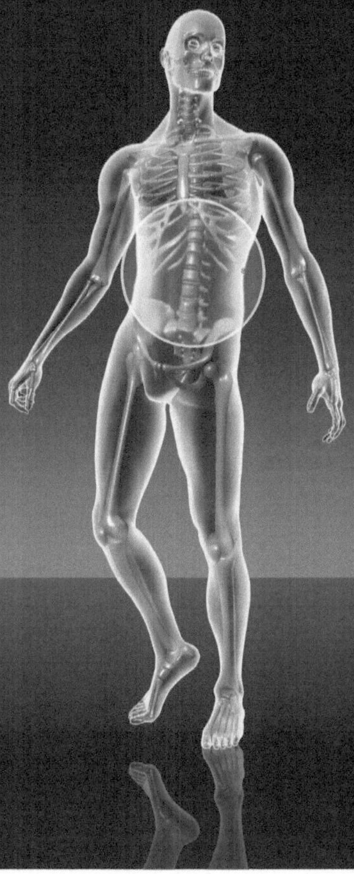

CHAPTER 8

# Thorax and Abdomen

## QUICK REFERENCE

CASE 8.1
**Traumatic Pneumothorax**

CASE 8.2
**Sudden Cardiac Arrest**

CASE 8.3
**Spleen Rupture**

CASE 8.4
**Rib Fracture**

CASE 8.5
**Costochondritis**

CASE 8.6
**Rectus Abdominis Strain**

CASE 8.7
**Breast Contusion**

CASE 8.8
**Scapular Fracture**

CASE 8.9
**Liver Injury**

CASE 8.10
**Kidney Contusion**

# ANSWERS TO CASE QUESTIONS

## CASE 8.1 Traumatic Pneumothorax

8.1 / **1.** *Based on the information presented in the case, determine (a) the differential diagnoses and (b) the clinical diagnosis.*

a. Differential diagnoses: clavicle fracture, rib fracture, scapular fracture, sternal fracture, punctured lung, heart contusion

b. Clinical diagnosis: traumatic pneumothorax

8.1 / **2.** *What is the immediate management for this condition?*

If the athletic trainer suspects a pneumothorax, immediate oxygen supplementation and immediate referral to the hospital is the best course of action. To confirm the diagnosis, a posteroanterior (PA) chest radiograph, or an expiratory or lateral decubitus film if the condition is relatively small, would be indicated. Usually, a pulmonologist will diagnosis a pneumothorax as a percentage of the lung affected, such as 20 to 30 percent pneumothorax. Depending on the severity, re-expansion of the lung with a chest tube (Heimlich chest valve drain) or thoracostomy is warranted,[3,6] along with monitoring in the hospital.

8.1 / **3.** *(a) What other signs and symptoms may be presented with this injury? (b) What precautions should an athletic trainer take?*

a. Traumatic pneumothorax may present with tachycardia, decreased breath sounds, tracheal deviation, distended neck veins, hypotension, breathing difficulties, pain radiating to the shoulder and neck on the affected side, pain in the chest with exertion, or tachypnea.[3,6,8]

b. Approximately 10 percent of traumatic pneumothorax conditions can be asymptomatic,[26] and systematic monitoring of the athlete is paramount. In addition, because symptoms may take hours or days to develop, any possible rib fracture or contusion should be followed up with x-rays, especially if symptoms do not appear to resolve or decrease over time.

8.1 / **4.** *After Billy is diagnosed and treated appropriately, (a) when should he be allowed to return to play? (b) Should any other restrictions be put in place?*

a. Because of the low incidence of this condition, return-to-play guidelines are speculative. It is recommended that return to play begin after full resolution of symptoms[8] or up to three weeks for a full contact-sport athlete.[3]

b. Air travel should also be restricted because of the potential for exacerbating or enlarging the pneumothorax through pressure changes when flying, but no specific guidelines are published.

8.1 / **5.** *This condition often is classified by two separate causes: one is spontaneous; the other traumatic. Please describe both.*

A spontaneous pneumothorax usually affects younger individuals between the ages of 20 and 40. The suspected cause is rupture of subpleural blebs or bullae as a result of family history; being tall and thin; smoking history; or sports activities involving pressure fluxuations, such as scuba diving, weight lifting, or jogging.[8]

A traumatic pneumothorax usually results from a blunt force that can cause a rib/sternal/clavicle fracture by pushing the rib inward to puncture the lung (rib fractures are not always associated with pneumothorax).

## CASE 8.2 Sudden Cardiac Arrest

8.2 / **1.** *Based on the information presented in the case, identify the clinical diagnosis.*

The athlete died as a result of sudden cardiac arrest. There are only about 100 cases of sudden cardiac arrest per year in athletics.[18] Although it occurs in low numbers, in the athletic population, sudden death from cardiac arrest is considered the leading cause of death among young athletes,[11,16,17,19,20,25] despite pre-participation physical exam screenings and emergency planning, including the availability of AEDs at athletic events.[11]

8.2 / **2.** *Andrew and Tara initiated immediate medical care, as identified in textbook Figure 8.2.1, after the primary assessment. Looking at the figure, (a) what is the name of this procedure? (b) Do they appear to be performing the procedure correctly?*

a. The procedure performed in textbook Figure 8.2.1 is two-rescuer cardiopulmonary resuscitation (CPR).

FIGURE A8.2.1 Correct hand placement for CPR.

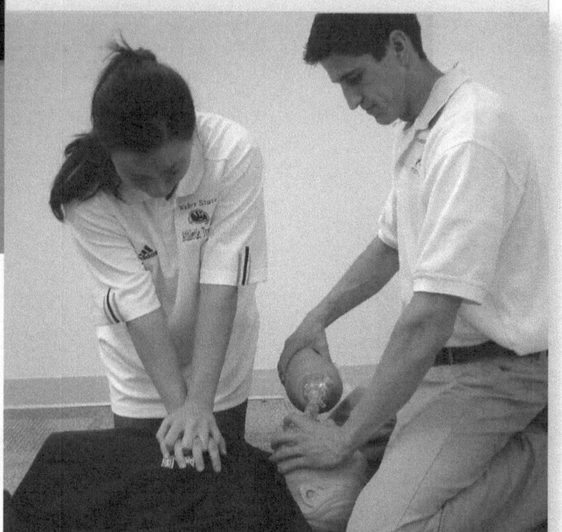

b. After the initial assessment that determined the need for CPR, Andrew and Tara did not correctly perform the procedure (at least based on the photo in the textbook). The first and biggest error was the hand placement for chest compressions. The hands appear to be at the level of the xiphoid process rather than on the center of the chest (shown in the correct position in Figure A8.2.1). Another incorrect or improper action is the lack of personal protective equipment (i.e., gloves). Personal protective equipment should be used at all times and is required, according the Bloodborne Pathogens Standard (29 CFR 1910.1030) outlined by the Occupational Safety and Health Administration (OSHA).[22] Finally, remember that during two-rescuer CPR, the cycles should continue for 2 minutes, or five total cycles, before changing positions, in order to prevent fatigue and poor mechanics.

8.2 / **3.** *(a) Did Andrew and Tara handle the situation appropriately? (b) Outline the management steps you would employ in this same situation.*

a. The athletic trainers should have requested before the event that an AED be available on site or brought one with them in case of medical emergencies. If an AED was available, the athlete should have been connected, and these steps followed: One shock followed by immediate chest compressions and rescue breathing (30:2) to help improve oxygen flow and to avoid interruptions of chest compressions while waiting for rhythm analysis.[11] In addition, CPR can be initiated while the second rescuer is connecting the AED.

b. A proper emergency action plan (EAP) should have been reviewed before Andrew and Tara covered the event. Specific elements should have included:

- Lines of communication (which was correctly done in this scenario)

- Pre-event review of other emergency responders at the event; location of all emergency medical equipment (especially an AED)
- Pre-event practice run of all trained medical personnel for such emergencies
- Identification of person(s) for initiating and conducting different parts of the EAP[11]

8.2 / **4.** *What are some associated medical conditions that may be involved in the outcome of the above scenario?*

Of the cardiovascular diseases that are most prevalent, hypertrophic cardiomyopathy and congenital coronary artery anomalies account for approximately 36 percent and 17 percent, respectively, of the athletes who experience sudden cardiac death (or survived cardiac arrest).[14,18] Blunt trauma to the chest (commotio cordis) is one of the leading causes of death from sudden cardiac arrest or ventricular arrhythmia. Hypertrophic cardiomyopathy (HCM) is a congenital disorder characterized by abnormal thickening of the left ventricle wall that develops before the age of 20. The thickened ventricle wall (normally >1 cm) leads to electrical problems and arrhythmia, including ventricular fibrillation. Congenital coronary artery anomalies such as congenital variations in right or left coronary anatomy are often associated with structural forms of congenital heart disease. The most common abnormality is a wrong origin of the left main coronary artery. Other conditions include Marfan syndrome, myocarditis, aortic stenosis, mitral valve prolapsed, long-QT syndrome.

8.2 / **5.** *It has been postulated that pre-participation examinations (PPE) should screen for heart-related irregularities. What are some screening questions and tests that should be used to help detect abnormalities? When should an athlete be restricted from athletic participation?*

Questions should be asked to determine the presence of the following conditions[14]:

- Syncope (fainting) during or after exercise
- Pain, pressure, or discomfort in chest while exercising
- Heart skipping beats during exercise
- High blood pressure, high cholesterol, murmur, heart infection
- Family history of cardiovascular disease
- Family history of Marfan syndrome

Screening tests

- Listen for a murmur that changes in sound with squatting or standing during a Valsalva maneuver.

Suspicions raised by screening questions are grounds for restricting participation until further diagnosis. Athletes with stage 2 hypertension (higher than 160/100) should be restricted until the condition is controlled.

## CASE 8.3 Spleen Rupture

8.3 / **1.** *Based on the information presented in the case, determine (a) the differential diagnoses and (b) the probable clinical diagnosis.*

a. Differential diagnoses: fractured ribs, flail chest, kidney injury, rib contusion, pneumothorax

b. Clinical diagnosis: spleen rupture/injury

8.3 / **2.** *The literature suggests that this injury is made worse if a specific illness is present before sustaining a traumatic event. What is the illness?*

Athletes with mononucleosis, commonly known as "mono," have an increased risk of traumatic spleen injuries, especially if the mono occurs within six weeks prior to the spleen rupture/injury.[10] Infectious mononucleosis is caused by the Epstein-Barr virus, frequently referred to as EBV. Literature is inconclusive concerning when to return to play after mononucleosis, but one month seems to be a common suggestion[27] as to when the spleen returns to normal size and/or compliance.

8.3 / **3.** *Management of injuries to the abdominal region is based on signs, symptoms, severity, location, and what other factor(s)?*

Answers to this question may vary among students; however, two issues to consider are time and shock. Some symptoms, such as hemorrhage may take several hours to manifest. Internal bleeding will cause the body to show signs and symptoms of shock, which must be monitored for any athlete struck with an abdominal blunt force or suffering abdominal trauma.[5,10]

8.3 / **4.** *What are the special tests or signs used to assess this injury?*

There are no specific special tests an athletic trainer can perform during an on-field assessment. An athletic trainer may observe for referred pain called the Kehr's sign, which transmits pain to the upper left shoulder/neck region (Figure 8.7). If the spleen is perforated or ruptured, bleeding within the abdominal cavity may result in discoloration and lowering of blood pressure, in which case monitoring of vital signs is of importance. Lastly, vomiting may also be present, and blood, bile, or other unusual substances in the vomit should be recorded.

8.3 / **5.** *After completing the physical examination, Will helped Suko to document her findings electronically and sent a copy of the report to Antwan's physician. Using your athletic training room's computer tracking software, document your findings electronically as if you were the treating clinician. If the report does not provide information you believe is pertinent to the clinical diagnosis, please add this information to your documentation. If you do not have access to injury tracking software, consider downloading a trial version from CSMI Solutions (Sportsware) by going to www.csmisolutions.com/cmt/publish/service_software_dl.shtml and following the on-screen directions.*

Answers will vary. Students should consider writing a SOAP note (see textbook Appendix B) using the ABCD format when writing the short- and long-term goals.

## CASE 8.4 Rib Fracture

8.4 / **1.** *Based on the information presented in the case, determine (a) the differential diagnoses and (b) the clinical diagnosis.*

a. Differential diagnoses: rib contusion, costochondral sprain, intercostal strain

b. Clinical diagnosis: rib fracture

8.4 / **2.** *What is the immediate management for this type of condition?*

Radiographs will be necessary to determine the severity of and presence of rib body (shaft) damage such as fracture. If no internal injury(s) is/are present, only bony trauma, then the most common treatment options are rest, NSAIDs, and protective padding or commercial vests, such as the Flak jacket (monitor for hypostatic pneumonia arising from not being able to inhale/exhale fully due to the rib support). Later on, core strength training exercises that include the serratus anterior and joint mobilization of the costovertebral and costotransverse joints can be utilized.

8.4 / **3.** *Injuries to this area often are associated with other potentially damaging injuries. Please list some possible associated or secondary injuries.*

The following is a list of possible secondary injuries to consider[21]:

- Fractures of the upper four ribs can injure or damage the subclavian artery, subclavian vein, aortic artery, or lung (pneumothorax, hemothorax).
- Damage to the first rib can also cause a diminished upper extremity pulse and brachial plexus entrapment or injury.
- Fractures of the lower two ribs may damage the kidneys or spleen.
- There is potential puncture injury to any internal organ.
- Flail chest, which is classified as a fracture of two or more ribs in two locations in which the rib segments "free-float" about the chest wall, can cause injury to the underlying abdominal organs, heart, lungs, and major arteries.

8.4 / **4.** *The literature reports two types of classifications for the injury.[21] Please name the two types and describe both the MOIs and sports that may be associated with each type.*

The two types of rib fractures are first-rib fractures and floating-rib fractures. First-rib fractures can result from direct trauma or from indirect trauma when an athlete falls on an outstretched and hyperabducted arm. Fractures of the first rib may also occur with forceful and powerful contraction of the scalene muscle, where the rib is the thinnest, such as heavy lifting and sudden scalene contraction, pitching, or throwing the head backward/sideways.[21] Possible sports include tennis, baseball, softball, rowing, and basketball.

Floating-rib fractures occur in the lower two ribs and result from a direct blow. The ribs are avulsed from the external oblique muscles. Possible sports include baseball and softball, especially pitchers and batters.

8.4 / **5.** *Apart from the clinical diagnosis, stress fractures can also occur within the bony segments of this region. Please describe the etiology of how these fractures develop.*

Stress fractures to the ribs occur at the point on the rib that is the smallest diameter or at the section where it changes direction.[24] They happen via muscle etiology when the muscle is weak and loses some of the shock absorption properties, placing stress on the ribs; muscle force across the rib; muscle imbalance (serratus anterior and external oblique).

## CASE 8.5 Costochondritis

8.5 / **1.** *Based on the information presented in the case, determine (a) the differential diagnoses and (b) the clinical diagnosis.*

a. Differential diagnoses: rib fracture/contusion, Tietze syndrome, heart attack, sternal fracture, abdominal injury, costochondral separation

b. Clinical diagnosis: costochondritis

8.5 / **2.** *This condition is sometimes confused with a similar disorder that affects the same region. (a) Please identify and describe this similar disorder. (b) How can a clinician differentiate between the two disorders?*

a. Costochondritis, an inflammatory condition of the costochondral or costosternal joint(s), causes localized pain and tenderness and is sometimes confused with Tietze syndrome.

b. Tietze syndrome is an inflammation of the costochondral cartilage that results in tenderness and swelling (while costochondritis typically does not present with any swelling) over the ribs and cartilage at the sternal/rib articulation. It mimics both myocardial pain and costochondritis, and many individuals experience very sharp pain that begins abruptly and radiates to the arms or shoulder (as with heart attacks). Many times, swelling from the syndrome is found at the second to third rib junctions with the sternum.

8.5 / **3.** *Aspegren, Hyde, and Miller[2] have found that several treatment methods have been effective for managing this disorder. Please (a) describe the methods, and (b) discuss which methods may be most appropriate in managing this condition.*

a. One treatment uses high velocity, low amplitude (HVLA) manipulation to the hypokinetic (loss of motion) costovertebral, costotransverse, and facet joints. Another approach applies the Graston Technique (GT) to the chondrosternal joints. The Graston Technique incorporates an instrument-assisted soft tissue mobilization to detect and treat restrictions that affect normal function. It often separates and breaks down collagen and stretches connective tissue and muscle fibers, increasing skin temperature and blood flow to and from the area. This is accomplished by having the clinician use stainless steel instruments to move over and "catch" fibrotic tissue, which identifies the areas of restriction in which the instruments are used to break up adhesions and the like. More information on this technique can be found at www.grastontechnique.com. A third method uses Kinesio taping. Kinesio taping involves taping over and around muscles in order to assist and give support or to prevent over-contraction. In this case, one strip should be applied over the chondrosternal segments and another strip over the fifth costocartilage.

b. Of the three techniques identified by Aspegren, Hyde, and Miller,[2] the first—HVLA manipulation—does not typically fall within the scope of practice of an athletic trainer. The second, the Graston Technique, requires advanced continuing professional education, which is available to athletic trainers and is BOC-approved. In fact, this technique is taught as part of many athletic training master's degree programs. More information on this technique can be found at www.grastontechnique.com. The third technique, Kinesio taping, does not require certification to purchase and utilize the tape, but a training course is recommended to gain proficiency in the use of the tape. More information on this technique can be found at http://www.kinesiotaping.com.

8.5 / **4.** *Palpation is an important part of the assessment of this condition. A good understanding of the anatomy is important for successful palpation. Describe the anatomy of the structures involved in this condition and the bony structures you would have palpated.*

Refer to the chapter's anatomical review, particularly the section on thoracic bones. Students can also turn to their preferred anatomical reference books.

8.5 / **5.** *Overall, do you believe Fernandez performed an adequate evaluation? What, if anything, would you as the evaluating clinician have done differently?*

The answers to this question will vary among students. Overall, Fernandez performed an adequate assessment. A couple of items that were not reported include a neurological assessment and examination for referred-pain patterns. Based on the information reported, the decision to refer Theresa to a medical facility was appropriate.

## CASE 8.6 Rectus Abdominis Strain

8.6 / **1.** *Based on the information presented in the case, determine (a) the differential diagnoses and (b) the clinical diagnosis.*

a. Differential diagnoses: hernia, visceral organ trauma, intercostal muscle strain, rib fracture, and rib contusion

b. Clinical diagnosis: rectus abdominis strain

8.6 / **2.** *What is the major function of the muscle(s) in this region?*

The rectus abdominis muscle is primarily responsible for trunk and core stability as well as trunk flexion. The external and internal abdominal obliques are responsible for trunk flexion and rotation; the transverses abdominis is responsible for compression of the abdominal content and core stability.

8.6 / **3.** *What is the major MOI for this injury and the associated signs and symptoms?*

The MOI is usually a sudden twisting motion when the arm(s) are overhead that stretches the muscle with eccentric forces.[12] In one study, 23 percent of injuries during a two-year period for NHL ice hockey were abdominal injuries, with 91 percent occurring with a combination of either a stretch, torsion, overuse, or other non-contact-related motion.[12] A decrease in muscle strength and/or muscular imbalance can also lead to injury.

Signs and symptoms include a hematoma, pain, noticeable muscle defect upon palpation, loss of ROM, and difficulty with deep respirations.

8.6 / **4.** *Based on the information presented in the case, (a) why didn't Placido perform any special tests? (b) What, if anything, would you have done differently as the evaluating clinician? (c) How would you manage this condition?*

a. There are no specific special diagnostic tests that could be used in this case, except to assess active and passive ROM and muscular strength.

b. Placido could have also questioned Jacque about any referred pain coming from the visceral organs; however, there was no report of a traumatic event, making the risk of internal trauma less likely. Palpation for abdominal rigidity and rebound tenderness is also possible.

c. Most of the time, the condition is managed with complete rest, ice, and bracing or wrapping (e.g., elastic wrap) the abdominal area for added pressure to stabilize the core. Muscle strengthening focusing on eccentric activities is recommended, along with a decrease in any muscle imbalance activities.

8.6 / **5.** *What are some common sports in which this injury occurs?*

Sports in which abdominal strains are more prevalent include ice hockey, tennis, football, volleyball, and racquetball. An abdominal muscle strain can take anywhere from several days to several weeks to heal properly.

## CASE 8.7 Breast Contusion

8.7 / **1.** *Based on the information presented in the case, determine (a) the differential diagnoses and (b) the clinical diagnosis.*

a. Differential diagnoses: pectoralis strain/contusion, rib contusion, rib fracture

b. Clinical diagnosis: breast contusion

8.7 / **2.** *Please describe the anatomy of the structure involved in the clinical diagnosis.*

It is a mammary gland, found over the pectoralis major muscle that extends approximately from the second to seventh rib. It has 15 to 25 lobes, connective tissue, nipple, and areola. The lobes have excretory ducts that drain to the nipple, and the lobes are separated by connective tissue. The breast has fascial planes or suspensory ligaments called Cooper's ligaments (not true ligaments in that they do not really support the breast) that are found in the upper breast that run from the fascia of the pectoralis major to the fascia of the skin on the outside of the breast and may limit some breast movement. Cooper's ligaments also hold the nipple at the fifth intercostal level. Cooper's droop is a condition that affects large-breasted women when their Cooper's ligament becomes stretched.[15]

8.7 / **3.** *Based on the clinical diagnosis, what are the most common athletic injuries to the involved anatomical structure, and how should they be treated?*

There are three common injuries to the mammary gland:

- Contusions: Contusions from a direct blow by another person or object can lead to the rupture of superficial capillaries. Edema and discoloration will usually occur and resolve in several weeks. Treatment consists of ice and analgesics for pain and discomfort. Proper support is also necessary to prevent unwanted movement. In some instances, a hematoma can occur, and aspiration may be needed if the condition or pain does not resolve over time. Mammography and a physical examination will be needed.
- Abrasions: Abrasions occur in common sports such as biking, skiing, and softball. They also occur from bra parts sliding or scraping over the breast tissue in these or other sporting activities. Bleeding occurs from the disruption of the soft tissue. Management is the same as for any abrasion.
- Nipple abrasions: These kinds of abrasions occur from tight-fitting clothing, rubbing of sports bras, shirts, or other types of clothing over the nipple. Cold weather, when the nipple becomes more prominent, may cause irritation with clothing. Friction while running (jogger's nipple) is another common mechanism that can also affect men. Prevention includes applying a bandage over the nipple while exercising, applying a type of lubrication (petroleum jelly), properly fitting clothing, and especially, using a properly fitted sports bra.

8.7 / **4.** *A contusion to the affected tissue can lead to a rare benign disease. Please describe this disease.*

Breast contusion can lead to Mondor's disease. Mondor's disease is characterized by thrombophlebitis that affects the superficial veins (lateral thoracic, thoracoepigastric, superior epigastric) of the chest wall. Clinical signs include tension of the lateral chest wall and pain related to a subcutaneous linear/winding cord-like structure associated with the affected vessel. In addition, the person can experience redness of the skin, edema, and sometimes retraction of the breast. In most cases, the disease will resolve over time, but surgical intervention (open-breast biopsy) may be necessary.[13,15]

8.7 / **5.** *Clearly, Brad engaged in an act that caught Leona off guard. Based on the information presented in the case, (a) what if anything did Brad do that was inappropriate or unethical? (b) How would you have handled the situation if you were the evaluating athletic trainer?*

a. The answers might vary among students and should be discussed with the classroom instructor. All should agree that Brad should not have palpated Jennifer's breast. In fact, his action could lead to a violation of code 3.11 of the Board of Certification's Standards of Professional Practice (see textbook Appendix B). This code states:

> "Does not take any action that leads, or may lead, to the conviction, plea of guilty or plea of nolo contendere (no contest) to any felony, or to a misdemeanor related to public health, patient care, athletics or education. This includes, but is not limited to: rape; sexual abuse of a child or patient; actual or threatened use of a weapon of violence; the prohibited sale or distribution of controlled substance, or its possession with the intent to distribute; or the use of the position of an athletic trainer to improperly influence the outcome or score of an athletic contest or event or in connection with any gambling activity."

b. Although Jennifer did not verbally object, Brad should have asked her permission to palpate her injury. Even if Jennifer had agreed to such an evaluation, Brad should have consulted his clinical supervisor before doing so. The supervisor would have referred Jennifer's care to a female athletic trainer or a female healthcare professional. Because of the nature of the injury, any palpation or inspection should have been done in privacy, away from other athletes, spectators, or coaches. A female athletic trainer or coach who works closely with gymnastics should have been asked to be present in the room in order to witness the medical treatment and to make sure nothing else happened.

If Jennifer objected to medical screening by the certified athletic trainer, referral to the health center at the college for evaluation or to a medical doctor should be made. Any unintentional touching of a female patient, even during routine medical examinations, can be construed as sexual harassment and can result in termination of employment. Always ask permission, have someone of the same sex as the patient present when evaluating a gender-specific injury, conduct the evaluation in a separate room, away from others, for privacy, and document thoroughly all your actions during the exam.

Had this been a high-school athlete, Brad's action could have had dire consequences if an allegation of inappropriate sexual contact was made, including criminal and civil actions.

## CASE 8.8 Scapular Fracture

8.8 / **1.** *Based on the information presented in the case, determine (a) the differential diagnoses and (b) the clinical diagnosis.*

a. Differential diagnoses: rotator cuff strain/impingement, rotator cuff contusion, AC joint separation

b. Clinical diagnosis: scapular fracture

8.8 / **2.** *What are the recommended diagnostic tests to confirm the condition?*

Diagnostic testing always begins with radiographic testing with anteroposterior (AP), axillary, and scapular Y views. However, because of the three-dimensional structure of the scapula, it is recommended that additional diagnostic tests, such as an MRI, be used. If there are still doubts, a CT scan of the structure can be performed.[7,9]

8.8 / **3.** *What is the average healing time for this injury, and why?*

Because of the mobility of the scapula and muscular support, most trauma (99%)[28] to the scapula that results in a fracture is not treated operatively, unless the fracture is displaced or found in the glenoid area. The average healing time is six to eight weeks. In addition, approximately 80 percent of patients have concomitant injuries with scapular fractures, but most of these injuries occur because of increased forces not associated with athletics (e.g., car accidents).[7,9] The rich blood supply from the suprascapular artery and circumflex scapular artery does help decrease the required healing time.

8.8 / **4.** *If the injury in this case is non-displaced, it can be treated non-operatively. Outline the treatment/management you would provide to Punch as the treating clinician.*

The answers to this question will vary among students; however, non-operative management would include:

- Use of a sling in the initial phases of rehabilitation or after the onset of the injury for comfort and support. This would be followed or completed in conjunction with the remaining measures.
- Use of shoulder and scapular passive ROM exercises, such as pendulums, wall walks, and manual therapy.
- Active ROM after pain-free movement is achieved using a variety of activities. Active exercises for the elbow and wrist are also encouraged.
- Resistive and functional strength training of the muscles acting on the scapula.

In some cases, electrical bone stimulation may be needed.

## CASE 8.9 Liver Injury

8.9 / **1.** *Based on the information presented in the case, determine (a) the differential diagnoses and (b) the clinical diagnosis.*

a. Differential diagnoses: ruptured appendix, rib contusion/fracture, flank contusion, intercostal injury, kidney contusion

b. Clinical diagnosis: liver trauma

8.9 / **2.** *What are the most common MOIs for this injury?*

Liver trauma usually occurs from a direct blow to the right upper quadrant, sudden deceleration, and/or rib fracture displacement. An enlarged liver as a result of hepatitis can be more easily damaged from a direct blow and would exacerbate the condition.[1]

8.9 / **3.** *Any injury to the abdominal region requires the athletic trainer to examine all internal organs for injury. List the organs of the abdominal region by quadrant, and indicate the referred-pain sites for the major organs.*

The following is a list of the major organs and referred-pain patterns of the abdominal and thorax cavity.

- Right upper quadrant organs include liver, head of the pancreas, kidney, gallbladder, and lung. Referred pain is as follows: liver/right shoulder; pancreas/upper left quadrant and middle abdomen around the umbilicus; kidney/lower right quadrant both anterior and posterior abdomen; lung/upper left shoulder, neck, chest, and posterior upper quadrants; gallbladder/upper right shoulder.
- Left upper quadrant organs include lung, heart, spleen, kidney, tail of the pancreas, and stomach. Referred pain is as follows: kidney/lower left quadrant both anterior and posterior abdomen; lung/upper left shoulder, neck, chest, and posterior upper quadrants; heart/middle chest, upper left shoulder, neck, and arm; spleen/upper left shoulder, neck, and upper left quadrant at spleen site; stomach/middle abdomen around the umbilicus.
- Right lower quadrant organs include appendix, ureter, bladder, colon, gonads, and small intestine. Referred pain is as follows: appendix/lower right quadrant and lower back; ureter/groin area and lower posterior back; bladder/groin area and upper thighs; colon/groin area and upper thighs; gonads/groin area and lower back; small intestine/below the umbilicus and lower right quadrant.
- Left lower quadrant organs include ureter, bladder, colon, gonads, and small intestine. Referred-pain patterns are the same as above.

For specific components of the large intestine (colon) and small intestine refer to a more in-depth source.

8.9 / **4.** *When an athlete is complaining of abdominal trauma, palpation of the area is recommended while the athlete assumes the hook-lying position in order to relax the abdominal muscles. In addition, palpation is conducted specifically to assess for what three items?*

Palpation is conducted first to determine the location and presence of referred-pain patterns. The next item to assess for is rebound tenderness. Pressing on the abdomen puts pressure on the peritoneum, which is sensitive to a stretch. While pushing down or applying pressure, the peritoneum should stretch relatively pain free; however, if inflamed due to trauma, pain will be elicited upon the "rebound" of the stretched tissue when pressure is taken away. Determination of rigidity is the final goal of palpation. In most cases, injury to an abdominal organ will signal the muscles in that area to spasm or tighten for a "splinting" action to protect the site. In addition, if the injury to the area caused some abdominal hemorrhaging, blood may accumulate and also cause a firm feeling. A firm feeling is a sign of possible abdominal trauma.

8.9 / **5.** *Clearly, Joey handled the situation inappropriately. If you were the evaluating clinician, what would you have done differently, and why?*

The answers to this question may vary among students. However, as alluded to in previous questions, trauma to the abdomen can result in internal bleeding and referred-pain patterns from the visceral organs. In this case, the right shoulder pain without trauma to the area should have been the symptom of main concern. Thus, Joey should have expected trauma to the liver, initiated the school's emergency action plan, and treated Tisha for shock. Joey could have also assessed for rib fractures and, most importantly, conducted follow-up evaluations every few minutes.

## CASE 8.10 Kidney Contusion

8.10 / **1.** *Based on the information presented in the case, determine (a) the differential diagnoses and (b) the clinical diagnosis.*

a. Differential diagnoses: rib fracture, costochondral separation/fracture, liver injury, diaphragm injury, transverse process fracture, ruptured appendix

b. Clinical diagnosis: kidney contusion

8.10 / **2.** *What is the recommended treatment for the injury, and what are some signs and symptoms to observe over time?*

Most kidney-contusion injuries resolve in several weeks with bed rest (usually until bleeding of the organ subsides)[23] and fluid intake. Brophy, et al,[4] state that most NFL players returned to competition after two weeks, but lacerations lasted approximately eight weeks. If a laceration is suspected, surgery will be indicated. Follow-up examinations should be conducted prior to competition.

As the condition progresses, if the athlete's condition is left untreated he will present with increased blood in the urine, discoloration of the flank, severe pain, and possible hypertension.[4] This situation requires immediate medical management.

8.10 / **3.** *According to the American Association for the Surgery of Trauma Grading System (AASTGS), what are the five injury classifications for this injury?*

- Grade 1: Minor—contusion and hematoma
- Grade II: Minor—<10 mm laceration
- Grade III: Minor—>10 mm laceration
- Grade IV: Major—laceration through the renal cortex, renal artery/vein injury with hemorrhage
- Grade V: Major—shattered kidney or renal hilum (part of the organ where nerves and vessels enter and leave) avulsion

8.10 / **4.** *If the organ of this player had to be removed, can he still play professional football or other contact sports after successful surgery and healing of the area?*

According to Brophy et al.,[4] professional football players can be allowed to participate since the incidence of traumatic kidney injury is rare in professional football. However, the authors state that the risk of injury in other contact sports cannot be determined and discretion should be used by the physician, the player, or the parent.

8.10 / **5.** *Neither the physician nor Amanda conducted a complete abdominal organ evaluation. If either had, what should he have done?*

The athletic trainer should have performed an abdominal percussion test to examine for any hard or echo sound in organs that normally produce a hollow sound.

# REFERENCES


1. Amaral JF. Thoracoabdominal injuries in the athlete. *Clin Sports Med.* 1997;16(4):739–753.
2. Aspegren D, Hyde T, Miller M. Conservative treatment of a female collegiate volleyball player with costochondritis. *J Manipulative Physiol Ther.* 2007;30:321–325.
3. Blecha K. Managing a traumatic pneumothorax. *Athl Ther Today.* 2006;11(5):51–53.
4. Brophy RH, Gamradt SC, Barnes et al. Kidney Injuries in professional American football: implications for management of an athlete with 1 functioning kidney. *Am J Sports Med.* 2008;36(1):85–90.
5. Buchta R. A ruptured spleen due to body surfing. *J Adolesc Health.* 1981;1(4):317–318.
6. Ciocca M. Pneumothorax in a weight lifter: the importance of vigilance. *Physician SportsMed.* 2000;28(4):97–103.
7. Cole PA. Scapula fractures. *Orthop Clin N Am.* 2002;33(1):1–18.
8. Curtin SM, Tucker AM, Gens DR. Pneumothorax in sports: issues in recognition and follow-up care. *Physician SportsMed.* 2000;28(8):23–32.
9. Curtis C, Sharma V, Micheli L. Delayed union of a scapular fracture: an unusual cause of persistent shoulder pain. *Med Sci Sports Exerc.* 2007;39(12):2095–2098.
10. Diamond D. Sports-related abdominal trauma. *Clin Sports Med.* 1989;8(1):91–99.
11. Drezner J, Courson R, Roberts W, Mosesso V, Link M, Maron B. Inter-Association Task Force recommendations on emergency preparedness and management of sudden cardiac arrest in high school and college aathletic programs: a consensus statement. *J Athl Train.* 2007;42(1):143–158.
12. Emery CA, Meeuwisse WH, Powell JW. Groin and abdominal strain injuries in the national hockey league. *Clin J Sport Med.* 1999;9(3):151–156.
13. Gatta G, Pinto A, Romano S, et al. Clinical, mammographic and ultrasonographic features of blunt breast trauma. *Eur J Radiol.* 2006;59(3):327–330.
14. Giese EA, O'Connor FG, Brennan FH, et al. The athletic preparticipation evaluation: cardiovascular assessment. *Am Fam Physician.* 2007;75(7):1008–1014.
15. Greydanus D, Patel DR, Baxter TL. The breast and sports: issues for the clinician. *Adolesc Med.* 1998;9(3):533–550.
16. Maron BJ. Heart disease and other causes of sudden death in young athletes. *Curr Probl Cardiol.* 1998;23(9):480–529.
17. Maron BJ. Sudden death in young athletes. *N Engl J Med.* 2003;349(11):1064–1075.
18. Maron BJ, Doerer JJ, Haas TS, Tierney DM, Mueller FO. Sudden deaths in young competitive athletes: analysis of 1866 deaths in the United States, 1980–2006. *Circulation.* 2009;119(8):1085–1092.
19. Maron BJ, Maron MS, Lesser RL, et al. Sudden cardiac arrest in hypertrophic cardiomyopathy in the absence of conventional criteria for high risk status. *Am J Cardiol.* 2008;101:544–547.
20. Maron BJ, Roberts W, McAllister H, Rosing D, Epstein S. Sudden death in young athletes. *Circulation.* 1980;62(2): 218–229.
21. Miles JW, Barrett GR. Rib fractures in athletes. *Sports Med.* 1991;12(1):66–69.
22. Occupational Safety and Health Administration. Bloodborne pathogens (29 CFR 1910.1030). United States Department of Labor. 2009; 1198. Available from: http://www.osha.gov/pls/oshaweb/owadisp.show_document?p_table=STANDARDS&p_id=10051. Accessed July 19, 2009.
23. Osias MB, Hale SD, Lytton B. The management of renal injuries. *J Trauma.* 1976;16(12):954–957.
24. Rumball JS, Lebrun CM, DiCiacca SR, Orlando K. Rowing injuries. *Sports Med.* 2005;35(6):537–555.
25. Van Camp S, Bloor C, Mueller F, Cantu R, Olson H. Nontraumatic sports death in high school and college athletes. *Med Sci Sports Exerc.* 1995;27:641–647.
26. Volk CP, McFarland EG, Hornsmon G. Pneumothorax: on-field recognition. *Physician and Sportsmedicine.* 1995; 23(10):43–46.
27. Waninger K, Harcke HT. Determination of safe return to play for athletes recovering from infectious mononucleosis: a review of the literature. *Clin J Sport Med.* 2005;15(6): 410–416.
28. Zlowodzki M, Bhandari M, Zelle BA, et al. Treatment of scapula fractures: systematic review of 520 fractures in 22 case series. *J Orthop Trauma.* 2006;20(3):230–233.

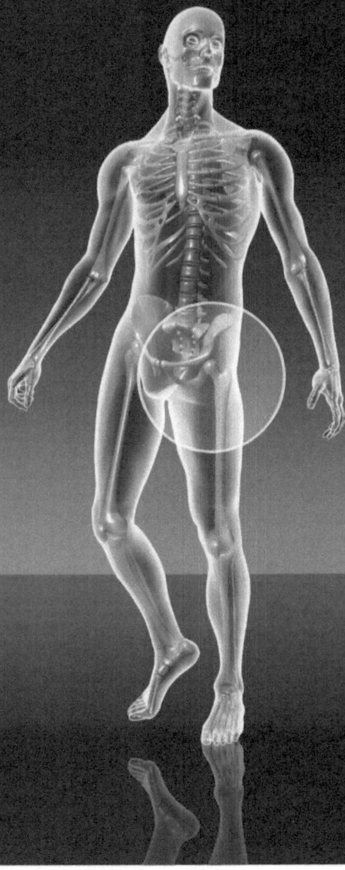

# CHAPTER 9

# Thigh, Hip, Groin, and Pelvis

QUICK REFERENCE

# ANSWERS TO CASE QUESTIONS

## CASE 9.1 Sacroiliac Joint Sprain

9.1 / **1.** *Based on the information presented in the case, determine (a) the differential diagnoses and (b) the clinical diagnosis.*

a. Differential diagnoses: lumbar disc pathology, facet syndrome, erector spinae or quadrates lumborum strain, sciatica, spondylosis, spondylolisthesis

b. Clinical diagnosis: sacroiliac (SI) joint sprain

9.1 / **2.** *The area in question has multiple ligamentous support structures. Please identify the major ligament structures and their function in the sacral region.*

- Pubic symphysis: This ligament is comprised of three bands/ligaments called the superior, arcuate, and interpubic that connect the pubis bones together anteriorly. They function to resist shear stresses, enable superior movements of the sacrum, and prevent pubis joint separations.[26,65]
- Sacrotuberous ligament: This ligament attaches on the posterior superior and inferior iliac spines, the sacrum, and coccyx and runs downward and inserts onto the ischial tuberosity.[66] It functions to limit sacral rotation.
- Anterior SI ligament: This ligament functions to limit movement of the sacrum superiorly or inferiorly and limits joint separation.[26] It is part of the anterior joint capsule and well defined.
- Posterior SI ligament: This ligament arises from the posterior aspect of the sacrum and attaches to the posterior aspect of the ilium. It limits joint separation.
- Sacrospinous ligament: This triangular shaped ligament originates on the ischial spine and inserts onto the sacrum and coccyx and lies in front of the sacrotuberous ligament. It helps to form the greater sciatic foramen and lesser sciatic foramen. Its function is to limit sacral rotation.[26]
- Iliolumbar ligament: The iliolumbar ligament runs from L4 and L5 to the iliac crest, merging with the interosseous ligament. It is designed to limit motion between the lumbar spine and the sacrum.[26]

9.1 / **3.** *What are the most common pain-referral sites for this injury?*

According to Slipman,[57] patients with SI joint pain have several pain-referral sites. Pain can be associated with subsequent trauma to the sciatic nerve and L5 nerve root, and pain intensity and referral patterns are highly variable, depending on severity and SI joint location. See Table A9.1.1 for pain-referral sites.

9.1 / **4.** *What are some of the provocative or diagnostic tests used to differentiate this pathology? Are these tests valid and reliable?*

There are a number of tests[11] used in diagnosing or differentiating SI joint pain (Table A9.1.2). However, the thigh thrust test, compression test, and three or more positive stress tests have the better discrimination power for an appropriate SI joint diagnosis.[60]

Other diagnostic tests, such as an MRI and/or CT scan are often used but may not be able to adequately diagnosis SI joint pathology.[57] Fluoroscopically guided SI joint intra-articular injection with an anesthetic has also become a popular diagnostic test used in diagnosing SI joint pathology.[57]

9.1 / **5.** *Do you think Shaun should have removed Tracey's leotard for inspection of the area?*

The answers will vary among students. Inspection of the area required removal of clothing, but Shaun should have taken Tracey to a private location or back to the designated athletic training room for evaluation. Although Tracey may be accustomed to frequent changes of clothing in front of others, especially during performances or shows, the evaluation of an injury warrants medical privacy, confidentiality, and consent.

TABLE A9.1.1 **Sacroiliac pain-referral sites and percentage of patients reporting pain.**

| PAIN-REFERRAL SITE | PERCENTAGE OF PATIENTS WHO FELT PAIN AT THIS SITE |
|---|---|
| Buttock | 91 |
| Lower lumbar region | 72 |
| Posterior thigh | 30 |
| Lateral thigh | 10 |
| Posterior lower leg | 18 |
| Lateral lower leg | 12 |
| Groin | 12 |
| Lateral foot | 8 |
| Abdomen | 2 |

TABLE **A9.1.2** **Provocative tests used to diagnose sacroiliac joint pathology.**[35,53,60]

| PROVOCATIVE TEST | TESTING PROCEDURES |
|---|---|
| Static palpation | Palpate SI joint for pinpoint tenderness. |
| Gillet standing flexion test | Ask the patient to stand. Place one thumb directly over the second sacral tubercle and the other thumb over left PSIS. Ask the patient to flex at the hip to 90°. If joint dysfunction is present, the left thumb will move in the cephalad direction. |
| Anterior and distraction/Gapping test | Ask the patient to lie supine. Place heels of the hands on the ASIS in a cross pattern and place pressure on heels of the hand in a downward and outward direction. If there is pain or discomfort, SI joint pathology is present. |
| Gaenslen's test | Place patient in a supine position with knee of affected side up to the chest and opposite leg fully extended. If the test is positive, this should increase stress and elicit pain. A positive test will result in pain. |
| Iliac crest compression test | Place patient on his side, and apply downward pressure on the iliac crest. Pain may indicate SI joint pathology. |
| Single leg stand | Ask the patient to stand on the leg of the affected side with opposite leg flexed at 90° at the hip and knee. After 30 to 60 seconds, stress on the leg of the affected side may produce SI joint pain. |
| Patrick's/FABER | Ask the patient to lie supine and place foot of test leg on opposite knee (in a "figure 4" position). In a positive test, the bent knee does not fall below the height of opposite leg and may cause SI joint pain. |
| Thigh thrust test | Ask the patient to lie supine, place the hip at 90° of flexion with the knee bent. Place posterior shearing stress on the SI joint through the femur of the flexed leg. Pain may indicate SI joint pathology. |

## CASE 9.2 Quadriceps Strain

9.2 / **1.** *Based on the information presented in the case, determine (a) the differential diagnoses and (b) the clinical diagnosis.*

a. Differential diagnoses: quadriceps tendon rupture, contusion, patella avulsion fracture, contusion

b. Clinical diagnosis: quadriceps femoris muscle strain

9.2 / **2.** *Judy discussed some immediate treatment care for the injury. Based on the information provided, what immediate care do you think she recommended to Sumpta?*

The answers will vary among students. Many acute muscle injuries are best treated with rest, ice, compression, and elevation (RICE)[6,53] and NSAIDs to block prostaglandin formation and to control edema, bleeding, and pain. Keep in mind that prolonged use of NSAIDs can adversely affect muscle recovery.[1]

9.2 / **3.** Based on the clinical diagnosis, what section of muscle(s) does this type of injury usually affect and why?

The most common site for muscular strains such as a quadriceps strain is at the myotendinous junction. This is because this transitional area between the muscle belly and tendon is subject to the greatest stress from transmitted forces directly applied to the tissue, based on its surface area, fiber orientation, and function.[6]

9.2 / **4.** Based on the clinical diagnosis, what type of muscles and muscle actions are usually associated with this type of injury?

Muscles most at risk are those that cross two joints, because of the angular positions of the muscle fibers and the velocity that these muscles can produce. Most of the injuries occur during eccentric action, when a muscle is attempting to decelerate joint motion.[6]

9.2 / **5.** Sumpta reluctantly agreed to the immediate course of action. When she asked about returning to play, what factors did Judy need to consider before allowing her to return to play?

The answers will vary among students, based on a variety of factors, including extent of trauma, location of injury, sport/activity, pain tolerance, and other factors. Many clinicians require strength and flexibility comparable to the non-injured side (90%) and require functional field tests of acceleration/deceleration and changes in direction to ensure that the athlete is not placing herself at risk for further injury.

# CASE 9.3 Myositis Ossificans

9.3 / **1.** *Based on the information presented in the case, determine and define the clinical diagnosis.*

The clinical diagnosis is myositis ossificans.

Myositis ossificans means inflammation of muscle leading to bone formation.[58] Many diseases share this commonality and are lumped under this name.[47] Today, the term "myositis ossificans" has been replaced with the term "heterotopic ossification" (HO) because primary muscle inflammation is not a necessary precursor for such ossification and the ossification does not always occur in muscle tissue.[47] There are several types of HO, and they are classified according to the clinical setting and location of the lesions.[47] In this case, Emerson's condition would be referred to as myositis ossificans traumatica (HO occurring after a blunt injury, surgery, or burn).[47]

9.3 / **2.** *Based on the information presented in the case, do you believe Lacretia took an adequate history? If not, what if any additional questions would you ask as the evaluating clinician?*

According to the clinical diagnosis, there may be several other questions Lacretia could have asked in addition to gathering information about the MOI. One specific question could have determined whether or not Emerson was wearing any type of thigh protection when he was kneed. Also, based on his occupation, identification of whether or not he had limited mobility and pain at work while kneeling or squatting could have been useful.

9.3 / **3.** *Based on the information presented in the case, the initial radiographs were unrevealing, yet the follow-up radiographs three weeks later were positive. Why do you suppose that was the case?*

The MOI, the blow to the thigh, produced a crushing of the underlying soft tissue against the bone (most often affecting the vastus intermedius). This resulted in muscle-bleeding, which triggered a cascade of cellular responses. This stimulated the dormant osteoprogenitor stem cells (mesenchymal cell that differentiates into an osteoblast) within the affected soft tissue. They converted into osteoblasts and began the process of osteoid formation,[38,47] eventually maturing into heterotopic bone. Development of the lesion at the periphery of the injury site occurs within seven to ten days, with faint calcification visible within two weeks[36,47] and a sharp view on plain film radiographs within six to eight weeks, or earlier in some cases.

9.3 / **4.** *During the initial history and physical examination, Lacretia could have provided some basic rehabilitation to help decrease the likelihood of developing this condition. If you were the evaluating clinician, what basic rehabilitation would you have recommended?*

Conservative treatment in the acute phase should consist of RICE, which helps to minimize additional trauma and decreases the likelihood of incapacitating bone formation.[34,38,41] When symptoms are severe, the use of NSAIDS will help to inhibit prostaglandin synthesis and decrease new bone formation.[34] This should be followed with passive ROM exercises, followed by active ROM exercises progressing to resistive exercises and, eventually, functional exercise as the pain is alleviated.[38,41]

9.3 / **5.** *Overall, do you believe Lacretia adequately evaluated Emerson's condition? Do you believe that Lacretia ever overstepped her boundaries as a certified athletic trainer? Why?*

The answers to this question will vary among students. The debate in most cases will be whether or not Lacretia should have recognized the possibility of HO at the initial visit and then made recommendations to minimize its development.

The bigger legal/ethical issue here was Lacretia's decision to order/acquire radiographs. The case makes no mention of physician supervision during the initial or follow-up evaluation, so the question of concern would be whether Lacretia violated any type of local, state, or national regulations regarding the ordering of radiographs. Did she act in a manner that could be deemed as practicing medicine without a license? As athletic trainers, our scope of practice according to the Board of Certification Role Delineation Study makes no mention of ability to order diagnostic imaging. We would refer you to your class instructor for further clarification and insight, because all state laws are different.

## CASE 9.4 Posterior Hip Dislocation

*by Dilip Patel, M.D., Michigan State University, Kalamazoo Center for Medical Studies*

9.4 / **1.** *Based on the information presented in the case, determine (a) the differential diagnoses and (b) the clinical diagnosis.*

a. Differential diagnoses: femoral neck fracture, femur shaft fracture, hip fracture, hip pointer, hip sprain[23]

b. Clinical diagnosis: posterior dislocated hip

9.4 / **2.** *Based on the clinical diagnosis above, identify two or three history questions you as the evaluating clinician may have asked.*

The answers to this question will vary among students; however, some questions that may help in the clinical diagnosis would include:

- Where is the location of your pain?
- Did you hear or feel anything "pop"?
- Did you have any changes in neurovascular status such as circulation, sensation, or movement?

9.4 / **3.** *(a) Do you believe Joseph and Stephanie performed a complete neurovascular exam? (b) What is the clinical significance of a neurovascular exam in this case? (c) What should the exam assess?*

a. Based on the information presented in the case, students should recognize that an adequate neurovascular screening was not completed. All that appeared to be completed was reflex testing.

b. With a hip dislocation, secondary damage to the nerves and blood vessels, particularly the sciatic nerve and femoral nerve, is possible. Therefore, a complete neurovascular examination should be conducted, followed by immediate transportation to appropriate medical care (reduction within 6 hours) in order to decrease the risk of avascular necrosis of the femoral head.[25,37]

c. If you were the evaluating clinician, it would be imperative to assess for[63]:
   - Pain in hip, buttock, and posterior leg
   - Loss of sensation in posterior leg and foot
   - Loss of dorsiflexion (peroneal nerve branch) or plantar flexion (tibial nerve branch)
   - Loss of deep tendon reflexes (DTRs) at the ankle (S1)
   - Loss of a distal pulse (popliteal, dorsalis pedis, and posterior tibial) and capillary refill

9.4 / **4.** *There is one common MOI for this injury that typically does not relate to athletics. Identify this MOI and the pathomechanics involved.*

Posterior hip dislocations are the most common type of dislocation; however, nearly 70 percent of these injuries are the direct result of high-velocity motor vehicle accidents[23] in which the victim's knee strikes the dashboard, causing the longitudinal force to be applied to the long axis of the femur when the hip is flexed 90°. Hip dislocations in athletics occur from an indirect blow to the hip joint when the foot is firmly planted and an internal rotation force is applied to the femur.[22] A direct blow causing a longitudinal force along the long axis of the femur when the hip is flexed 90° and slightly adducted (e.g., falling on the knee) can also result in a posterior hip dislocation and possible concomitant knee injuries from the force on the knee. Hip dislocations and the rare fracture-dislocation have been reported in football,[25] rugby, skiing,[46] gymnastics,[45] and basketball.[62]

9.4 / **5.** *As the evaluating clinician, what if anything would you have done differently in managing the case, particularly on the field?*

The answers to this question will vary among students; however, Juan clearly should have not been removed from the field prior to the arrival of EMS. The possibility of concomitant injuries exists with a hip dislocation, so stabilization is paramount. Attempts to reduce the dislocation on the field are ill advised[63] and should occur only in the hospital setting. When a hip dislocation is suspected, establish and monitor the ABCs, limit any excessive movement to prevent additional trauma, watch for changes in the neurovascular status, and immobilize the hip using a vacuum splint or mattress or a soft splint and spine board, allowing the leg to assume a position of comfort.

9.4 / **6.** *If there are no complications, that is, no concomitant injuries, how long will it take before Juan can return to full sports participation?*

After a successful reduction, Juan will have to undergo several weeks of rehabilitation. The current practice is to allow early weight bearing. Over the first three to four weeks after reduction, crutch assisted walking may be allowed as tolerated. When the pain is resolved, the athlete can begin ROM exercises, starting with abduction and extension. Ambulation is allowed if assisted by use of a walking aid. The total rehabilitation plan may last from four to eight weeks, and it may be three months before the athlete can return to full sports participation.

## CASE 9.5 Femoral Head/Neck Stress Fracture

9.5 / **1.** *Based on the information presented in the case, determine (a) the differential diagnoses and (b) the clinical diagnosis.*

a. Differential diagnoses: iliopsoas bursitis/tendinitis, osteitis pubis, snapping hip syndrome, adductor strain, piriformis syndrome, SI joint injury, slipped capital femoral epiphysis[15]

b. Clinical diagnosis: stress fracture to the femoral head

9.5 / **2.** *Based on the information presented in the history portion of the case, what is one of the hallmark signs indicating this clinical diagnosis?*

Several pieces of information presented in the history would suggest a stress fracture to the femoral neck, including:

- Gender and location of pain (anterior groin or thigh)
- Type of pain (diffuse or localized achy pain in the anterior groin or thigh during weight-bearing activities)
- Pain that increases with activity and can persist for hours afterward
- Pain that is relieved with rest
- Night pain that wakes the patient

9.5 / **3.** *What significance does the low iron play in this case?*

Low iron levels in the body indicate a potential for osteoporotic bones that would be more susceptible to stress fractures than healthy bones.

9.5 / **4.** *What, if any, special tests could a clinician perform to aid in the physical examination and clinical diagnosis?*

One test that would be indicative of a stress fracture, demonstrating increased pain with a single-leg stance, is the stork standing test. Another special test that would aid in the diagnosis of a stress fracture to the femoral head would be percussion of the greater trochanter.

9.5 / **5.** *Where should Sarah have referred Jenny in order to confirm the clinical diagnosis?*

Based on the history and high index of suspicion presented in the case, Sarah would be wise to refer Jenny to the team's orthopedic surgeon for further evaluation[61] and diagnostic imagining. Imaging modalities such as plain radiography, scintigraphy, computed tomography (CT scan), and magnetic resonance imaging (MRI) may provide confirmation of the clinical diagnosis.[4]

# CASE 9.6 Iliac Crest Apophysitis

*by Dilip Patel, M.D., Michigan State University, Kalamazoo Center for Medical Studies*

9.6 / **1.** *Based on the information presented in the case, determine (a) the differential diagnoses and (b) the clinical diagnosis.*

a. Differential diagnoses: localized contusion (hip pointer), osteomyelitis, anterior iliac crest apophyseal avulsion, internal or external oblique strain, osteosarcoma[2,49]

b. Clinical diagnosis: iliac crest apophysitis

9.6 / **2.** *Overall, do you believe Eric adequately evaluated JJ's condition? If not, what would you have done differently? Would you have added any additional tests?*

Given JJ's history, physical examination, and diagnostic imaging, Eric appears to have completed a relatively complete clinical evaluation. In most cases, no further evaluation is necessary when the clinician gathers a complete history. In addition to a thorough history, plain film radiographs are the first line of diagnostic testing,[49] followed by an MRI if radiographs are inconclusive.[29]

9.6 / **3.** *Because JJ is a minor, Eric must share the results of the physical examination with JJ's mother. She has a medical background and asks Eric to explain the pathophysiology involved in this condition. If you were the evaluating clinician, how would you describe the condition?*

The iliac crest has its own ossification center and does not fully fuse with the rest of the iliac bone until the age of 15 to 17 years (sometimes later than that). The anterior third is the last part to fuse. An apophysis is structurally similar to the growth plate, except that the apophysis does not contribute to the longitudinal growth of an extremity. Apophyses are the sites for various tendon insertions (e.g., internal and external obliques at the iliac crest, Achilles tendon at the posterior calcaneal, patellar tendon at the tibial tubercle), and acute avulsions can occur from a sudden violent muscle contraction. More commonly though, chronic stress from intense repetitive activity results in local periostitis and inflammation leading to apophysitis. Apophysitis is most common during rapid adolescent growth spurts.

9.6 / **4.** *As the evaluating clinician, describe how you would consider treating JJ's condition.*

JJ should respond well to a short period of protected weight bearing. This will be followed with a period of rest, application of ice, and a course of anti-inflammatory medication. Concurrently, stretching and mobilization of soft tissue according to the patient's pain tolerance is necessary, followed by AROM exercises, progressing to isometric and progressive resistance exercises. As activity is restored, a focus on proper mechanics and correction of any biomechanical deficiencies will be necessary. An avulsion fracture treated conservatively could take four to eight weeks to heal.[49]

9.6 / **5.** *After completing the physical examination, Eric documented his findings electronically. Using your athletic training room's computer tracking software, document your findings electronically as if you were the treating clinician. If the case did not provide information you believe is pertinent to the clinical diagnosis, please add this information to your documentation. If you do not have access to injury-tracking software, consider downloading a trial version from CSMI Solutions, (Sportsware) by going to www.csmisolutions.com/cmt/publish/service_software_dl.shtml and following the on-screen directions.*

Answers will vary. Students should consider writing a SOAP note (see textbook Appendix B) using the ABCD format when writing the short- and long-term goals.

# CASE 9.7 Osteitis Pubis

by Joel Beam, Ed.D., ATC, University of North Florida, Jacksonville

9.7 / **1.** *Based on the information presented in the case, determine (a) the differential diagnoses and (b) the clinical diagnosis.*

a. Differential diagnoses: adductor strain, pelvic stress fracture, hernia, iliopsoas strain, intra-articular hip pathology, snapping hip syndrome, nerve impingement (ilioinguinal or gentiofemoral), inferior pubic ramus stress fractures[3,43]

b. Clinical diagnosis: osteitis pubis

9.7 / **2.** *This injury/condition can be exacerbated by repetitive stresses for athletes in which sports?*

Osteitis pubis often affects athletes in sports such as soccer, hockey, football, and sprinting, basically any sports in which there is a great deal of running, rapid change of direction, repetitive kicking motion, or advancing of the leg forward.[3,12,51,56]

9.7 / **3.** *According to research by Mandelbaum and Mora, there are four primary clinical types of this condition. Please identify them.*

Osteitis pubis is an inflammatory condition of the pubic symphysis and surrounding muscular insertions.[12] Although the exact etiology of osteitis pubis is unknown, the following are four clinical types that can develop in this patient population[43]:

- Noninfectious osteitis pubis, associated with urologic, gynecologic procedures
- Infectious osteitis pubis, associated with local or distant infection loci
- Degenerative or rheumatologic
- Sports-related, particularly in sports requiring sprinting and sudden changes of direction, as seen in this case

9.7 / **4.** *It has been suggested that the major etiology of this condition is muscle imbalance. Please describe the muscle imbalance relationship and possible rationale behind it.*

Muscle imbalance has been reported as a factor in the development of osteitis pubis,[3,40,42,44] particularly in sports in which there is a great deal of shear forces across the pubic symphysis. To understand the etiology, one must understand the functions of the muscles that attach to the pubic rami. The hip adductors (i.e., gracilis, adductor longus, adductor brevis, and adductor magnus) originate at the inferior pubic ramus. In addition, the pectineus (adductor) and rectus abdominis muscles, along with the inguinal ligament, insert superiorly on the pubis. The rectus abdominis and the adductor longus are attached to the pubis symphysis, which means these muscles act antagonistically to each other during kicking sports (e.g., soccer, football). Coupled with multiple repetitions and cumulative stress, weakness of the adductor allows for greater development of cumulative stress on the pubic symphysis.

9.7 / **5.** *Overall, do you believe Al adequately evaluated Sara's condition? Are there any another special tests a clinician could perform to help guide the physical examination?*

The answers to this question will vary among students. Overall, the physical examination was adequate. More emphasis could have been placed on examining for muscular imbalances. There are several special tests that could be used to help diagnose this condition:

- Rocking cross-leg test: The athlete sits with one knee crossed over the other knee. The clinician applies a pressure downward on the crossed knee while holding the opposite iliac crest to elicit pain in the pubis region.[9]
- Lateral pelvis compression test: The athlete lies on her side while the clinician presses on the iliac crest to compress them together.
- Pubic symphysis gap test: The athlete is placed in a 90° hip/knee flexed position with the legs supported by the athletic trainer. The athlete performs an isometric adductor contraction against the clinician, who has his fist/hand on the side of the leg at the knee.
- Valsalva maneuver: The clinician can also provoke the symptoms by asking the athlete to increase her internal abdominal pressure by performing a Valsalva maneuver.[40]

9.7 / **6.** *The signs and symptoms of this condition often mimic other common injuries in this region, do you therefore think all athletes who present with the above scenario should be immediately referred for diagnostic imaging?*

The answer to this question will depend on the type of sport and etiology. If you have a football or soccer player who does a lot of sprinting and kicking activities and the athlete is young, he might warrant diagnostic testing, although the incidence of osteitis pubis is about 0.5–6.4 percent.[56] Therefore, a clinician should first manage the symptoms for several weeks, and if there is no improvement, another course of action is warranted, which should include medical referral and diagnostic imaging.

## CASE 9.8 Athletic Pubalgia

9.8 / **1.** *Based on the information presented in the case, determine (a) the differential diagnoses and (b) the clinical diagnosis.*

a. Differential diagnoses: adductor strain, osteitis pubis, stress fracture of the femoral head/pubis area, bursitis, intra-abdominal disorders, genitourinary, referred lumbosacral pain abnormalities, hip joint disorders[48]
b. Clinical diagnosis: athletic pubalgia

9.8 / **2.** *(a) In most cases, the pain experienced by Montclair in and around the pubic tubercle suggests injury to which structure(s)? (b) What mechanism is most likely responsible?*

a. The pain localized around the pubic tubercle could suggest involvement of the rectus abdominis tendon at its insertion, the anterior fibers of the adductor longus and brevis tendons at their origin, and the joint capsule of the pubic symphysis.[67]
b. The MOI often described for athletic pubalgia is repetitive hyperextension of the trunk with hyper-abduction of the hip when pivoting on the pelvis and pubic symphysis. This causes the muscles and tendons to pull away from the pubic bone. Athletes, particularly males who participate in sports that involve repetitive twisting and turning while moving, such as soccer, ice hockey, rugby, field hockey, tennis, or track, are often at greatest risk.

9.8 / **3.** *What is the name of the special test performed in textbook Figure 9.8.2? What is considered a positive finding? Was it appropriate to perform in this case?*

The special test performed in Figure 9.8.2 is commonly referred to as the Patrick's or FABER (Flexion, ABduction, and External Rotation) test. It is a screening test for pathology of the hip or sacroiliac joint.[35] The test is performed by first placing the athlete in the supine position. The involved leg is then flexed, and the foot is placed on the opposite knee, creating the motion of flexion, abduction, and external rotation at the hip. The clinician slowly presses down on the superior aspect of the tested knee joint, lowering the leg into further abduction and external rotation. The test is positive if there is pain at the hip or sacral joint, or if the leg cannot lower to the point of being parallel to the opposite leg.

9.8 / **4.** *If you were the treating clinician, what treatment or rehabilitation protocols would you suggest to treat the injury/condition?*

Conservative care would consist of:

- RICE
- Anti-inflammatory medications and possible corticosteroid injection
- Therapeutic modalities to control pain
- Restoration of any muscular hip imbalances and strengthening of pelvic stabilizers; stretching of hip flexors and low back muscles
- Abdominal muscle strengthening
- Avoidance of massage over the abdominal or inguinal musculature

Note that conservative treatment is rarely successful.[48] If several weeks of conservative treatment fails or if symptoms persist, the athlete should undergo surgical exploration and repair.[30,39]

9.8 / **5.** *Why is this type of injury/condition difficult to diagnose?*

Many of the signs and symptoms of athletic pubalgia are consistent with other injuries such as distal rectus abdominis strain/avulsion and groin disruption, and most injuries have an insidious onset.[48] However, the pain of athletic pubalgia is usually located more laterally and proximally than that of a groin disruption.

## CASE 9.9 Hip Trochanteric Bursitis with ITB Syndrome (Snapping Hip Syndrome)

9.9 / **1.** *Based on the information presented in the case, determine (a) the differential diagnoses, and (b) identify the final clinical diagnosis made by the orthopedic surgeon.*

a. Differential diagnoses: hip flexor strain, adductor strain, osteitis pubis, femoral neck stress fracture, femoral head avascular necrosis, acetabular labral tear, apophysitis[24,48,50]

b. Clinical diagnosis: hip trochanteric bursitis with ITB syndrome (snapping hip syndrome)

9.9 / 2. *Based on the physical examination, what was Jill's initial clinical diagnosis? How do you think this initial condition resulted in the final condition?*

The initial diagnosis Jill made was hip flexor/adductor strain. How the case spiraled into the development of trochanteric bursitis with snapping hip syndrome could not have been anticipated. The most logical conclusion is that the initial injury resulted in an alteration in Lisa's biomechanics, eventually leading to subsequent development of trochanteric bursitis. Paluska[52] identifies several factors that may contribute to the onset of greater trochanter bursitis, including gluteus medius insertional dysfunction, hip osteoarthritis, lumbar spondylosis, excessive or rapidly increased mileage, frequent training on hard or banked running surfaces, poorly cushioned shoes, excessive pronation, leg length discrepancies and ITBFS, and adduction of hips beyond midline while running. Combined with a history of ITBFS and a tight ITB, the result was snapping hip syndrome, which continued to perpetuate the bursitis.

9.9 / **3.** *(a) What is the purpose of the special test in textbook Figure 9.9.1? (b) Is there a modification to this special test? (c) If so, what is the reliability of this modified test?*

a. The special test shown is the Ober's test, which is used to assess for ITB contractures.[7,35]

b. Kendall[32] recommends performing a modified Ober's test when assessing the length of the ITB. This test is completed with the knee in an extended position instead of the flexed position in an Ober's test. A modified Ober's test places less strain on the knee and less tension on the patella and involves less interference from the tight rectus femoris.[32]

c. Reese and Bandy's[54] examination of intra-rater reliability of ITB flexibility assessment using an inclinometer to measure the hip adduction angle found interclass correlation (ICC) values of 0.90 for the Ober's test and 0.91 for the modified Ober's test. They also found significantly greater ROM of the hip in adduction using the modified Ober's test than with the Ober's test. Because of the increase in ROM, Reese and Bandy[54] recommend not using the test interchangeably to measure flexibility of the ITB.

9.9 / **4.** *What caused Lisa's snapping sensation to occur?*

The term "snapping hip" has become a catch-all phrase to describe a palpable or audible snap that occurs at the hip as the ITB passes over the greater trochanter. The friction between the ITB and greater trochanter is the most prevalent cause of snapping hip syndrome, though a variety of conditions may be responsible for producing the "snapping." Intra-articular pathologies include loose bodies, synovial chondromates, osteocartilaginous exostosis, and subluxating hip. Extra-articular causes of snapping hip include stenosing tenosynovitis of the iliopsoas muscle near its insertion on the femur, crossing of the iliopsoas tendon over the iliopectineal eminence of the pelvis, crossing of the iliofemoral ligament over the head of the femur, and crossing of the long head of the biceps femoris over the ischial tuberosity.[52]

9.9 / **5.** *In this case, the coach became very upset at both Lisa and Jill. If you were the evaluating athletic trainer, how would you respond to a coach's comments that you are not doing your job? If another athlete told you that Lisa was out dancing at a club during the time when she was supposedly suffering from the lateral hip pain, would you use this information to defend yourself against the coach?*

The answers to this question will vary greatly among students. In fact, this question is best answered in a group discussion, because there is not necessarily one correct answer. Certainly the actions of the coach were at best inappropriate; however, how the situation is handled could have significant consequences for Jill or another clinician. The development of positive working relationships is paramount to the success of the athletes, coaches, and athletic trainers, but at the same time, coaches must understand that athletic trainers have certain foundational behaviors and ethics to which they are bound. This includes the concept of "do no harm" and the primacy of the athlete. Athletic trainers need to be advocates for their athletes, ensuring that a certain level of care be provided by the most qualified individuals.

Regarding the information related to Lisa's extracurricular activity, until this information can be verified, it offers little value to Jill's situation.

## CASE 9.10 ITB Friction Syndrome

9.10 / **1.** *Based on the information presented in the case, determine (a) the differential diagnoses and (b) the clinical diagnosis.*

a. Differential diagnoses: lateral meniscus tear, lateral collateral knee sprain, myofacial pain, patellofemoral pain syndrome, popliteal tendinopathy, stress fracture

b. Clinical diagnosis: ITB friction syndrome (ITBFS)

9.10 / **2.** *What are some common causative factors for the development of this condition?*

There are many plausible causative factors for the development of ITBFS. In fact, development of ITBFS is most likely multi-factorial and includes both internal and external causes.[33,52] The following are some of the possible factors:

- Leg length discrepancies, genu varum, ITB tightness
- Regional muscle weakness, including knee extensor/flexor and hip abductor muscle weakness
- Cavus feet or excessive pronation resulting in tibial internal rotation that increases stress placed on the ITB
- High weekly running mileage, running on a banked track or uneven surfaces, or inappropriate footwear

9.10 / **3.** *What two common special tests are used to assist in determining the clinical diagnosis? How would you perform them on Dewalt?*

Two common special tests are the Renne's and Ober's test. To perform a Renne's test, ask the patient to stand, palpate the femoral epicondyle, and then ask the patient to squat and return to a starting position while pressing the epicondyle. Pain elicited over the site will suggest irritation and tightness of the ITB. A non–weight-bearing test would be the Noble's test.

To perform an Ober's test, place the patient lying on his unaffected side, knee/hip at about 90°. Stabilize the pelvis, be sure the gluteus medius has cleared the greater trochanter, and abduct and extend the hip, allowing the thigh to adduct passively toward the midline. A positive finding occurs when the thigh does not return to at least a neutral position or lateral hip pain/tightness is reproduced. A modified Thomas test may also be helpful in measuring ITB tightness with a positive J-sign.[28]

9.10 / **4.** *What is the usual course of conservative therapy for this condition?*

The prognosis for ITBFS is generally good with conservative rehabilitation and correction of biomechanical or causative factors.[52] Rehabilitation programs should focus on correcting regional strength and flexibility deficits. In one study of three types of ITB stretching, an overhead arm extension ITB stretch significantly increased the average ITB length change and average external adduction moments in elite athletes.[20] Other forms of conservative care would consist of[19,33]:

- RICE
- Anti-inflammatory medications and possible corticosteroid injection if the pain persists
- ITB massage (i.e., myofascial release, deep friction)

- Stretching and strengthening of muscles around the hip and knee joint, especially the gluteus medius muscle
- Limiting knee-flexion activities
- Gradual increases in activity after initial rest

9.10 / **5.** *What is the common procedure to alleviate the tension/stress of the ITB if surgery is indicated?*

A procedure to alleviate tension on the ITB would be a posterior release of 2 cm of the ITB as it crosses over the epicondyle of the femur. Approximately 84 percent of patients reported good results with this technique.[13]

## CASE 9.11 Piriformis Syndrome

9.11 / **1.** *Based on the information presented in the case, determine (a) the differential diagnoses and (b) the clinical diagnosis.*

a. Differential diagnoses: disk herniation, SI joint pathology, sciatic nerve pathology, hamstring and hip external rotator tightness, lumbosacral facet syndrome, spondylolisthesis, spondylolysis

b. Clinical diagnosis: piriformis syndrome

9.11 / **2.** *What other observations or special tests could be used to help diagnose this injury? Please explain what indicates a positive finding and what information you would gain from performing the test.*

Answers to this question may vary among students; however, some special tests include the following:

- Freiberg test: In this test, pain is elicited during passive internal rotation of the affected hip.
- Lasegue sign: Pain is elicited when pressure is placed on the piriformis muscle when the hip is flexed to 90° with the knee in full extension.
- Piriformis sign: A positive sign occurs when the patient is in a supine relaxed position and the affected limb rests in external rotation from the hip.
- FAIR (Flexion, Adduction, Internal Rotation) test: With this test, the athlete is placed on the unaffected side. The affected hip is then flexed to 60°, adducted and internally rotated by placing downward pressure on the lateral knee. If sciatic symptoms are recreated, the test is considered positive. This test was found to have a specificity of 0.83 and a sensitivity of 0.88.[17]

9.11 / **3.** *(a) What population seems more likely to suffer from this condition? (b) Why is this condition likely to cause sciatic nerve symptoms?*

a. Individuals age 40 to 50 seem more likely to have symptoms of piriformis syndrome, with the incidence in women greater than in men. This is possibly related to the wider Q-angle associated with child bearing.[5]

b. In a majority of the population, the sciatic nerve exits inferior to the piriformis muscle; however, in 22 percent of the population the sciatic nerve actually pierces the piriformis muscle.[55] In some instances, the sciatic nerve splits—with one portion, usually the fibular portion, piercing the sciatic nerve and the tibial portion exiting inferior to the piriformis. Local inflammation can cause compression and disruption of the blood vessels and nerves that can also cause sciatic symptoms.[5]

9.11 / **4.** *As the treating clinician, (a) how would you treat this condition? (b) What methods, including those used by other health care professionals, can be implemented to relieve this condition if conventional therapy does not work?*

a. Answers to this question will vary among students. Some answers may include the use of ultrasound, electric stimulation, heat, ice, stretching exercises, or strengthening of the hip adductors and abductors. Muscle energy can also be used if the piriformis is tight enough to cause pelvic misalignment. Iontophoresis and/or phonophoresis may also be considered for treatment. If conservative treatment is not successful, a physician may consider an injection of lidocane in conjunction with a corticosteroid. Botulinum toxin has been shown to have a 40–90 percent improvement rate.[17]

b. NSAIDs, muscle relaxants, ice, and rest have been shown to be an effective means of reducing symptoms.[16] Even acupuncture may be used by a licensed acupuncturist. Surgical intervention is a last resort in treating piriformis syndrome, by removing restrictions on the sciatic nerve and exploring the sciatic notch for restrictions.[5]

# CASE 9.12 Legg-Calve-Perthes Disease

*by Dilip Patel, M.D., Michigan State University, Kalamazoo Center for Medical Studies*

9.12 / **1.** *Based on the information presented in the case, determine (a) the differential diagnoses and (b) the clinical diagnosis.*

a. Differential diagnoses: septic arthritis, transient infectious synovitis, toxic synovitis, slipped capital femoral epiphysis, stress fracture

b. Clinical diagnosis: Legg-Calve-Perthes disease (LCPD)

9.12 / **2.** *(a) Please explain why you ruled out at least two of your differential diagnoses. (b) Explain the clinical diagnosis.*

a. A child with acute inflammatory and infectious conditions that include septic arthritis, transient infectious synovitis, toxic synovitis, and juvenile arthritis will generally present with a more painful and inflamed joint. Slipped capital femoral epiphysis is generally seen in pubertal children and can present with acute or chronic hip pain. Stress fracture of the femoral neck can result from high intensity activity over a longer period of time, and the child will have moderate, continuous pain in the hip and pain upon bearing weight; typically, ROM is maintained.

b. Idiopathic osteonecrosis of the femoral head, or Legg-Calve-Perthes disease (LCPD), is typically seen in a child between four and eight years of age, with a range between two years and twelve years. Known causes of osteonecrosis of the femoral head include Gaucher disease, hypothyroidism, multiple epiphysial dysplasia, sickle cell disease, spondyloepiphyseal dysplasia, and some genetic causes. All will have associated signs and symptoms of the underlying disease. A relatively painless limp in a young child with the given examination findings, who is in excellent general health and has had no history of acute trauma, will most likely point to LCPD.

9.12 / **3.** *(a) How can the clinical diagnosis be confirmed? (b) What will you advise the athlete and his parents to do at this time?*

a. The diagnosis can be confirmed in most cases by plain film radiographs of the hip in Lauenstein (frog-leg) and anteroposterior views. Radiographs are also used to determine the stage of the disease and monitor the healing process. The physician/radiologist can determine the head-at-risk signs for the femoral head which include:

- Gage's sign and calcifications lateral to the epiphysis. Gage's sign is a noticeable convexity of the upper border of the proximal femoral neck.[21]
- Lateral subluxation of the femoral head. Lateral calcification is described as calcification just lateral to the epiphysis.[8] A hip is considered laterally subluxed if there is 2 mm of lateral movement greater than the opposite side.
- The presence of a horizontal growth plate. If a horizontal growth plate is present, the angle between the femoral shaft and the physis is measured. A growth plate with a physeal angle >73° is considered horizontal.[18]
- Metaphyseal cystic changes.[18] Metaphyseal cystic changes are cysts around radiotranslucent areas with a well defined edge.[59]

Also within the case study, it is reported that AJ had a 1-inch leg length discrepancy. To accurately assess the growth rate of the affected leg, Knemometry can be used.[10]

Knemometry is a technique that measures knee to heel length under standardized pressure.[64] This technique can be used to verify the clinical diagnosis.

b. At this time, the father should be advised that AJ should refrain from further sport participation and be seen by his pediatrician and orthopedic surgeon (pediatric orthopedic surgeon or one with similar expertise) for further evaluation and definitive treatment.

9.12 / **4.** *What is the etiology of this condition?*

The exact etiology of LCPD has not been clearly elucidated. Disruption of the blood supply to the capital femoral epiphysis is a widely held hypothesis. The deformity in LCPD probably stems from a combination of factors that include growth disturbance of the capital femoral epiphysis and the physis; asymmetric growth of the femoral head, neck, and trochanter during the repair process; overgrowth of the articular cartilage relative to the underlying bone; and complications from treatment aimed at containing the femoral head in the acetabulum.

9.12 / **5.** *Describe the treatment, course, and prognosis of this condition.*

Over a period of 12 to 18 months, gradual healing occurs that involves the processes of revascularization of the femoral head, replacement of the devitalized bone with new bone, and eventual remodeling. Most children follow this typical course of healing over time. During this time, various management strategies have been applied that vary, depending on the prognostic factors, the age of the child, acuity of symptoms, and the development of deformities. Some children can simply be observed without active intervention. All children need periodic orthopedic follow-up and radiographic evaluation.

Containment of the femoral head within the acetabulum during the healing process is the primary goal of treatment. The goals of containment are to prevent deformity and allow functional ROM and remodeling to occur. Various specific criteria are used to decide if containment is appropriate, and one of the prerequisites is full hip range of motion prior to initiating containment. Containment is achieved by the use of abduction orthoses; a widely used one is the Scottish Rite Abduction Orthosis. Various orthopedic surgical procedures are used to correct residual chronic deformities. Children younger than six years of age at the time of presentation have a relatively better prognosis for recovery. Prognosis also depends on the duration of the disease and the extent of involvement of the capital femoral epiphysis at the time of the diagnosis.

9.12 / **6.** *(a) Who is most affected by this condition? (b) What are the potential complications of the condition?*

a. Legg-Calve-Perthes disease affects children between the ages of four and ten, with a greater incidence occurring in boys.

b. Deformity of the femoral head and neck, shortening of the affected leg, limping, and delayed or no healing are all potential complications of LCPD. A child with Legg-Calve-Perthes disease may develop osteoarthritis of the hip as an adult.

# CASE 9.13 Slipped Capital Femoral Epiphysis

9.13 / **1.** *Based on the physical findings, determine (a) the differential diagnoses and (b) the clinical diagnosis.*

a. Differential diagnoses: femur fracture, adductor strain, iliofemoral ligament sprain

b. Clinical diagnosis: slipped capital femoral epiphysis (SCFE). An SCFE occurs when there is separation of the proximal femoral epiphysis through the growth plate. The head of the femur remains in the acetabulum, but the neck slips anteriorly.

9.13 / **2.** *Diagnostic imaging can help confirm and classify the severity of the condition. Please identify the three classifications and the amount of movement that may occur with each classification.*

Classification of the SCFE is characterized by the amount of femoral head slippage. The condition is classified as mild when there is less than 33 percent slippage of the epiphysis or less than a 30° slip angle. A slippage is considered moderate when there is 33–50 percent slippage of the epiphysis or a 30°–60° slip angle. Finally, a slippage is classified as severe when the there is greater than 50 percent slippage of the epiphysis or greater than a 60° slip angle. For a visual representation see Hart, Grottkau, and Albright.[27]

9.13 / **3.** *Why is the pain associated with this condition often felt elsewhere than the specific place of injury?*

Even though the pathology has occurred in the hip, the obturator and femoral nerves provide sensory distribution down the leg into the knee, therefore causing referred symptoms (Figure A9.13.1).[14] So a patient with SCFE can have medial knee/thigh pain attributable to obturator or femoral nerve entrapment.

FIGURE A9.13.1

Sensory distribution of femoral and obturator nerves.

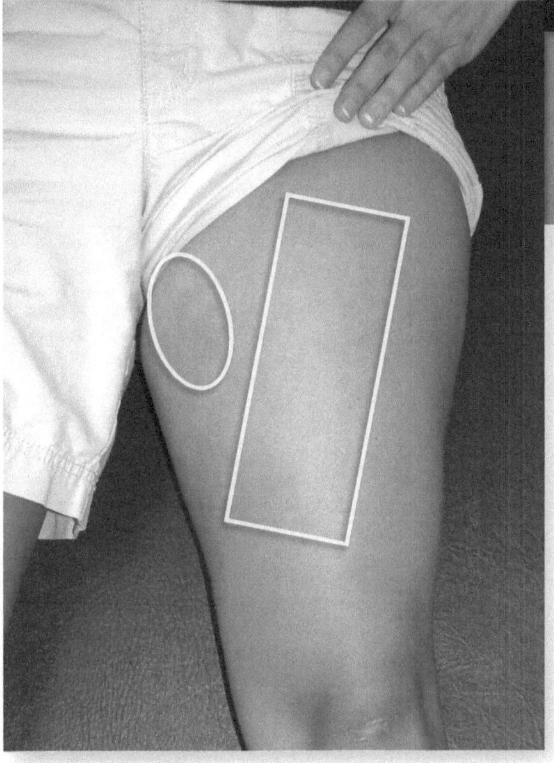

Circle indicates obturator nerve entrapment. Rectangle indicates femoral nerve entrapment.

9.13 / **4.** *(a) Where do you think Joshua should refer Adalyn for a further diagnostic workup? (b) If you were the evaluating clinician, what do you think the best course of treatment for this condition might include?*

a. Joshua would be prudent to refer Adalyn to a pediatric orthopedist to order the necessary radiographs for a proper diagnosis.

b. First and foremost, the epiphysis needs to be stabilized to prevent further slippage. Crutches and/or a wheelchair should be used immediately upon diagnosis to prevent weight bearing on the affected hip. It is vital that both the child and the child's parents be educated in the importance of maintaining a non–weight bearing status on the affected side, because this will assist in preventing further slippage of the epiphysis. The standard treatment is surgical correction of the slipped capital femoral epiphysis. A screw is placed through the neck of the femur and into the central aspect of the proximal femoral epiphysis.[27]

9.13 / **5.** *What population and risk factors are most commonly associated with this condition?*

The most significant risk factor for SCFE is childhood obesity. Children with growth plate disorders, who have retroversion of the femur, or open growth plates in youngsters who are still growing are also at risk for SCFE.[14,31]

9.13 / **6.** *Overall, do you believe Joshua adequately evaluated Adalyn's condition? If you were the evaluating clinician, what would you have done differently?*

The answers to this question will vary among students. More emphasis could have been placed on assessing active and passive ROM. There is no mention of a neurological assessment, which in this case may have demonstrated areas of altered sensitivity, particularly the sensory distribution of the femoral and obturator nerves. An assessment of deep tendon reflexes is also warranted.

# REFERENCES


1. Almekinders L. Anti-inflammatory treatment of muscular injuries in sport: an update of recent studies. *Sports Med.* 1999;28:383–388.
2. Adkins S, Figler R. Hip pain in athletes. *Am Fam Physician* [electronic version]. 2000;61:2109–2118 Available from: http://www.aafp.org/afp/20000401/2109.html.
3. Batt M, McShane J, Dillingham M. Osteitis pubis in collegiate football players. *Med Sci Sports Exerc.* 1995;27(5):629–633.
4. Boden BP, Osbahr DC. High-risk stress fractures: evaluation and treatment. *J Am Acad Orthop Surg.* 2000;8(6):344–353.
5. Boyajian-O'Neill L, McClain R, Coleman M, Thomas P. Diagnosis and management of Piriformis Syndrome: an osteopathic approach. *J Am Osteopath Assoc.* 2008;108(11):657–664.
6. Brothers A, Alamin T, Pedowitz R. Basic clinical management of muscle strains and tears. *J Musculoskel Med.* 2003;20:303–307.
7. Browning K. Hip and pelvis injuries in runners: careful evaluation and tailored management. *Physician Sportsmed.* 2001;29(1):23–34.
8. Catterall A. The natural history of Perthes's disease. *J Bone Joint Surg Br.* 1971;53-B(1):37–53.
9. Coventry M, William M. Osteitis pubis: observations based on a study of 45 patients. *JAMA.* 1961;178:898–905.
10. Crofton P, Macfarlane C, Wardhaugh B, et al. Children with acute Perthes' disease have asymmetrical lower leg growth and abnormal collagen turnover. *Acta Orthop.* 2005;76(6):841–847.
11. DeMann JL. Sacroiliac dysfunction in dances with low back pain. *Man Ther.* 1997;29(1):2–10.
12. Disabella V. Osteitis pubis. *eMedicine* [electronic version]. 2008. Available from: http://emedicine.medscape.com/article/87420-overview. Accessed June 24, 2009.
13. Drogset J, Rossvoll I, Grontvedt T. Surgical treatment of iliotibial band friction syndrome: a retrospective study of 45 patients. *Scand J Med Sci Sports.* 1999;9:296–298.
14. Eldridge J. Slipped capital femoral epiphysis. In: Sponseller P, ed. *Orthopaedic Knowledge Update: Pediatrics.* Rosemont, IL: American Academy of Orthopaedic Surgeons; 2002:143–151.
15. Finn S. Femoral neck stress fracture. *eMedicine* [electronic version]. 2007. Available from: http://emedicine.medscape.com/article/86808-overview. Accessed June 23, 2009.
16. Fishman L, Dombi G, Michaelsen C, Ringel S, Rozbruch J, Rosner B, et al. Piriformis syndrome: diagnosis, treatment, and outcome-a 10-year study [review]. *Arch Phys Med Rehabil.* 2002;83:295–301.
17. Fishman L, Schaefer M. The piriformis syndrome is underdiagnosed. *Muscle Nerve.* 2003;28(5):646–649.
18. Forster M, Kumar S, Rajan R, Atherton W, Asirvatham R, Thava V. 2006; Head-at-risk signs in Legg-CalvÈ-Perthes disease: poor inter- and intra-observer reliability. *Acta Orthop.* 77(3):413–417.
19. Fredericson M, Cookingham C, Chaudhari A, Dowdell B, Oestreicher N, Sahrmann S. Hip abductor weakness in distance runners with iliotibial band syndrome. *Clin J Sport Med.* 2000;10:169–175.
20. Fredericson M, White J, Macmahon J, Andriacchi T. Quantitative analysis of the relative effectiveness of 3 iliotibial band stretches. *Arch Phys Med Rehabil.* 2002;83(5):589–592.
21. Gage H. A possible early sign of Perthes' Disease. *Br J of Radiol.* 1933;6:295–297.
22. Gallaspy JB, May JD. *Signs and Symptoms of Athletic Injuries.* St. Louis, MO: Mosby; 1996.
23. Gammons M. Hip dislocation. *eMedicine* [electronic version]. 2009. Available from: http://emedicine.medscape.com/article/86930-overview. Accessed June 23, 2009.
24. Garry J, Jenkins W. Snapping hip syndrome. *eMedicine* [electronic version]. 2006. Available from: http://emedicine.medscape.com/article/87659-overview. Accessed June 23, 2009.
25. Giza E, Mithofer K, Matthews H, Vrahas M. Hip fracture-dislocation in football: a report of two cases and review of the literature. *Br J Sports Med* [electronic version]. 2004;38, e17. Available from: http://bjsm.bmj.com/cgi/content/abstract/38/4/e17. Accessed August 1, 2004.
26. Harrison D, Harrison D, Troyanovich, S. The sacroiliac joint: a review of anatomy and biomechanics with clinical implications. *J Manipulative Physiol Ther.* 1997;20(9):607–617.
27. Hart E, Grottkau B, Albright M. Slipped capital femoral epiphysis: don't miss the pediatric hip disorder. *Nurse Pract.* 2007;32(3):14–21.
28. Harvey D. Assessment of flexibility of elite athletes using the modified Thomas test. *Br J of Sports Med.* 2002;32:68–70.
29. Hebert KJ, Laor T, Divine JG, Emery KH, Wall EJ. MRI appearance of chronic stress injury of the iliac crest apophysis in adolescent athletes. *Am J Roentgenol.* 2008;190(6):1487–1491.
30. Holmich P, Uhrskou P, Ulnits L, et al. Effectiveness of active physical training as treatment for long-standing adductor-related groin pain in athletes: randomized trial. *Lancet.* 1999;353:439–443.
31. Kehl D. Slipped capital femoral epiphysis. In Morrissy R, Weinstein S, eds. *Lovell & Winter's Pediatric Orthopedics* (5th ed.). Lippincott Williams and Wilkins. 2001;999–1033.
32. Kendall F, McCreary E, Provance P. *Muscles: Testing and Function* (4th ed.). Baltimore, MD: Lippincott Williams and Wilkins; 1993.
33. Khaund R, Flynn S. Iliotibial band syndrome: a common source of knee pain. *Am Fam Physician.* 2005;71:1545–1550.
34. King J. Post-traumatic ectopic calcification in the muscles of athletes: a review. *Br J Sports Med.* 1998;32(4):287–290.

35. Konin JG, Wiksten D, Isear JA, Brader H. *Special Tests for Orthopedic Examination* (3rd ed.) Thorofare, NJ: Slack; 2006.
36. Kransdorf MJ, Meis JM. From the archives of the AFIP. Extraskeletal osseous and cartilaginous tumors of the extremities. *RadioGraphics.* 1993;13(4):853–884.
37. Lam F, Walczak J, Franklin A. Traumatic asymmetrical bilateral hip dislocation in an adult. *Emerg Med J* [electronic version]. 2001;18:506–507. Available from: http://emj.bmj.com/cgi/content/abstract/18/6/506. Accessed June 18, 2007.
38. Larson C, Almekinders L, Karas S, Garrett W. Evaluating and managing muscle contusions and myositis ossificans. *Physician Sportsmed.* 2002;30(2):41–50.
39. Larson C, Lohnes J. Surgical management of athletic pubalgia. *Oper Tech Sports Med.* 2002;10(4):228–232.
40. Lentz S. Osteitis pubis: a review. *Obstet Gynecol Surv.* 1995;50:310–315.
41. Lipscomb A, Thomas E, Johnston R. Treatment of myositis ossificans traumatica in athletes. *Am J Sports Med.* 1976;4(3):111–120.
42. Major N, Helms C. Pelvis stress injuries: the relationship between osteitis pubis (symphysis pubis stress injury) and sacroiliac abnormalities in athletes. *Skeletal Radiol.* 1997; 26:711–715.
43. Mandelbaum B, Mora S. Osteitis pubis. *Oper Tech Sports Med.* 2005;13:62–67.
44. Miller J, Schultz A, Anderson G. Load displacement behavior of the sacroiliac joints. *Orthop Res.* 1987;5:92–101.
45. Mitchell JC, Giannoudis PV, Millner PA, Smith RM. A rare fracture-dislocation of the hip in a gymnast and review of the literature. *Br J Sports Med* [electronic version].1999;33:283–284. Available from: http://bjsm.bmj.com/cgi/content/abstract/33/4/283. Accessed June 18, 2007.
46. Mohanty K, Gupta SK, Langston A. Posterior dislocation of hip in adolescents attributable to casual rugby. *Emerg Med J* [electronic version]. 2000;17(16):429. Available from: http://emj.bmj.com. Accessed June 18, 2007.
47. Moore D, Cho G. Heterotopic ossification *eMedicine* [electronic version]. 2007. Available from: http://emedicine.medscape.com/article/390416-overview. Accessed June 22, 2009.
48. Morelli V, Smith V. Groin injuries in athletes. *Am Fam Physician.* 2001;64(8):1405–1414.
49. Naude M, Lindeque B, Rensburg D. Avulsion fractures of the pelvis. *S Afr J Sports Med.* 2003;(June):18–24.
50. O'Kane JW. Anterior hip pain. *Am Fam Physician.* 1999;60:1687–1696.
51. Orchard J, Seward H. AFL injury report 2002. *Sport Health.* 2003;21(2):18–23.
52. Paluska S. An overview of hip injuries in running. *Sports Med.* 2005;35(11):991–1014.
53. Prentice WE. *Arnheim's Principles of Athletic Training: A Competency-Based Approach* (13th ed.). Boston, MA: McGraw Hill Publishing; 2009.
54. Reese N, Bandy W. Use of an inclinometer to measure flexibility of the iliotibial band using the Ober test and the modified Ober test: differences in magnitude and reliability of measurements. *Orthop Sports Phys Ther.* 2003;33(6):326–330.
55. Robinson D. Piriformis muscle in relation to sciatic pain. *Am J Surg.* 1947;73:356–358.
56. Rodriguez C, Miguel A, Lima H, Heinrichs K. Osteitis pubis syndrome in the professional soccer athlete: a case report. *J Athl Train.* 2001;36(4):437–440.
57. Slipman C, Patel R, Whyte W, et al. Diagnosing and managing sacroiliac pain. *J Musculoskel Med.* 2001;18:325–332.
58. Sloan R. Quadriceps contusions and hip pointers in football. *Hughston Health Alert* [electronic version]. 1998;10(3). Available from: http://www.hughston.com/hha/a.quad.htm. Accessed June 22, 2009.
59. Smith S, Ions G, Gregg P. The radiological features of the metaphysis in Perthes Disease. *J Pediatr Orthop.* 1982;2(4):401–404.
60. Szadek K, van der Wurff P, van Tulder M, Zuurmond W, Perez R. Diagnostic validity of criteria for sacroiliac joint pain: a systematic review. *J Pain.* 2009;10(4):354–368.
61. Talbot J, Townen C, Langham M, Parker P. Femoral neck stress fractures in military personnel: a case series *J R Army Med Corps.* 2007;154(1):47–50.
62. Tennent TD, Chambler AF, Rossouw DJ. Posterior dislocation of the hip while playing basketball. *Br J Sports Med* [electronic version]. 1998;32:342–343. Available from: http://bjsm.bmj.com/cgi/content/abstract/32/4/342. Accessed December 1, 1998.
63. Tham E, Doty C. Dislocation, hip. *eMedicine* [electronic version]. 2008. Available from: http://www.emedicine.com/emerg/topic144.htm. Accessed June 23, 2009.
64. Wales J, Milner R. Knemometry in assessment of linear growth. *Arch Dis Child.* 1987;62:166–171.
65. Willard F. The anatomy of the lumbosacral connection. *Spine: State of the Art Rev.* 1995;9:333–355.
66. Woodley S, Kennedy E, Mercer S. Anatomy in practice: the sacrotuberous ligament. *Physiother.* 2005;33(3):91–94.
67. Zoga AC, Kavanagh EC, Omar IM, et al. Athletic pubalgia and the "sports hernia": MR imaging findings. *Radiol.* 2008;247(3):797–807.

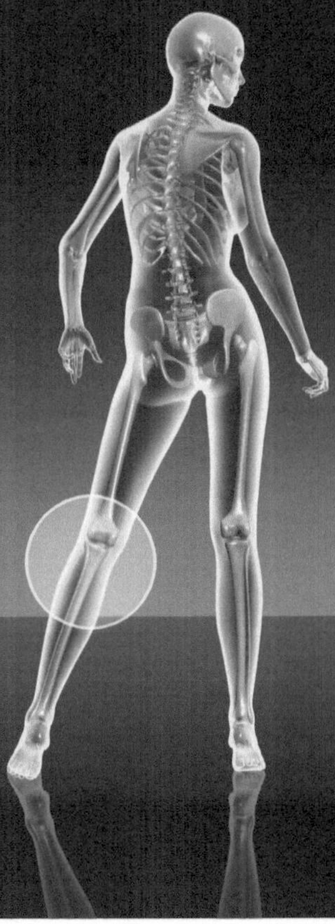

CHAPTER 10

# Knee and Lower Leg

## QUICK REFERENCE

CASE 10.1
**Unhappy Triad**

CASE 10.2
**Lateral Collateral Ligament Sprain with Secondary Peroneal Nerve Damage**

CASE 10.3
**Tibial Plateau Stress Fracture**

CASE 10.4
**Plica Syndrome**

CASE 10.5
**Medial Tibial Stress Syndrome**

CASE 10.6
**Posterior Cruciate Ligament Sprain**

CASE 10.7
**Patellar Tendon Rupture with Patella Avulsion Fracture**

CASE 10.8
**Patella Dislocation**

CASE 10.9
**Quadriceps Tendon Rupture**

CASE 10.10
**Patella Tendinopathy**

CASE 10.11
**Patellofemoral Pain Syndrome**

CASE 10.12
**Knee Dislocation (Tibiofemoral Dislocation with Vascular Compromise)**

CASE 10. 13
**Fibular Dislocation**

CASE 10.14
**Pes Anserine Bursitis**

CASE 10.15
**Compartment Syndrome**

CASE 10.16
**Osgood-Schlatter Disease**

# ANSWERS TO CASE QUESTIONS

## CASE 10.1 Unhappy Triad

**10.1 / 1.** *Based on the information presented in the case, determine (a) the clinical diagnosis and (b) the common name for this condition.*

a. Clinical diagnosis: ACL, MCL, and medial meniscus damage

b. Common name: unhappy triad or "terrible triad," typically involving a valgus stress to the knee[40]

**10.1 / 2.** *(a) Identify the bony and soft tissue structures that should have been palpated as part of the physical examination. Then (b) identify two or three other observations Tyler could have made during the initial assessment. (c) Why was the flexed carrying position noted sometime later during the evaluation and not initially?*

a. Possible bony and soft tissue structures that can be palpated include:
- Bony: proximal tibia and fibula, distal femur, patella, condyles, joint line
- Soft: MCL, LCL, patellar tendon, gastrocnemius, biceps femoris, semimembranosus, semitendinosus.

b. Other observations may include deformity, redness, patella alignment, gait, and symmetry of the knee.

c. The flexed carrying angle was noticed later because increased joint effusion causes the knee to flex to its open pack position to allow for the greatest accumulation of the effusion. Immediate gross effusion (within 2 hours), which limits function, may indicate significant knee trauma and may suggest some degree of ACL trauma.[19,67]

**10.1 / 3.** *Based on Jim's MOI and his signs and symptoms, identify at least three ligamentous tests that could have been performed to assist in determining the clinical diagnosis. Describe how to perform each test.*

There are several ligamentous testing procedures that could be used in determining the clinical diagnosis. These may include, but are not limited to, the anterior draw, Lachman's test, lateral pivot shift, Solcum and Hughston's test, and valgus stress test.

**10.1 / 4.** *According to the evidence-based literature, which ligamentous tests used by clinicians are the most accurate in diagnosing this condition?*

According to Scholten,[82] examination of the accuracy of diagnostic testing for assessing trauma to the anterior cruciate ligament found the Lachman's test a more accurate overall test for assessing the ACL, followed by the lateral pivot shift test. The anterior draw test, according to authors, appears to be of little value due to guarding of the hamstring muscles. The position of the anterior draw test places the knee in less of an open-pack position during the test.

**10.1 / 5.** *Jim questions you as to why the doctor wants to see him tomorrow and why he needs an MRI. How do you answer him?*

The answer should focus on the need for further evaluation by a medical physician. In states where an athletic trainer works under the direct supervision of a licensed physician, it will often be necessary for a physician to determine the final medical diagnosis and assess the need for, as well as order, the appropriate diagnostic imaging.

In this case, the MRI is used to detect soft tissue lesions (i.e., ligaments). As a diagnostic modality, an MRI uses a powerful magnetic field and radiofrequency waves to visualize anatomical structures (e.g., joint, tendons, ligaments). A patient is placed within a magnetic field as radiowaves are introduced, absorbed, and released by the tissues. The intensity of the signals differs, based on the make-up of the involved tissues, and the signals are then converted into a set of tomographic images by using field gradients in the magnetic field, all of which permits a three-dimensional localization of the point sources of the signals.[75,87]

## CASE 10.2 Lateral Collateral Ligament Sprain with Secondary Peroneal Nerve Damage

10.2 / **1.** *Based on the information presented in the case, determine (a) the differential diagnoses and (b) the clinical diagnosis.*

a. Differential diagnoses: osteochondral fracture, tibial plateau fracture, extensor mechanism rupture, patellofemoral injury

b. Clinical diagnosis: lateral collateral ligament sprain with secondary peroneal nerve damage

10.2 / **2.** *Figure 10.2.1 demonstrated a positive knee ligamentous test. The test revealed instability at 0° and 20° of knee flexion. What is the name of the test performed, and what is the diagnostic accuracy of this test?*

The name of the test is a varus stress test, which assesses the stability of the lateral collateral ligament. Positive findings included increased laxity, decreased quality of the end point, and increased pain compared with the uninvolved knee.

According to McConagy,[58] there is no data examining the accuracy of the medial or lateral collateral ligamentous tests.

10.2 / **3.** *What is the clinical significance of varus ligamentous instability at both 0° and 20° of knee flexion?*

The lateral collateral ligament (LCL) is the primary static stabilizer of the lateral knee. Damage to the LCL is typically sustained when a varus force is applied to the knee. Ligamentous testing for the stability of the LCL is accomplished through a varus stress test. Laxity or a decreased end-point when the knee is in 15°–20° indicates damage to the LCL, while significant laxity in full extension may indicate concomitant injury to the joint capsule, posterior cruciate ligament, and possibly, the anterior cruciate ligament[46] and other related soft-tissue structures.[49,86]

10.2 / **4.** *Why was a deficit in ankle dorsiflexion and eversion noted?*

Concomitant common peroneal nerve injury can occur with an LCL injury because of a traction force[54] applied to the nerve as it wraps around the fibula head. As the LCL is stretched, so is the common peroneal nerve. The traction injury can result in drop foot (from weakness of the dorsiflexor muscles of the foot, which are enervated by the deep peroneal nerve) and numbness in the dorsum of the foot, as well as other neurological issues.[54]

10.2 / **5.** *How would you respond to Sam if he asks, "How is the doctor going to determine exactly what is wrong with me?"*

The answers to this question will vary among students. The answer should include a statement that initially the physician will correlate the findings of the history and physical examination. From there, the physician will determine the need for further diagnostic testing if the history and physical examination do not clearly determine the clinical diagnosis. In this case, a physician would most likely order diagnostic testing, such as an MRI or electrophysiological testing (electromyography or nerve conduction studies). Consult your team physician to determine how she would manage this patient in her medical practice.

## CASE 10.3 Tibial Plateau Stress Fracture

10.3 / **1.** *Based on the information presented in the case, determine (a) the differential diagnoses and (b) the clinical diagnosis.*

a. Differential diagnoses: medial meniscus tear, osteochondritis dissecans, pes anserine bursitis, femoral condyle contusion

b. Clinical diagnosis: tibial plateau stress fracture

10.3 / **2.** *(a) Overall, do you feel Deb performed an adequate history in this case? (b) Identify three or four history questions you as the evaluating clinician may have asked about extrinsic risk factors involved in the development of this condition.*

a. The answers to this question will vary among students. Given the information presented in the case though, it would be fair to state that Deb did not really perform a complete history assessment.

b. Some of the history questions that could have guided the examination include:

- Questioning the patient about training errors such as, but not limited to, an abrupt increase in training frequency, duration, or intensity or changes in an individual's training techniques.
- A clinician may ask about the training surfaces, such as running on stairs, banked surfaces, and irregular surfaces (grass, sand, and/or gravel).
- Questioning the patient about his running shoes, such as the use of insoles and orthotics, and current distance used. Running shoes lose ability to absorb shock after 300 to 500 miles.
- Questioning the patient about his general health and dietary habits.[10]

10.3 / **3.** *The findings of Deb's physical examination in this case are not well identified, except for the statement that "After Deb completes her physical examination of Mike, she determines that he is suffering from pes anserine bursitis." As the evaluating clinician, identify the steps you would have to follow to arrive at the initial clinical diagnosis of per anserine bursitis. Would you have considered the diagnosis of pes anserine bursitis, given the location of Mike's pain?*

Answers to this question will vary among students and should be discussed with the classroom instructor. In fact, this question is best answered as a group discussion, because there is not necessarily only one correct answer. Many different evaluation techniques could have been used to arrive at the diagnosis.

10.3 / **4.** *Based on the case's clinical diagnosis, identity the possible intrinsic risk factors for the development of this condition.*

In the physically active population, the etiology of stress fracture formation typically begins with a change or increase in physical activity.[78] However, the development of a stress fracture is a multi-factorial process with a number of risk factors, including intrinsic (Table A10.3.1), extrinsic (Table A10.3.2), nutritional, and hormonal factors, to name a few.[9] Clinicians should pay particular attention to intrinsic risk factors (e.g., age, bone composition and density) when dealing with non-college-age recreational athletes, such as in this case, because stress fractures occurring as a result of physical activity are less common than those occurring from other causes.[10]

Intrinsic factors include bone geometry,[17,31,78] age,[13,66,84] and muscular fatigue.[50,60]

TABLE A10.3.1

**Intrinsic risk factors associated with the development of a stress fracture.**[10]

| RISK FACTOR | CLINICAL PRESENTATION/ACTIVITY |
|---|---|
| Anatomical factors | ■ Excessive subtalar pronation<br>■ Hindfoot varus and forefoot varus<br>■ Pes planus and pes cavus<br>■ Genu varus and varum<br>■ Leg-length discrepancies<br>■ Excessive Q-angle |
| Muscular fatigue | ■ Weak or fatigued muscles unable to dissipate mechanical stress effectively; bone failure on tensile, compressive, or both sides |
| Physiological factors | ■ Rapid bone turnover rate<br>■ Poor flexibility<br>■ Overall conditioning<br>■ Obesity, poor nutrition<br>■ Menstrual disturbance<br>■ Bone cysts |
| Bone characteristics | ■ Geometry<br>■ Low mineral density |

TABLE A10.3.2

**Extrinsic risk factors associated with the development of a stress fracture.**[10]

| RISK FACTOR | CLINICAL PRESENTATION/ACTIVITY |
|---|---|
| Training errors | ■ Abrupt increases in frequency, duration, or intensity<br>■ High total mileage<br>■ Changes in training technique<br>■ Aggressive increases in total mileage in runners |
| Training surface | ■ Stairs, sloped or banked surfaces, curbs and irregular surfaces (grass, sand, and gravel) increase strain<br>■ Abrupt changes in surfaces, which increase external loading |
| Shoe type | ■ Shock absorption properties of footwear; shoes lose the ability to absorb shock after 300 to 500 miles<br>■ Insoles and orthotics |
| Unaccustomed activities | ■ Sedentary lifestyle |

It has long been thought that low bone mineral density (BMD) may also be a risk factor for the development of stress fractures because it reduces bone strength, thereby increasing the accumulation of microtrauma with repetitive cyclical loading.[14] However, studies examining athletes and military recruits are mixed at best, mostly because of differences in research methodology.[6,8,18,74]

Age is also a possible risk factor, particularly as it relates to BMD, because studies have shown that bone becomes less resistant to fatigue failure with decreases in BMD and bone tissue size.[60,84]

10.3 / **5.** *(a) Do you believe that Deb made a bad decision regarding the use of the therapeutic ultrasound? (b) Why did the therapeutic ultrasound produce intense pain at the injury site?*

a. No, Deb's decision was justifiable. It is conceivable that Mike's initial pain was caused by pes anserine bursitis. Given this information, therapeutic ultrasound would be an appropriate treatment. Terminating the treatment because of the increased pain was also the appropriate clinical decision.

b. Use of therapeutic ultrasound to identify stress reactions has been reported with mixed opinions in the literature.[35,63,65,79] Moss and Mowatt's examination of tibial shaft stress fractures with radiographs and ultrasound (.75 MHz, intensity 1.0 and 2.0 W/cm$^2$) demonstrated that ultrasound was successful in identifying 96 percent of the radiographically confirmed fractures.[63] Giladi found that ultrasound testing identified 38 of the 51 (75%) confirmed tibial stress fractures.[35] Ultrasound was found to have less sensitivity and specificity than bone scans, but greater sensitivity than radiographs alone. An examination of therapeutic ultrasound by Romani to identify stress fractures refutes the findings of other studies. They found that none of the subjects found to have a stress fracture according to the MRI were correctly identified by the use of continuous ultrasound (1 MHz, increasing intensity from 0 to 2.9 W/cm$^2$ every 30 s), thus having a sensitivity of 0 percent.[79]

Mike's intense pain was probably produced because of coinciding therapeutic ultra-sound longitudinal and transverse waves. When the two waves are in phase, they produce a summated energy level resulting in a standing wave that produces heating of the tissue.[35] In the presence of damaged bone (mircofractures), the heating of the perisoteum produces intense pain within the sensitized damaged tissue.

## CASE 10.4 Plica Syndrome

*by William Holcomb, Ph.D., ATC, CSCS-D, University of Nevada, Las Vegas*

10.4 / **1.** *Based on the information presented in the case, determine (a) the differential diagnoses and (b) the clinical diagnosis.*

a. Differential diagnoses: torn medial meniscus, patellofemoral pain syndrome (PFPS), fat pad syndrome (FPS), chondromalacia patella[32,33]

b. Clinical diagnosis: medial plica syndrome

10.4 / **2.** *(a) What is the name of the special test shown in textbook Figure 10.4.1? (b) As the evaluating clinician how would you perform the test? (c) What is a positive finding?*

a. The special test in Figure 10.4.1 is known as a Stutter test.

b. To perform the test, place the athlete in short sitting position with the legs hanging over the edge of the table. The clinician should stand or sit lateral to the affected leg, placing the hand over the patella. The athlete then actively extends the knee while the clinician notes the tracking of the patella.[49]

c. A positive indication is irregular movement of the patella. Typically, with medial synovial plica present, the patella motion "stutters" between 40° and 60° of flexion.

10.4 / **3.** *What other special tests, if any, could be performed to assist in determining the clinical diagnosis?*

A second test for plica would be the Hughston's plica test. To perform this, examine the athlete in the supine position with his knee flexed to 90°. The clinician internally rotates the tibia and moves the patella medially, palpating the anteromedial capsule (Figure A10.4.1a). The athlete's knee is then flexed and extended from 90° to 0° while the tibia is rotated internally (Figure A10.4.1b). A positive sign is pain or palpable clicking, also indicative of medial synovial plica.

FIGURE **A10.4.1** Hughston's plica test.

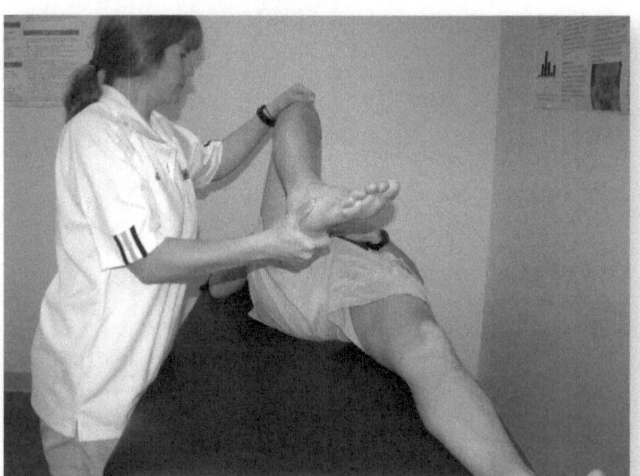

(a) Start position for the plica test. The athlete is supine with the knee flexed to 90°.

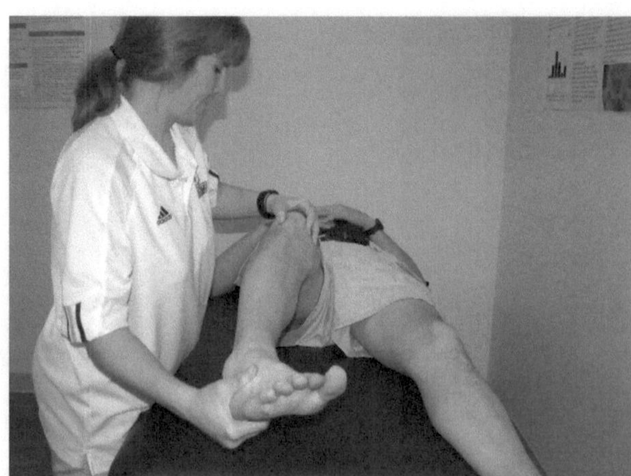

(b) The clinician then flexes and extends the athlete's knee while internally rotating the tibia.

10.4 / **4.** *Discuss the etiology of this condition. Include the following in your answer: (a) the definition of the condition, (b) the MOI, (c) a description of the asymptomatic condition, and (d) a description of the symptomatic condition.*

a. Plica is defined as an embryonic remnant of developmental knee chambers where incomplete absorption of the chamber walls leaves synovial folds. Three synovial folds, superior, inferior, and medial are typically described by most authors.[23]

b. The most commonly affected plica is the medial plica. The most common MOI would be a direct blow to the medial femoral condyle or dramatic increases in the duration of activity.

c. Normal plica is a thin almost translucent, pliable band of synovium, normally offering few problems.

d. These mechanisms can cause the plica to become inflamed and fibrotic, which is the basic description of symptomatic plica. Continued activity causes the plica to thicken and become unyielding. Friction as the band slides over the femoral condyle during flexion and extension of the knee can lead to erosion of the medial condyle.[23,81]

10.4 / **5.** *(a) Describe the goals for management of this condition and the techniques that have been shown to be effective, including conservative methods. (b) Describe more aggressive treatments to be used should the conservative treatment methods fail.*

a. The goal of treatment should be to decrease inflammation and make the plica more pliable to reduce the effects of friction. Rest has been shown to be beneficial, but rest is difficult during the competitive season. Conservative management of inflammation includes cryotherapy and NSAIDS. When inflammation is under control, thermotherapy such as ultrasound can be used to make the plica more pliable.[81]

   A lateral tracking patella and tight lateral retinaculum have been implicated as contributing factors to medial plica syndrome.[32,33] If lateral tracking is identified, isometric quadriceps strengthening to correct patellar alignment should be used. Medial gliding of the patella can also be used to stretch the lateral retinaculum. If the IT band is tight, IT band stretching should be used.

b. If conservative management fails, a combined injection of an anti-inflammatory agent and a long-acting local anesthetic directly into the plica have been shown to provide complete relief.[81] If the plica becomes fibrotic and erosion of the femoral condyle is occurring, then arthroscopic excision and debridement is warranted.[23,32]

# CASE 10.5 Medial Tibial Stress Syndrome

*by William Holcomb, Ph.D., ATC, CSCS-D, University of Nevada, Las Vegas*

10.5 / **1.** *Based on the information presented in the case, determine (a) the differential diagnoses and (b) the clinical diagnosis.*

a. Differential diagnoses: stress fracture, chronic exertional compartment syndrome (chronic ECS), popliteal artery entrapment syndrome (PAES), nerve entrapment[25,29,51]

b. Clinical diagnosis: medial tibial stress syndrome (MTSS)

10.5 / **2.** *Explain how each of the differential diagnoses could be eliminated with confidence based on the physical examination and diagnostic tests.*

The answers will vary among students, based on what they have determined to be the differential diagnoses. Based on the diagnoses listed above:

- Negative radiograph and bone scans should eliminate stress fracture.[25]
- Pain for chronic ECS is typically lateral to the tibia and symptoms subside with rest.[25] Gaines experienced pain on the medial tibial, and as the condition progressed, pain was experienced even at rest.
- Normal peripheral nerve testing and a negative Tinel's sign would not indicate nerve entrapment, but EMG testing would be required for a definitive assessment.[25]
- Pain at rest and palpable tenderness, along with normal pedal pulse even with provocation, eliminate PAES.[25]

10.5 / **3.** *The clinical diagnosis is often graded based on the single criteria of pain. Describe what the four grades would be, based on the clinical diagnosis.*

The following are the grades of medial tibial stress syndrome.

- Grade 1: pain following activity
- Grade 2: pain before and after activity that subsides after warm-up
- Grade 3: pain before, during, and after activity
- Grade 4: pain so severe that activity is not possible

10.5 / **4.** *(a) When Gaines reported to the athletic training clinic, what grade, based on question 10.5/3, was she experiencing? (b) What does that mean for her participation in cross-country?*

a. Based on the presentation of pain along the anterior-medial border, Gaines' MTSS would be grade 3.

b. Because she is at this grade, she should be restricted from activity to allow the condition to calm down. However, this often is not practical for competitive athletes who must remain fit. In addition to the management described for controlling inflammation, other interventions (see question 10.5/5) may help to relieve the stress causing this injury.

10.5 / **5.** *If you were the treating clinician in this case, identify the possible interventions you may use to treat Gaines.*

The answers to this question will vary according to the students' experience, and classroom discussion regarding this question would be appropriate. However, some of the recommended interventional steps include:

- Correct lower extremity anomalies such as hyperpronation and pes planus with orthotics.[6,51,70] Assess the sacroiliac joint for innominate rotation causing increased leg length and compensatory pronation to shorten the leg.
- Correct improper running techniques that may increase tibial loading.[51]
- Strengthen posterior and anterior tibialis muscles. Increase the flexibility of the triceps surae.[51]
- Avoid dramatic changes in training that would cause the tibia to be exposed to unaccustomed forces.[51]
- Wear lightweight, shock-absorbing footwear, and change shoes every 300 to 500 miles.[6,51]
- Run on level, uniform surfaces of moderate firmness, such as asphalt.[6]

## CASE 10.6 Posterior Cruciate Ligament Sprain

**10.6 / 1.** *Based on the information presented in the case, determine (a) the differential diagnoses and (b) the clinical diagnosis.*

a. Differential diagnoses: anterior cruciate ligament (ACL) sprain, lateral collateral ligament (LCL) sprain, medial collateral ligament (MCL) sprain, quadriceps strain

b. Clinical diagnosis: posterior cruciate ligament (PCL) sprain

**10.6 / 2.** *What other MOI(s) can cause this injury?*

Falling on a flexed knee is a common MOI, but two other mechanisms include forced hyperextension of the knee and a flexed knee striking a dashboard during an automobile accident.[86]

**10.6 / 3.** *(a) In your opinion, and based on the information in the case, explain whether you think Sue took an appropriate history. (b) What other questions would you have asked as the evaluating clinician?*

a. Based on the above case scenario, Sue did appear to perform a thorough history.

b. Some examples of other history questions that could have been asked by a clinician include:

- What is your pain level, specifically during activity?
- What makes the pain better or worse?
- Was there an audible pop or snap at the time of injury?
- If the injury occurred with a rotatory force, what position was your foot in when the injury occurred? In this case, what position was the foot in when landing on the knee? Studies have shown that most PCL injuries occur with a force of the tibia in a posterior direction, as in the above situation, with the foot in a plantar flexed position, causing hyperflexion of the knee.[37,94]

**10.6 / 4.** *According to the case, it was reported that there was an antalgic gait pattern, but Jeannette's location of pain was not addressed. In what area do you think Jeannette would complain most about pain?*

The pain would most likely be located in the posterior aspect of the knee.

**10.6 / 5.** *What could Sue have done to address the antalgic gait pattern?*

Sue should have fitted Jeannette with crutches and instructed her in their proper use in order to decrease the antalgia and to limit gait and mechanical abnormalities. According to Wind, one of the treatments for a low grade PCL sprain is limiting weight-bearing activities with the use of crutches.[94]

**10.6 / 6.** *The clinical diagnosis can be classified into one of three different grades. Describe the classification of each grade.*

A PCL tear is typically graded in a 90° flexed position of the knee. The tibial plateau position is compared with the medial femoral condyle. The tibia typically is 1 cm anterior to the femoral condyles in this 90° position.[53,94] The three grades of PCL damage include:

- Grade I: tibia lies anterior to femoral condyles (0–5 mm of patholaxity)
- Grade II: tibia is flush with femoral condyles (5–10 mm patholaxity)
- Grade III: tibia no longer has a medial step-off and can be pushed beyond medial femoral condyle (>10 mm patholaxity)

10.6 / **7.** *Overall, do you believe that Sue managed the condition appropriately? What else could have been done to assist with Jeannette's recovery?*

The answers to this question will vary among students. However, Sue could have done a better job on the initial management of the injury. She could have initiated quadriceps (quad) sets to assist with decreased posterior translation of the tibia.[71] Crutches could have assisted in pain control, and bracing or wrapping could have assisted with the antalgic gait and any joint effusion.

## CASE 10.7 Patellar Tendon Rupture with Patella Avulsion Fracture

10.7 / **1.** *Based on the information presented in the case, determine (a) the differential diagnoses and (b) the clinical diagnosis.*

a. Differential diagnoses: quadriceps tendon rupture, patella fracture, patella dislocation

b. Clinical diagnosis: patellar tendon rupture with an avulsion fracture of the inferior pole of the patella

10.7 / **2.** *Why do you believe that Melissa was unable to actively extend her knee?*

The patellar tendon, which inserts onto the tibial tuberosity, is part of the quadriceps muscle group and is therefore responsible for active knee extension. With the report that there was moderate effusion of the knee and an abnormality in the anterior thigh, it is likely the patellar tendon is no longer attached to the rest of the quadriceps.[27] When this occurs, the result is a loss of active knee extension.

10.7 / **3.** *(a) Overall, do you believe that Sara managed the situation appropriately? (b) What if anything could she have done better to manage the situation?*

a. Although Sara activated EMS in a timely fashion, she should have stayed with Melissa while she activated her EAP. If Sara had properly reviewed the facility's EAP, she would have been more prepared.[4]

b. It may have been prudent for Sara to ask a coach to call EMS—or even another athlete or athletic training student; this way, she could have splinted Melissa while EMS was being activated. Sara also did not attempt to monitor vital signs while waiting for EMS or to check vascular or neurological status of the lower extremity after noticing a defect in the anterior thigh.[2] By not initiating splinting, Sara allowed Melissa to stay on the field longer, which kept Melissa in the center of attention longer and delayed the game longer.

10.7 / **4.** *What are some possible consequences of Sara's on-scene actions?*

Answers will vary among students but may include the following:

- Because Sara did not perform a neurovascular assessment, Melissa could have ended up with more serious injuries, including impaired blood flow to the lower extremity, which could have required amputation.

10.7 / **5.** *After Melissa arrived at the hospital, how do you think this case was managed medically?*

At the hospital, initial diagnostic testing would most likely include radiographs to reveal the extent of the injury, which showed an avulsed inferior pole of the patella. When the nature of the injury is discovered, an open reduction internal fixation (ORIF) would be needed to re-attach the avulsed inferior patella to the main body of the patella and place the patella in its normal position. Post-operatively, Melissa would be placed in a straight leg cast for immobilization for six weeks[26] or in a hinged knee brace. However, medical management varies among physicians. Some physicians place individuals in a hinge brace for six weeks, allowing passive extension and active flexion to 45°, to assist in the healing process.[56]

10.7 / **6.** *Now that Melissa is cleared to begin rehabilitation, what should be the first thing Sara should concentrate on in Melissa's rehabilitation? Please explain your reasoning.*

Improving the ROM could be an option. However, 120° of flexion is functional, and Melissa already has the full extension necessary for proper gait. Melissa is unable to actively contract the quadriceps, which is also necessary for gait and other functional activities. Therefore, quad sets with the use of a biofeedback machine or with use of self biofeedback through education of what to look for in a quad contraction might be a good way to start. This would entail use of her own hand to try to educate the quadriceps to activate. Neuromuscular re-education with electrical stimulation is also an option to help improve overall muscle contraction and strength of the quadriceps.[11] After quadriceps contraction has been initiated, SLRs are appropriate, without the use of weight in the beginning. Other strengthening exercises can be initiated for the hamstrings and the gastrocnemius.

Answers will vary depending on the exercises chosen. The remaining explanations will vary among students depending on their initial answer, and they should be discussed with the classroom instructor. In fact, this question is best answered as a group discussion because there is not necessarily only one correct answer.

## CASE 10.8 Patella Dislocation

10.8 / **1.** *Based on the information presented in the case, determine (a) the differential diagnoses and (b) the clinical diagnosis.*

a. Differential diagnoses: ACL sprain, MCL sprain, meniscal tear, patella fracture, tibia fracture, patella subluxation, patella instability
b. Clinical diagnosis: patella dislocation

10.8 / **2.** *Based on the information presented above, do you think Samantha took a thorough history and physical examination? What else could have Samantha asked or performed to help make the diagnosis?*

The answers will vary among students. Samantha could have asked for a pain rating and then asked for a description of the pain. Samantha could also have performed simple palpation along the knee to assess the injury further. Areas to palpate would have been the medial and lateral borders of the patella, the femoral condyles, the tibia, the MCL, and the LCL. A tap test along the plantar aspect of the foot could have been performed to assist in ruling out a fracture.

10.8 / **3.** *Do you believe that Samantha performed the necessary immediate care steps? Explain your answer.*

Based on the above information, Samantha could have braced/splinted Sandy's right leg/knee to ensure proper stabilization while waiting for EMS. However, in most cases simple stabilization of the joint may be enough, because EMS will need to evaluate the injury before transport.

Even though the case scenario states that Sandy is medically stable, it does not state how Samantha came to this conclusion; therefore, baseline and ongoing vital signs should have been taken to ensure that Sandy was medically stable.[2]

10.8 / **4.** *At the emergency room, Sandy underwent several radiographs to rule out bony trauma. The radiographs were negative for fractures, but an Insall-Salvati ratio of 1.4 did show up, along with proper alignment of the patella in the femoral groove. What is an Insall-Salvati ratio, and why is it significant?*

Insall-Salvati, also known as Insall-Salvati index, is a measurement of the patellar tendon length from the inferior pole of the patella to the tibial tubercle, divided by the patella height. An Insall-Salvati ratio greater than 1.2 is indicative of patella alta, and a ratio of less than 0.8 is indicative of patella infra or patella baja.[21,26,88]

The ratio is significant because patella alta (a more proximal x-ray position of the patella than anticipated, resulting from a longer patellar tendon) predisposes an individual to instability of the patella and/or dislocation.

10.8 / **5.** *(a) What is the significance of knowing that the patella is in proper alignment within the femoral groove? (b) What are some other factors that may contribute to a patella dislocation?*

a. A properly aligned patella within the femoral groove suggests that the patella is no longer dislocated and probably spontaneously reduced as the athlete tried to actively extend the knee.

b. Some of the factors contributing to a patella dislocation include:
   - Increased Q-angle (the angle formed by the line of traction of the quadriceps tendon on the patella and the line of traction of the patellar tendon on the tibial tubercle)[87]
   - An abnormally shallow femoral groove
   - Hypermobile patella attributable to weak medial stabilizers and tight lateral stabilizers
   - Deficits in medial quadriceps (VMO) muscle strength
   - Patella alta

10.8 / **6.** *(a) What is the name of the test in textbook Figure 10.8.2? (b) What does it assess?*

a. The test is the patella apprehension test.

b. In the patella apprehension test, the examiner stresses the medial patellar retinaculum by placing a force on the medial side of the patella in a lateral direction in an attempt to replicate the pain and apprehension caused by a dislocation (Figure A10.8.1). One must take care not to actually cause dislocation. A positive test is indicated by pain or muscle contraction to guard the patella from dislocating.[49,86] Tanner suggests a modified patellar apprehension test using a distal lateral force to appropriately test the integrity of the medial patellofemoral ligament.[88]

FIGURE A10.8.1 Patella apprehension test.

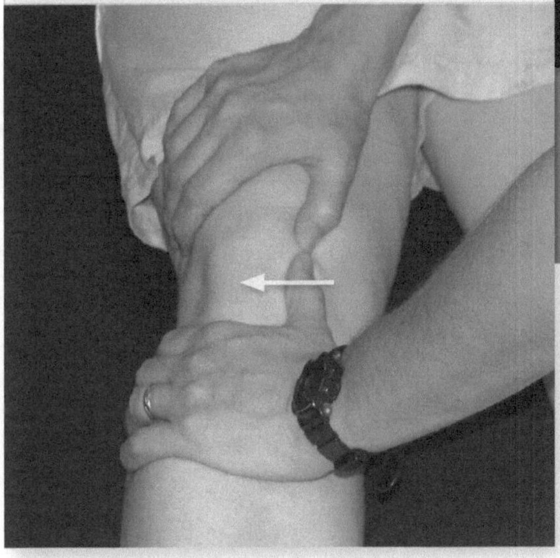

Arrow indicates direction of force applied by the thumbs.

10.8 / **7.** *After completing each physical examination, Samantha documented her findings. Please document your findings from both examinations as if you were the treating clinician. If the case did not provide information you believe is pertinent to the clinical diagnosis, please feel free to add this information to your documentation.*

Answers will vary. Students should consider writing a SOAP note (see textbook Appendix B) using the ABCD format when writing the short- and long-term goals.

# CASE 10.9 Quadriceps Tendon Rupture

10.9 / **1.** *Based on the information presented in the case, determine (a) the differential diagnoses and (b) the clinical diagnosis.*

a. Differential diagnoses: patellar tendon rupture, jumper's knee, patella fracture, knee dislocation, osteochondral fracture[55]

b. Clinical diagnosis: quadriceps tendon rupture

10.9 / **2.** *What questions might Jessica have asked in this particular situation to help establish the proper clinical diagnosis?*

The answers to this question may vary among students. However, some possible questions include the following:

- Do you have any previous complaints of knee pain or pathology?
- Do you use any anabolic steroids?
- Do you have any metabolic conditions, significant medical conditions, or past medical history?

Quadriceps tendon ruptures are more common in the healthier population with the presence of a metabolic disorder, renal insufficiency, and anabolic steroid use.[44,55]

10.9 / **3.** *Describe how you think Jessica should have immobilized Antonio's knee.*

Trauma to the knee joint will often require that the bones above and below (femur and tibia) be immobilized. The easier method in this case would have been the use of a straight leg knee immobilizer. However, if one is unavailable or in cases in which the knee cannot be moved because of increased risk of injury, a SAM SPLINT® with an elastic wrap or a vacuum splint may be used to stabilize the knee.

10.9 / **4.** *What medical studies or diagnostic imaging may be ordered for this injury upon evaluation at the emergency room?*

Antonio will most likely have a set of plain film radiographs to rule out any fractures. This may be followed by an MRI to assess the integrity of the soft tissue structures. Ultrasonography, according to Heyde, is a very useful tool to quickly and accurately diagnose a quadriceps tendon rupture.[39] A CT scan could also be used to rule out the possibility of bone or soft tissue trauma.

10.9 / **5.** *Based on the information presented in the case, what if anything should have been done differently?*

Had Jessica recognized the palpable defect during the on-scene physical examination, she could have immobilized and boarded Antonio right there, rather than immobilizing him and asking two competitors to carry him to the sideline, where EMS still had to board him before taking him to the hospital.

10.9 / **6.** *What medical management do you think is required for the above injury?*

For the best result, surgical intervention is usually indicated for a complete quadriceps tendon rupture. Typically, immobilization with a full leg cast is necessary for four to six weeks. The patient is usually allowed to bear weight as tolerated with crutches or a walker. Rehabilitation begins with gentle quad ROM and strengthening exercises after the cast is removed. Some physicians allow isometric quad contraction while the patient is still immobilized in the straight leg cast. A hinge brace may be used to provide stability, while flexion is increased progressively over time. Rehabilitation is continued until both legs are equal in motion and strength.

Incomplete tears usually receive more conservative treatment, requiring immobilization in full extension for three to six weeks. Straight leg raises are initiated late in the immobilization phase. When straight leg raises become pain free for 10 days, immobilization can be discontinued gradually. Range of motion exercises are then started. Quadriceps strengthening is continued until bilateral strength is equal. Aggressive swelling management is also indicated to reduce effusion because effusion can limit the quad strength.[77]

## CASE 10.10 Patella Tendinopathy

10.10 / **1.** *Based on the information presented in the case, determine (a) the differential diagnoses and (b) the clinical diagnosis.*

a. Differential diagnoses: knee osteochondritis dissecans, meniscus injuries, Osgood-Schlatter disease, patellar injury and/or dislocation, PFPS, pes anserine bursitis, quadriceps injury

b. Clinical diagnosis: patella tendinopathy

10.10 / **2.** *What other history questions could Jonathan have asked to help with his differential diagnoses and to assist him in determining which special tests to perform?*

Answers will vary among students. Some questions Jonathan could ask are as follows:

- Which other activities besides running increase pain?
- Which positions bother the knee (e.g., kneeling, squatting, ascending and descending stairs)?
- What makes the knee feel better?
- What is the reaction of the knee to stair climbing (better or worse)?
- What, if any, home treatment has she used?

10.10 / **3.** *What, if any, other special tests could you as the evaluating clinician perform to assist in determining the differential diagnoses?*

The clinician could use the decline squat test, also called the patellar tendon load response (Figure A10.10.1). According to Purdam, the decline squat test increases the load on the patellar tendon by decreasing the activity of the gastrocnemius during the squat.[76] The angle of decline is best at 25°, with the angle of knee flexion between 50° and 55°, to decrease the involvement of any patella–femoral symptoms that may be present, because the maximal patellofemoral loading occurs at 70° and beyond. A painful response is a positive test.[76,93]

10.10 / **4.** *What would be the most effective rehabilitation program for Eva so that she may participate in her marathon training with the least amount of pain?*

Answers may vary among students. Answers may include use of therapeutic modalities to control pain and swelling and therapeutic exercises to improve the quadriceps musculature. It has been suggested that the use of eccentric quadriceps exercises, while using a decline board to decrease the involvement of the gastrocnemius during the squatting motion, assists in strengthening of the quadriceps and patellar tendon.[20,45,93] Hamstring stretching and corrections of biomechanical abnormalities such as pronation of the foot should be employed as necessary.

10.10 / **5.** *Based on the history that Jonathan acquired from Eva, what stage of the injury is Eva presently experiencing?*

A classification system of patellar tendon injury by stages, which was developed by Blazina, identifies four stages of injury.[5,12]

- Stage 1: pain after activity only, with no functional limitations or impairment
- Stage 2: pain at the initiation of activity, which disappears but recurs after activity

- Stage 3: pain during and after activity that limits function and activity
- Stage 4: complete rupture to the tendon

Based on this classification system, Eva presents as Stage 2 patellar tendonitis.

10.10 / **6.** *If you were Jonathan, what would you advise Eva do regarding her marathon training?*

Answers could include resting from marathon training and continuing with pool workouts that consist of swimming and running within the water or, alternatively, cardiovascular training that is less stressful on the patellar tendon. This question is best left as a class discussion.

FIGURE A10.10.1

Decline squat test.

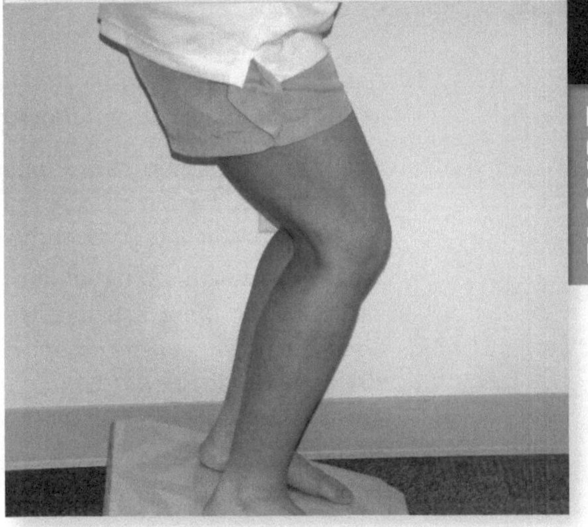

# CASE 10.11 Patellofemoral Pain Syndrome

10.11 / **1.** *Based on the information presented in the case, determine (a) the differential diagnoses, and (b) the likely clinical diagnosis.*

a. Differential diagnoses: malalignment, chonromalacia patellae, Osgood-Schlatter syndrome, Larsen disease, plica disorders, osteoarthritis of the patella, tendonitis, bursitis, radicular pain, tumor, infection of the knee joint[30,73,83]

b. Clinical diagnosis: patellofemoral pain syndrome

10.11 / **2.** *Overall, do you believe an appropriate physical examination was performed? What else, if anything, would you do as the evaluating clinician to determine the clinical diagnosis? Describe how to perform these evaluative techniques and the significance they would have on your findings.*

The answers will vary among students; however, several items that could be added to the assessment include the following:

- Assess the Q-angle. The Q-angle is measured by placing Sandra supine with her left knee extended. A goniometer is used to measure the Q-angle, with the fulcrum being the mid-patellar region. The stationary arm is placed over the line from the ASIS to the patella, and the movement arm is placed over the line from the patella to the tibial tuberosity. It is known that women are at greater risk of patellofemoral pain with an increased Q-angle. An increased Q-angle can cause patella maltracking by placing increased lateral forces on the patella. The normal Q-angle for males is 14°, and for females it is 17°.[83]
- Perform an Ober's test. The IT band connects to the lateral portion of the patella through the lateral retinaculum. A tight IT band can cause poor patella tracking and decreased muscle balance.
- Assess overall flexibility of the hamstrings, quads, IT band, and calf muscles should be assessed as they all contribute to proper tracking of the patella.
- Perform repetitive movements such as squatting to assess Sandra's pain level during squatting, as squatting typically provokes pain with patellofemoral pain syndrome.[73]
- Examine the hip for ROM and strength deficits.[85]

10.11 / **3.** *Based on the clinical diagnosis, what do you think is the best course of action to take as far as treatment?*

Several items need to be considered when treating patellofemoral pain syndrome:

- Rest from the activity (volleyball) that aggravates symptoms, specifically squatting and jumping.
- Stretching of the tight structures should be performed immediately. Medial glides of the patella will decrease tightness of the lateral retinaculum.
- Quadriceps strengthening should be performed, with emphasis on the VMO. Roush suggests performing a modified straight leg raise, with the hip in external rotation.[80] This technique, also known as the Muncie method, is said to cause greater activation of the VMO; however, Mirzabeigim concluded that the VMO was not activated to a greater degree than the vastus lateralis.[61]

- Kerri may want to consider evaluating, or having Sandra further evaluated, for positive foot pronation and provide correction for this problem with orthotics if appropriate.

10.11 / **4.** *Many individuals use McConnell taping to assist in managing this condition. (a) What is McConnell taping? (b) What is its efficacy in treating the condition?*

a. Patella taping (McConnell taping) is a taping method developed by Jenny McConnell. It is a taping technique that realigns, in theory, the patella so the patella can track correctly within the femoral grove. The technique is performed by pulling the patella medially with Leukotape P and a Cover-Roll tape (Beiersdorf AG, Hamburg, Germany). This is done because in PFPS the patella tracks laterally secondary to the tight structures. With McConnell taping, one can also correct the rotation, tilt, and glide, depending on what is needed for the particular client (Figures A10.11.1, A10.11.2, and A10.11.3).

b. It is difficult to say why it assists with PFPS. Studies show that McConnell taping assists with relief of pain but does not change the magnitude of activation of the VMO.[3,61,72] For muscle activation, McConnell taping is not effective; however, for pain reduc tion, it is effective, allowing pain-free exercise and activity.[3]

FIGURE A10.11.1

**McConnell taping preparation.**

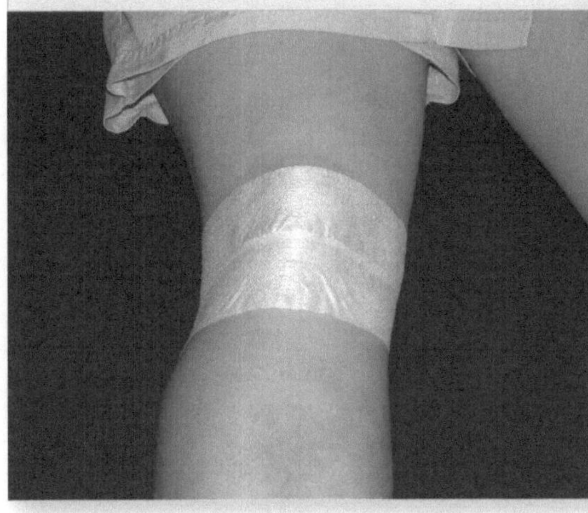

Apply "cover roll" tape 1/2 to 1/3 overlapping from medial to lateral aspect of joint. No force is needed at this time.

FIGURE A10.11.2

**McConnell taping medial glide.**

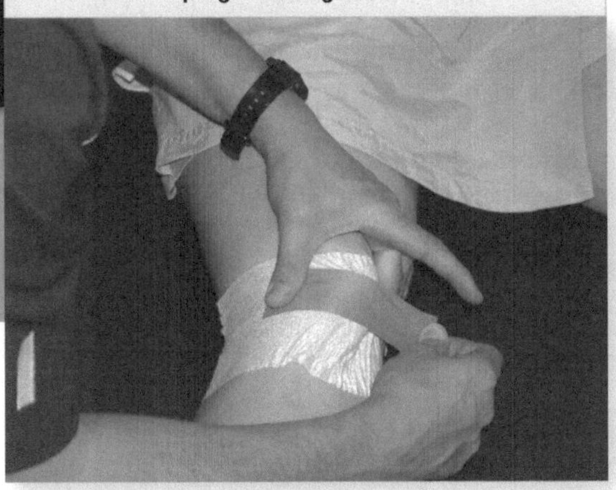

Identify lateral aspect of the superior patella, place edge of Leukotape at this point, and pull medially.

FIGURE A10.11.3

**McConnell secondary strip.**

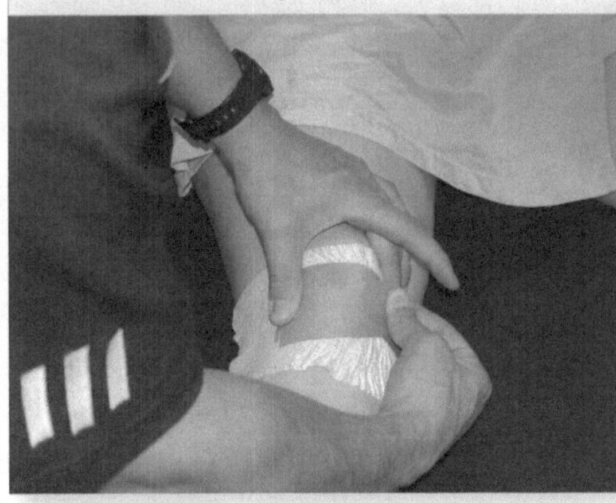

Locate inferior lateral portion of the patella, place edge of the Leukotape at this point and pull laterally. A superior force can also be applied to assist with any rotation or tilt the patella may have. The two strips of Leukotape should be overlapped by 1/2 to 1/3.

## CASE 10.12 Knee Dislocation (Tibiofemoral Dislocation with Vascular Compromise)

10.12 / **1.** *Based on the information presented in the case, determine (a) the differential diagnoses and (b) the clinical diagnosis.*

a. Differential diagnoses: tibia fracture, fibula fracture, femur fracture
b. Clinical diagnosis: posterior knee dislocation

FIGURE A10.12.1 Assessment of the dorsal pedal pulse.

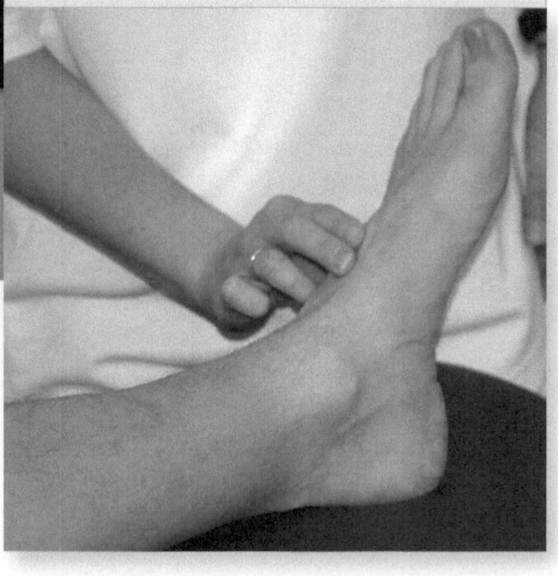

Dorsal pedal pulse is located lateral to the extensor hallucis longus tendon and medially to the extensor digitorum tendons along the dorsal surface of the foot, distal to the dorsal-most prominence of the navicular bone.[64]

10.12 / **2.** *Based on the information provided in the case, is there anything else that Doug should have assessed further?*

Based on the clinical assessment, John's distal foot was grayish-bluish, indicating possible neurovascular involvement. Doug, however, did not assess the dorsal pedal pulse or popliteal pulse (Figure A10.12.1). It is important that the vascular structures be evaluated, because the major arteries of the popliteal artery pass posterior to the knee. Reports have suggested that trauma occurs to the popliteal artery in 20 to 40 percent of knee dislocations.[47,59] David should also have continued to check John's vital signs to ensure that John was not going into shock while waiting for the EMS to arrive.

10.12 / **3.** *In what position was the knee when Doug splinted the injury? What materials do you think were used?*

David most likely splinted the knee in the position it was found, based on the deformity that he saw. Doug would just attempt to stabilize the joint in the most effective manner, without moving the joint a great amount, to avoid further injury. Materials used would include a vacuum splint or even a soft splint (with a bandage) and a spineboard.

10.12 / **4.** *(a) What other types of injuries does Doug need to be concerned with in addition to vascular damage? (b) How might he assess the problems?*

a. Another tissue that could be involved in the injury is nerve tissue, specifically the tibial and common peroneal nerves.
b. These nerves could be assessed generally for light-touch sensation and two-point discrimination.

10.12 / **5.** *(a) Based on the clinical diagnosis, what if any ligamentous structures could be affected? (b) What is the most likely treatment?*

a. The posterior cruciate ligament was probably involved and fully torn by the extreme force of the injury. Patellar tendon rupture may have occurred, as well as retinacular and capsule tears. The anterior cruciate ligament and the medial and lateral collateral ligaments may also be damaged.[68] In essence, any and all ligamentous structures could be and probably were involved.

b. Treatment depends on the extent of the injury and the involved tissues. First and foremost, the dislocation will need to be reduced, which will most likely be attempted under sedation in the ER. If that is not successful, then reduction under anesthetic will be appropriate. If there is vascular compromise, vascular surgery will be necessary to correct the injury.[36] Depending on the extent of the injury, surgical repair consisting of ligamentous reconstruction of the tissues may be necessary.[36,92]

## CASE 10.13 Fibular Dislocation

10.13 / **1.** *Based on the information presented in the case, determine (a) the differential diagnoses and (b) the clinical diagnosis.*

a. Differential diagnoses: lateral collateral sprain, tibiofemoral dislocation, proximal tibiofibular sprain, fibular fracture, lateral ankle sprain

b. Clinical diagnosis: fibular head dislocation with spontaneous reduction

10.13 / **2.** *Identify (a) the four classifications of this injury and (b) the most common MOI.*

a. The Ogden classification system for tibiofibular dislocations identifies four types of dislocation. The first is subluxation; the second is anterolateral dislocation; the third is posteromedial; and the fourth is superior.[1] This particular case study was an anterolateral dislocation of the fibula, which is the most common dislocation.

b. The MOI is usually a fall on a flexed knee and an inverted foot, which results in a sudden inversion strain and places increased tension on the peroneal muscles. This increased tension on the peroneal muscles can cause dislocation of the fibula in an anterior direction.[16,22,89]

10.13 / **3.** *If you were the evaluating athletic trainer, what other questions, if any, would you have asked?*

The answers will vary among students. Possible questions could include the following:

- Did you experience any altered sensations such as numbness or tingling?
- Describe your pain.
- What makes the pain better or worse?
- Have you experienced any previous injuries that may be related to this incident?

10.13 / **4.** *If you were evaluating this injury, which anatomical structures would you have palpated/tested, and why?*

The peroneal nerve needs to be tested to be sure there is no palsy occurring. In this particular incident, no palsy was present. The ankle joint also needs to be thoroughly examined to detect if there is involvement of the syndesmotic ligaments and the interosseous membrane. This would present as acute tenderness over the anterolateral joint line.[89] This is significant because the proximal fibula rotates during ankle motion.

10.13 / **5.** *What is the normal treatment for this condition?*

This condition is easily missed because it rarely occurs. A good history is important in catching this injury. Treatment, from an athletic trainer's perspective, should be immediate referral to an orthopedic physician, especially if the peroneal nerve is involved. Treatments vary, from closed reduction with immobilization and avoidance of weight bearing for a period of time, to open reduction with internal fixation followed by immobilization. Jennifer could consider performing modalities for pain control; however, she should be cautious about using ultrasound, because of the possibility of a fracture. Jennifer should refer Susie for radiographs to rule out a fracture and then, possibly, to an orthopedist for further evaluation if needed.

10.13 / **6.** *What underlying causes could have influenced this injury?*

The answers may vary from student to student. Some possible causes are (1) hypermobile joints resulting from laxity of ligaments and (2) pregnancy that causes ligamentous laxity. These two conditions can increase the mobility of the proximal tibiofibular joint, specifically the anterosuperior and posterosuperior tibiofibular ligaments. These ligaments are merely a thickening of the joint capsule with the anterior being thicker than the posterior.[89]

## CASE 10.14 Pes Anserine Bursitis

10.14 / **1.** *Based on the information presented in the case, determine (a) the differential diagnoses and (b) the clinical diagnosis.*

a. Differential diagnoses: prepatellar bursitis, hamstring (semitendinosus, semimembranosus) strain, jumper's knee, patellofemoral pain syndrome, plica, Osgood-Schlatter disease, osteochondritis dissecans[52]

b. Clinical diagnosis: pes anserine bursitis

10.14 / **2.** *What, if anything, did you recognize in the case that was inaccurate?*

The muscles attaching to the pes anserine are the semitendinosus, gracilis, and sartorius—not the semimembranosus. The semimembranosus inserts into the posterior aspect of the tibia.

10.14 / **3.** *What is the most appropriate way to manually test the muscles involved in this injury?*

This could vary depending on the reference source utilized.[15,48] The against-gravity position for the sartorius would be in a supine or sitting position, and the patient flexes, abducts and externally rotates the hip by bringing the heel of the affected foot up the shin of the unaffected side (Figure A10.14.1). Resistance is placed on the anterolateral surface of the distal thigh in the direction of extension, adduction, and medial rotation and against the lower medial leg in the direction of medial rotation.[15,48] Although the gracilis cannot be isolated from the rest of the adductor muscles, it can be tested collectively in the resisted gravity eliminated position.[15] This position is the supine position, and the athlete moves the hip toward midline while the clinician resists the hip into abduction from the medial aspect of the thigh just proximal to the knee. Alternatively, the adductors may be tested while the athlete is lying on the affected side with his body in a straight position with the lumbar spine and lower extremities straight. The clinician then holds the unaffected leg into abduction, and the athlete then adducts the affected leg while the clinician resists toward abduction against the medial aspect of the distal end of the thigh.[48] Finally, the semitendinosus would be tested in the prone position and, to isolate the medial hamstrings, the clinician resists flexion and internal rotation of the tibia. The athlete brings the heel toward the lateral aspect of the same buttock, and the clinician places resistance in the direction of knee extension and tibial external rotation.[15]

FIGURE A10.14.1 Sartorius manual muscle testing.

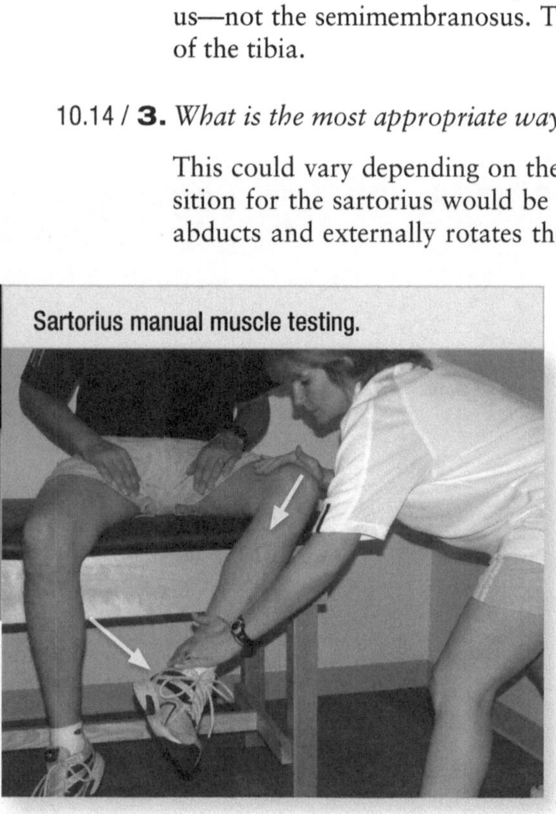

Clinician resists lateral rotation, abduction, and flexion of the hip.

10.14 / **4.** *If you were the evaluating clinician, what would be your treatment recommendations?*

Answers may include ice, ice massage, ultrasound, electric stimulation, and/or iontophoresis for pain and inflammation control. Referral to a physician may be considered for an injection. Stretching of the hamstrings and the adductor muscles and inclusion of the D2 LE PNF pattern may be useful.[90] Strengthening of the hip and knee joint may be useful as well.

10.14 / **5.** *What diagnostic imaging could be performed to help determine the clinical diagnosis?*

An MRI can be performed to confirm the clinical diagnosis. Because of the diffuse medial knee pain, pes anserine bursitis can be mistaken for a medial meniscal tear and/or medial collateral ligament injuries. An MRI can be performed to differentiate between medial mensical tears and pes anserine bursitis, which can result in the avoidance of unnecessary arthroscopic surgery.[28]

## CASE 10.15 Compartment Syndrome

10.15 / **1.** *Based on the information presented in the case, determine (a) the differential diagnoses and (b) the clinical diagnosis.*

a. Differential diagnoses: medial tibial stress syndrome, deep vein thrombosis, tibial stress fracture[57]

b. Clinical diagnosis: exercise-induced anterior compartment syndrome

10.15 / **2.** *Was everything performed during the physical examination that could or should have been performed?*

A neurovascular screening should be considered because compartment syndrome can affect the neurovascular structures located within each space.

10.15 / **3.** *(a) What diagnostic test can be done to confirm the clinical diagnosis? (b) What are the normal ranges of pressure in the area of the injury? (c) What is the treatment for the abnormal ranges?*

a. Intracompartment pressures are measured using various methods. The injection technique was the first to be used, but it is limited to resting measurements. The infusion technique is used for both dynamic and resting measurements. The non-infusion technique is the most ideal technique, but it is not readily available. There is also a micro-tip transducer technique.

b. Normal intracompartmental pressure ranges from 0 to 8 mm Hg.[96]

c. Abnormal ranges above 30 mm Hg require a fasciotomy.[38] Some researchers suggest more precise measurements, such as when pressures are above 15 mm Hg at rest, 30 mm Hg after a 2-minute exercise test, and/or more than 20 mm Hg after a 5-minute exercise test.[24]

10.15 / **4.** *(a) What do you believe would be the most appropriate treatment in Lisa's case after she presented to Hugh? (b) What are some alternative activities that could be performed to allow for proper cardiovascular training but not worsen the condition?*

a. Conservative treatment usually consists first of resting, ice, and stretching.[57] One may try modalities such as ice and electric stimulation to assist with pain control. Stretching of the anterior muscles of the leg may also be attempted. Probably the most important treatment would be holding Lisa from practice to allow for the inflammatory process to subside and to assist with a reduction of symptoms.

b. To allow for continued cardiovascular training during three-a-days, pool running may be beneficial as a non–weight-bearing activity. Other non-weight-bearing activities can also be used, such as the bike and upper body ergometer.

10.15 / **5.** *(a) Why do you think Hugh pulled Lisa out of practice? (b) What are the risks if she continues to play? (c) How long would you keep Lisa out of three-a-days? (d) What would be your response to the coach if she told you she was not happy with the decision presented in this case?*

a. Answers may include that Hugh pulled her out of practice to allow for the symptoms and inflammation to subside.

b. If playing or the activity that increases pain continues, increased pressure of the compartment increases, therefore causing vascular and neurological compromise. The increased pressure results in decreased blood flow to the muscles, causing decreased nourishment to the muscle and nerves. This in turn causes ischemic pain and paresthesia.[38,69,91]

c. Lisa should remain on the sidelines during three-a-day practices until her symptoms cease altogether and do not return during activity.

d. This answer will vary among students, depending on the student's education, clinical training, and other experiences. In fact, the question should be discussed with the classroom instructor. This question works well as a group discussion because there is not necessarily only one correct answer.

10.15 / **6.** *(a) How would you approach the coach and suggest that the training regime be changed? (b) If the coach were not receptive to Hugh's suggestions, what other course of action could he take?*

a. The answers will vary among students. Consider discussing this question with a coach you feel comfortable talking to or with your classroom instructor as a group activity. Some suggestions may include educating the coach on the implications of the injury. Use current research to show that conservative treatment is not always effective. Educate the coach on what compartment syndrome is and the long-term effects of the injury.

b. Some suggestions may be to speak to the coach's supervisor, which may be the Athletic Director. This should be done only as a last resort. Remember that the athletic trainer is responsible for the athlete's well-being and he needs to be an advocate for his injured athletes. Hugh may want to set up a meeting between himself, the athletic director, and the coach if problems continue.

## CASE 10.16 Osgood-Schlatter Disease

10.16 / **1.** *Based on the information presented in the case, determine (a) the differential diagnoses and (b) the clinical diagnosis.*

a. Differential diagnoses: slipped capital femoral epiphysis, patellar tendonitis, tibial stress fracture, pes anserine bursitis, infrapatella bursitis, prepatellar bursitis, patellofemoral pain syndrome, iliotibial tract friction syndrome, sepsis, trauma, tumor[43]

b. Clinical diagnosis: Osgood-Schlatter disease

10.16 / **2.** *Identify the etiology for this clinical diagnosis.*

Osgood-Schlatter disease is a condition that affects younger athletes, males more than females, from the ages of 10 to 15 years.[41] This disease is caused by repetitive trauma that causes part of the patellar tendon to avulse from the tibial tuberosity. Symptoms for this condition usually begin at the onset of a growth spurt.[41,42] This is when the attachment of the patellar tendon to the tibial tuberosity is most vulnerable and more likely to pull away from its attachment at the tibial tuberosity.[41,62]

10.16 / **3.** *What are the three classifications for this clinical diagnosis?*

Based on radiographs, Osgood-Schlatter disease can be classified into three types:

- Type I: The tibial tuberosity is prominent and irregular.
- Type II: The tibial tuberosity is prominent and irregular with a small free bone particle that is anterior and superior to the tuberosity.
- Type III: A free particle of bone is present that is located anterior and superior to the tuberosity. The tibial tuberosity appears normal in this type.[41,95]

10.16 / **4.** *(a) What else, if anything, could Nate have asked in his history to assist with determining the differential diagnosis? (b) Is there anything else Nate should have evaluated?*

a. Nate could have asked Jayden which foot he primarily jumps off of when playing basketball. With Osgood-Schlatter disease, pain is typically in the dominant knee. If Jayden reports that his right foot is dominant, then this would help support Nate's suspicion that Jayden is suffering from Osgood-Schlatter disease.[34] Nate could have asked about everyday activities and the cause of pain, particularly when negotiating stairs and squatting activities without jumping. It may be necessary to elaborate more on whether it is the jumping that causes pain, whether it is the stretch of the quadriceps muscles, or whether it is the eccentric phase of the quadriceps contraction that is causing the pain.

b. Nate did not perform palpation at the tibial tuberosity, the sight at which the abnormality was evident. With Osgood-Schlatter disease, the tibial tuberosity is typically point tender. If Nate palpated the site, this would have assisted him in determining the clinical diagnosis. Nate may want to examine the flexibility of the quadriceps/rectus femoris muscle and hamstrings to determine if the knee musculature is unbalanced.

10.16 / **5.** *What would be an appropriate treatment?*

The answers may vary among students. Answers should suggest that activity should be modified, resting the knees as much as possible. Ice, compression, and the use of an NSAID should also be considered. Bedigrew has found that it is helpful to place a homemade knee strap along the knee to ease pain levels. The knee strap compresses the patellar tendon, which allows the contraction of the quadriceps with less force placed on the tibial tuberosity.[7] The knee strap is made of a piece of rubber tubing, a shell of a pen, and athletic tape.[7] Consider performing hamstring and quadriceps stretching exercises and exercises to strengthen the vastus medialis oblique. Avoidance of hyperextension and flexion exercises greater than 90° would also be appropriate in the early phases of rehab.[41]

10.16 / **6.** *Jayden and his parents ask Nate if Jayden is able to continue playing basketball, because he has a tournament this weekend that he wants to compete in. What would be your response to this question? Would you allow Jayden to continue playing? Why or why not? When would you allow Jayden to return to playing if you feel he should not play?*

The answers may vary among students. As stated above, the best treatment for Osgood Schlatter disease is rest and/or modification of activity. It may be necessary to sit out this weekend to allow the inflammation to dissipate. Pain should be a good indicator of when he can return to play.

10.16 / **7.** *If conservative treatment does not work, what would be an alternative treatment?*

If the patient does not respond to cryotherapy, modification of activity, compression, and the use of NSAIDs, then casting is an option.[62] If the symptoms continue to persist, then surgical intervention may be necessary to remove the bony or cartilaginous ossicles or, in some cases, remove the tibial tuberosity.

# REFERENCES


1. Aladin A, Lam KS, Szypryt EP. The importance of early diagnosis in the management of proximal tibiofibular dislocation: a 9- and 5-year follow-up of a bilateral case. *Knee.* 2002;9(3):233–236.
2. American Red Cross. *Emergency Response.* Yardley, PA: Staywell; 2001.
3. Aminaka N, Gribble P. Patellar taping, patellofemoral pain syndrome, lower extremity kinematics, and dynamic postural control. *J Athl Train.* 2008;43(1):21–28.
4. Anderson JC, Courson R, Kleiner D, McLoda T. National Athletic Trainers' Association Position Statement: emergency planning in athletics. *J Athl Train.* 2002;37(1): 99–104.
5. Bazluki J. Surgical intervention and rehabilitation of chronic patellar tendinitis. *J Athl Train.* 1996;31(1):65–67.
6. Beck BR. 1998; Tibial stress injuries: an aetiological review for the purposes of guiding management. *Sports Med.* 1998;26(4):265–279.
7. Bedigrew S. Injury management update. Inexpensive Osgood-Schlatter management. *Athl Ther Today.* 2003;8(3):54–55.
8. Bennell KL, Malcolm SA, Thomas SA, Wark JD, Brukner PD. The incidence and distribution of stress fractures in competitive track and field athletes: a twelve-month prospective study. *Am J Sports Med.* 1996;24(2):211–217.
9. Bennell K, Matheson G, Meeuwisse W, Brunker PD. Risk factors for stress fractures. *Sports Med.* 1999;28(2):91–122.
10. Berry DC. Diagnosis of a medial tibial stress fracture by ultrasound. *Athl Ther Today.* 2007;12(2):16–20.
11. Bircan C, Senocak O, Peker O, et al. Efficacy of two forms of electrical stimulation in increasing quadriceps strength: a randomized controlled trial. *Clin Rehabil* [serial online]. 2002;16(2):194–199.
12. Blazina ME, Kerlan RK Jobe, FW, Carter, VS, Carlson, G J. Jumper's knee. *Orthop Clin N Am.* 1973;4(3):665–678.
13. Brunker P, Bradshaw C, Bennell K. Managing common stress fractures: let risk level guide treatment. *Physician Sportsmed.* 1998;26(8):39–48.
14. Carter DR, Caler WE, Spengler DM, Frankel VH. Uniaxial fatigue of human cortical bone. The influence of tissue physical characteristics. *J Biomech.* 1981;14(7):461–70.
15. Clarkson, H. *Musculoskeletal Assessment: Joint Range of Motion and Manual Muscle Strength.* Philadelphia, PA: Lippincott Williams & Wilkins; 2000.
16. Clews AG. Dislocation of the upper end of the fibula. *Can Med Assoc J.* 1968;98(3):169–170.
17. Couture C, Karlson KA. Tibial stress injuries. *Physician Sportsmed.* 2002;30:29–36.
18. Crossley K, Bennell KL, Wrigley T, Oakes BW. Ground reaction forces, bone characteristics, and tibial stress fracture in male runners. *Med Sci Sports Exerc.* 1999;31(8):1088–1093.
19. Cutts S, Edwards A. Clinical review. *GP: Gen Pract.* 2006;49–50.
20. Dale RB, Caswell C. Functional rehabilitation for "jumper's knee". *Athl Ther Today.* 2007;12(5):7–10.
21. Dath R, Chakravarthy J, Porter KM. Patella dislocations. *Trauma.* 2006;8:5–11.
22. Delaney RJ, MIB, Macnab I. Simple dislocation of the superior tibio-fibular joint; report of two cases. *Can Med Assoc J.* 1956;74(11):906–908.
23. Dupont JY. Synovial plicae of the knee: controversies and review. *Clin Sports Med.* 1997;16(1):87–122.
24. Edmundsson DG, Toolanen, Sojka P. Chronic compartment syndrome also affects nonathletic subjects: a prospective study of 63 cases with exercise-induced lower leg pain. *Acta Orthop.* 2007;78(1):136–142.
25. Edwards PH, Wright ML, and Hartman JF. A practical approach for the differential diagnosis of chronic leg pain in the athlete. *Am J Sports Med.* 2005;33(8):1241–1249.
26. Enad JG. Patellar tendon ruptures. *South Med J.* 1999; 92(6):563–566.
27. Felson DT, Niu J, McClennan C, et al. Knee buckling: prevalence, risk factors, and associated limitations in function. *Ann Intern Med.* 2007;147(8):534–540.
28. Forbes JR, Helms CA, Janzen DL. Acute pes anserine bursitis: MR imaging. *Radiology.* 1995;194(2):525–527.
29. Fredericson M, Wun C. Differential diagnosis of leg pain in the athlete. *J Am Podiat Med Assoc.* 2003;93(4):321–324.
30. Galea A, Albers J. Patellofemoral pain. *Physician Sportsmed.* 1994;22(4):48.
31. Gardner PJ. Injury prevention & performance enhancement: shin splints. *Athl Ther Today.* 2003;8(2):52–53.
32. Gerbino PG. Adolescent anterior knee pain. *Oper Tech Sports Med.* 2006;14(3):203–211.
33. Gerbino PG, Griffin ED, d'Hemecourt PA, et al. Patellofemoral pain syndrome: evaluation of location and intensity of pain. *Clin J Pain.* 2006;22(2):154–159.
34. Gigante A, Bevilacqua C, Bonetti MG, Greco F. Increased external tibial torsion in Osgood-Schlatter disease. *Acta Orthop Scand.* 2003;74(4):431–431.
35. Giladi M, Ziv Y, Aharonson Z, Nili E, Danon YL. Comparison between radiography, bone scan, and ultrasound in the diagnosis of stress fractures. *Mil Med.* 1984;149(8): 459–451.
36. Green JR, Shahrdar C, Owens BD. Knee dislocations. *eMedicine* [electronic version]. 2008. Available from: http://www.emedicine.com/orthoped/TOPIC409.HTM. Accessed July 19, 2009.
37. Harner C, H^her J. Evaluation and treatment of posterior cruciate ligament injuries. *Am J Sports Med.* 1998;26(3): 471–482.
38. Hayakawa H, Aldington DJ, Moore AR. Acute traumatic compartment syndrome: a systematic review of results of fasciotomy. *Trauma.* 2009;11(1):5–35.
39. Heyde CE, Mahlfeld K, Stahel PF, Kayser R. Ultrasonography as a reliable diagnostic tool in old quadriceps tendon ruptures: a prospective multicentre study. *Knee Surg Sports Traumatol Arthrosc.* 2005;13(7):564–568.
40. Hubble MW, Hubble JP. *Principles of Advanced Trauma Care.* Clifton Park, NY: Delmar-Thompson Learning; 2002.
41. Huie G, Math KR, Bruno PJ. Osgood-Schlatter disease. *Physician Assist.* 2003;27(1):39.

42. Ishida K, Kuroda R, Sato K, et al. Infrapatellar bursal osteochondromatosis associated with unresolved Osgood-Schlatter disease: a case report. *J Bone Joint Surg Am.* 2005;87-A(12):2780–2783.

43. Jamil T. Could youngster's knee pain be 'something serious'? *Pulse.* 2005;65(3):56–56.

44. Johnson AE, Rose SD. Bilateral quadriceps tendon ruptures in a healthy, active duty soldier: case report and review of the literature. *Mil Med.* 2006;171(12):1251.

45. Jonsson P, Alfredson, H. Superior results with eccentric compared to concentric quadriceps training in patients with jumper's knee: a prospective randomized study. *Br J Sports Med.* 2005;39(11):847–850.

46. Kakarlapudi TK, Bickerstaff DR. Knee instability: isolated and complex. *Br J Sports Med.* 2000;34(5):395–400.

47. Kaufman SL, Martin LG. Arterial injuries associated with complete dislocation of the knee. *Radiology.* 1992;184:153–155.

48. Kendall FP, McCreary EK, Provance PG. *Muscle Testing and Function.* Baltimore MD: Lippincott Williams & Wilkins; 1993.

49. Konin JG, Wiksten D, Isear JA, Brader H. *Special Tests for Orthopedic Examination* 3rd ed. Thorofare NJ: Slack; 2006.

50. Korpelainen R, Orava S, Karpakka J, Siira P, Hulkko A. Risk factors for recurrent stress fractures in athletes. *Am J Sports Med.* 2001:29:304–310.

51. Kortebein PM, Kaufman KR, Basford JR, Stuart MJ. Medial tibial stress syndrome. *Med Sci Sports Exerc.* 2000;32(3 supplement):S27–S33.

52. LaPrade RF, Flinn SD. Pes anserine bursitis. *eMedicine.* October 2007. Available from; http://www.emedicine.com/sports/topic100.htmpercent20October percent202007. Accessed August 14, 2008.

53. Logan M, Williams A, Lavelle J, Wady Gedroyc W, Freeman M. The effect of posterior cruciate ligament deficiency on knee kinematics. *Am J Sports Med.* 2004;32(8): 1915–1922.

54. Lorei MP, Hershman EB. Peripheral nerve injuries in athletes: treatment and prevention. *Sports Med.* 1993; 16(2):130–147.

55. Lyle J, Crosby LA. Quadriceps tendon rupture. *eMedicine.* March 7, 2008. Available from: http://www.emedicine.com/orthoped/topic274.htm. Accessed January 2, 2009.

56. Marder RA, Timmerman LA. Primary repair of patellar tendon rupture without augmentation. *Am J Sports Med.* 1999;27(3):304–307.

57. Mazerolle SM, McDermott B, Silverberg E. Bilateral exertional compartment syndrome: a case report. *Athl Ther Today.* 2008;13(3):20–23.

58. McConaghy JR. What is the diagnostic accuracy of the clinical examination for meniscus or ligamentous knee injuries? *J Fam Pract.* 2002 Jan;51(1):85.

59. Merrill KD. Knee dislocations with vascular injuries. *Orthop Clin N Am.* 1994;25:707–713.

60. Milgrom C, Giladi M, Simkin A, Rand N, Kedem R, Kashtan H, Stein M, Gomori M. The area moment of inertia of the tibia: a risk factor for stress fractures. *J Biomech.* 1989;22(11–12):1243–8.

61. Mirzabeigim E, Jordan C, Gronley J, Rockowitz N, Perry J. Isolation of the vastus medialis oblique muscle during exercise. *Am J Sports Med.* 1999;27(1):50–53.

62. Moore M. "Coach my knees hurt!" *Virginia J.* 2006; 28(2):6–7.

63. Moss A, Mowatt AG. Ultrasonic assessment of stress fractures. *BMJ.* 1983;286:1479–1480.

64. Mowlavi A, Whiteman J, Wilhelmi BJ, Neumeister MW, McLafferty RD. Dorsalis pedis arterial pulse: palpation using a bony landmark. *Postgrad Med J.* 2002;78(926): 746–747.

65. Nitz A, Scoville C. Use of ultrasound in early detection of stress fractures of the medial tibial plateau. *Mil Med.* 1980;145(12):844–846.

66. Nordin M, Frankel VH. *Basic Biomechanics of the Musculoskeletal System.* 3rd ed. Philadelphia Pa: Lippincott Williams & Wilkins; 2001.

67. Noyes FR, Bassett RW, Grood ES, Butler DL. Arthroscopy in acute traumatic hemarthrosis of the knee: incidence of anterior cruciate tears and other injuries. *J Bone Joint Surg Am.* 1980;62-A(5):687–695,757.

68. Ozkan C, Kalaci A, Tan I, Sarpel Y. Bilateral dislocation of the knee with rupture of both patellar tendons: a case report. *Knee.* 2006;13(4):333–336.

69. Padhiar N. Chronic compartment syndrome of the leg. *SportEX Med.* 2009;(40):16–22.

70. Pell RF, Khanuja HS, Cooley GR. Leg pain in the running athlete. *J Am Acad Orthop Surg.* 2004;12(6):396–404.

71. Petersen W, Loerch S, Schanz S, Raschke R, Zantop T. The role of the posterior oblique ligament in controlling posterior tibial translation in the posterior cruciate ligament deficient knee. *Am J Sports Med.* 2008;36(3):495–501.

72. Pfeiffer R, DeBeliso M, Shea K., Kelley L, Irmischer B, Harris C. Kinematic MRI assessment of McConnell taping before and after exercise. *Am J Sports Med.* 2004;32(3): 621–628.

73. Potter P. Patellofemoral syndrome. *eMedicine.* March 16, 2006. Available from: http://emedicine.medscape.com/article/308471-overview. Accessed August 8, 2008.

74. Pouilles JM, Bernard J, TremolliËres F, Louvet JP, Ribot C. Femoral bone density in young male adults with stress fractures. *Bone.* 1989;10(2):105–8.

75. Prentice WE. *Arnheim's Principles of Athletic Training: A Competency-Based Approach.* 13th ed. Boston MA: McGraw Hill Publishing; 2009.

76. Purdam CR, Cook JL, Hopper DM, Khan KM, Group VTS. Discriminative ability of functional loading tests for adolescent jumper's knee. *Phys Ther Sport.* 2003;4(1):3–9.

77. Rizzotto JB. Postsurgical rehabilitation of a quadriceps tendon rupture. *J Sports Chiropr Rehabil.* 1997;11(4): 147–150,181–142.

78. Romani W, Gieck J, Perrin D, Saliba E, Kahler D. Mechanisms and management of stress fractures in physically active persons. *J Athl Train.* 2002;37(3):306–314.

79. Romani W, Perrin DH, Dussault RG, Ball DW, Kahler DM. Identification of tibial stress fractures using therapeutic continuous ultrasound. *J Orthop Sports Phys Ther.* 2000; 30(8):444–452.

80. Roush M, Sevier T, Wilson J, et al. Anterior knee pain: a clinical comparison of rehabilitation methods. *Clin J Sport Med.* 2000;10(1):22–28.
81. Rovere GD, Adair DM. Medial synovial shelf plica syndrome: treatment by intraplical steroid injection. *Am J Sports Med.* 1985;13(6):382–386.
82. Scholten RJ, Opstelten W, van der Plas CG, Bijl D, Deville WL, Bouter LM. Accuracy of physical diagnostic tests for assessing ruptures of the anterior cruciate ligament: a meta-analysis. *J Fam Pract.* 2003 Sep;52(9):689–94.
83. Servi JT. Patellofemoral joint syndromes. *eMedicine.* March 22, 2008. Available from: http://emedicine.medscape.com/article/90286-overview. Accessed August 8, 2008.
84. Shaffer RA, Brodine SK, Almeida SA, Williams KM, Ronaghy S. Use of simple measures of physical activity to predict stress fractures in young men undergoing a rigorous physical training program. *Am J Epidemiol.* 1999;149(3):236–42.
85. Souza RB, Powers CM. Predictors of hip internal rotation during running: an evaluation of hip strength and femoral structure in women with and without patellofemoral pain. *Am J Sports Med.* 2009;37(3):579–587.
86. Starkey C, Ryan J. *Evaluation of Orthopedic and Athletic Injuries.* 2nd ed. Philadelphia PA: F.A. Davis; 2002.
87. Steadman's Concise Medical Dictionary. *Steadman's Medical Dictionary.* Philadelphia PA: Lippincott Williams & Wilkins; 2001.
88. Tanner SM, Soileau R, Lemons JE. A modified test for patellar instability: the biomechanical basis. *Clin J Sport Med.* 2003;13(6):327–338.
89. Van Seymortier P, Ryckaert A, Verdonk P, Almqvist KA, Verdonk R. Traumatic proximal tibiofibular dislocation. *Am J Sports Med.* 2008;36(4):793–798.
90. Voss D, Ionta M, Myers B. *Proprioceptive Neuromuscular Facilitation: Patterns and Techniques.* 3rd ed. Philadelphia PA: Harper & Row; 1985.
91. Warrington G. A case of increased pressure. *Nurs BC.* 2009;41(1):27–28.
92. Werier J, Keating JF, Meek RN. Complete dislocation of the knee: the long-term results of ligamentous reconstruction. *Knee.* 1998;5(4):255–260.
93. Wilson J, Best, T. Common overuse tendon problems: a review and recommendations for treatment. *Am Fam Physician.* 2005;72(5):811–818.
94. Wind W, Bergfeld J, Parker R. Evaluation and treatment of posterior cruciate ligament injuries: revisited. *Am J Sports Med.* 2004;32(7):1765–1775.
95. Woolfrey BF, Chandler EF. Manifestations of Osgood-Schlatter's disease in late teen age and early adulthood. *J Bone Joint Surg Am.* 1960;42, 327–369.
96. Wright E. Neurovascular impairment and compartment syndrome. *Paediatr Nurs.* 2009;21(3):26–29.

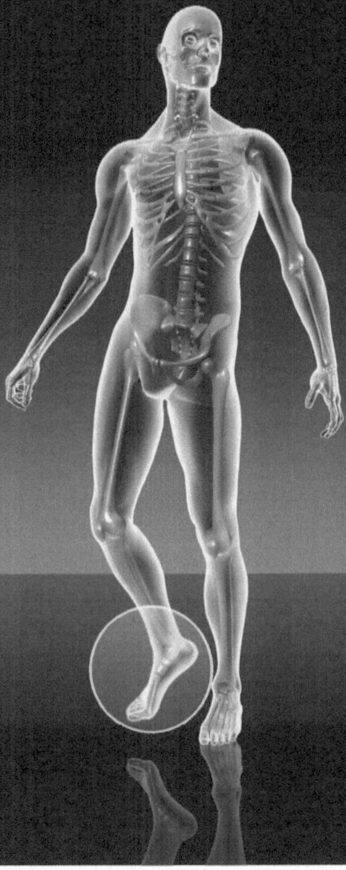

CHAPTER 11

# Ankle, Foot, and Toes

## QUICK REFERENCE

CASE 11.1
**ATF and CF Ligament Sprain with Peroneal Tendon Strain**

CASE 11.2
**Deltoid Sprain with Fibula Fracture**

CASE 11.3
**Syndesmosis Sprain**

CASE 11.4
**First MTP Joint Sprain (Turf Toe)**

CASE 11.5
**Posterior Tibialis Tendonitis with Spring Ligament Instability/Sprain**

CASE 11.6
**Achilles Tendon Rupture (Third Degree)**

CASE 11.7
**Plantar Heel Contusion**

CASE 11.8
**Ankle Dislocation**

CASE 11.9
**Peroneal Tendon Subluxation**

CASE 11.10
**Calcaneus Fracture**

CASE 11.11
**Metatarsal (Jones Fracture)**

CASE 11.12
**Sesamoid Fracture**

CASE 11.13
**Metatarsal (March Fracture)**

CASE 11.14
**Medial Tibial Stress Syndrome (MTSS) with Posterior Tibialis Tendonitis**

CASE 11.15
**Retrocalcaneal Bursitis**

CASE 11.16
**Tarsal Tunnel Syndrome**

CASE 11.17
**Plantar Fasciitis**

CASE 11.18
**Plantar Neuroma (Morton's Neuroma)**

# ANSWERS TO CASE QUESTIONS

## CASE 11.1 ATF and CF Ligament Sprain with Peroneal Tendon Strain

11.1 / **1.** *Based on the information presented in the case, determine (a) the differential diagnoses and (b) the clinical diagnosis.*

a. Differential diagnoses: ankle fracture, foot fracture, peroneal tendon subluxation, Achilles tendon rupture, tendonitis, tenosynovitis[93]

b. Clinical diagnosis: sprain of the anterior talofibular ligament (ATFL) and calcaneofibular ligament (CFL) with concomitant peroneal strain (caused by an excessive eccentric force)

11.1 / **2.** *Based on the information presented in the case, do you believe Josh took an adequate history? If not, what, if any, additional questions would you ask as the evaluating clinician?*

Answers will vary among students. They should remember that when assessing an acute lateral ankle sprain, determining the MOI and position of the joint at the time of injury is really the first step in a good clinical assessment.[4,151] It is often easier for the patient to demonstrate the position of the involved ankle with the uninvolved ankle rather than trying to explain the position. As the evaluating clinician, remember to phrase the questions as open-ended, rather than forced-choice (e.g., Ask, "Can you explain what position your foot was in?" instead of, "Was your foot turned inward?"). Also, determine if the injury was unprovoked or if it occurred in a situation that normally does not result in ankle injury, because the patient's condition may be result of another pathology, such as tarsal coalition, osteochondritis, or peroneal tendon dislocation.[4] The history should include the location of pain, presence of swelling, and functional capacity, including the ability to bear weight, walk, run, and jump. Additional questions that should be asked include ones about any prior injuries, treatments, impairments,[59] or joint weaknesses. If there was a feeling that the ankle gave way,[127] age, general health status, occupation (e.g., in the setting outside of collegiate or high school sports), and leg dominance should be ascertained.

11.1 / **3.** *Overall, do you believe Josh adequately evaluated Jasmine's condition given the clinical presentation? If not, what would you have done differently as the evaluating clinician?*

The answers to this question will vary among students. Overall, Josh appeared to perform an adequate clinical examination; however, one issue of concern is related to Figure 11.1.2. Assessment textbooks commonly recommend placing the ankle in a plantarflexed position between 15° and 20° when performing an anterior drawer.[69,106,124,131] However, Josh decided to place the ankle in a neutral position, which can yield questionable results, even though in this case it was reported as a positive finding.

The ability of stress tests such as the anterior draw and talar tilt to differentiate between specific ligaments has been reported as debatable.[47] A cadaver biomechanical analysis aimed at quantifying the instability of the hindfoot complex during the anterior displacement of the hindfoot by five clinicians under three conditions (intact ligaments, after sectioning the ATF ligament in an isolated ATFL injury, then after sectioning the CF ligament in a combined ATFL/CFL injury) found greater anterior displacement in

**TABLE A11.1.1** ATFL and CFL displacement under three conditions.[47]

| CONDITION | NEUTRAL POSITION | 20° PLANTARFLEXION |
|---|---|---|
| Intact ATFL | 15.1 mm (± 4.0 mm) | 8.3 mm (± 4.0 mm) |
| Sectioned ATFL | 19.0 mm (± 3.0 mm) | 10.3 mm (± 4.4 mm) |
| Combined ATFL and CFL section | 19.2 mm (± 3.2 mm) | 10.9 mm (± 3.8 mm) |

**TABLE A11.1.2** ATFL and CFL force during 80-Newton anterior drawer testing with foot at different flexion angles.

| POSITION | ATFL IN NEWTONS | CFL IN NEWTONS |
|---|---|---|
| 10° Dorsiflexion | 33 (SE, 6) | 40 (SE, 6) |
| Neutral | 23 (SE, 5) | 15 (SE, 5) |
| 10° Plantar flexion | 34 (SE, 6) | 6 (SE, 3) |
| 20° Plantar flexion | 53 (SE, 24) | –3 (SE, 2) |

the neutral position (Table A11.1.1).[47] It is believed, however, that when the foot is in plantarflexion, the ATFL orients itself parallel to the long axis of the fibula, acting as the main collateral ligament.[24] This then supports the result of Bahr,[9] who found greater force application to intact cadaver ATFL when in 20° of plantarflexion (Table A11.1.2). Bahr also noted a small increase in anterior translation between the intact and cut ATFL in 10° and 20° of plantarflexion. When both ligaments were transected, cadaveric anterior translation increased at all flexion angles used during testing.[9] In a more recent study, researchers found that knee and ankle position influences anterior drawer laxity and stiffness of the ankle complex.[71] Specifically, they found that anterior drawer testing of the ankle complex with the knee positioned at 90° of flexion and 10° of ankle plantarflexion produced the most laxity and the least stiffness. This suggests that this position permits better isolation of the ankle ligamentous structures than knee extension or a neutral ankle position. Clinically, these three studies provide very different results; however, two of the three studies used cadaver sections of the lower leg, while Kovaleski[71] used human subjects. This fact suggests that other factors may affect the sensitivity of the test, including (1) variations in individual tissue properties and bony structures, (2) torque and axial load application by a clinician, (3) joint position (knee and ankle), and (4) the effects of other structures such as the gastrocnemius-Achilles tendon complex.[47,48,71,75]

11.1 / **4.** *(a) What is the name of the ligamentous stress test performed in textbook Figure 11.1.3? (b) Why is it used, and what is considered a positive finding?*

a. The stress test performed in Figure 11.1.3 is commonly referred to as the talar tilt or inversion stress maneuver.

b. It is commonly used to evaluate injuries of the lateral ligaments of the ankle joint,[48,78] particularly the stability of the CFL. The test is typically performed with the patient lying supine or side-lying, with the foot relaxed. The ankle is held in a neutral position while the clinician supports the calcaneus and tries to invert the calcaneus with respect to the tibia.[78] The difficulty with the test is that there ". . . is no standardized value for the degree of talar tilt, which indicates instability" and that the test cannot evaluate isolated pathologies of the lateral ankle ligaments (i.e., CFL).[48] Gaebler found that reports of talar tilt values more than 5° greater than those of the involved side indicate significant injury, even though a tilt of 15° to 30° indicates only moderate instability.[48] Lynch sites reports that talar tilt values between 5° and 23° are normal, but a 10° difference between ankles is considered abnormal.[78]

11.1 / **5.** *Josh assessed active and passive ROM as part of the on-field assessment; however, his clinical findings do not list any specific ROM limitations. (a) Why do you believe this is the case? (b) If you were doing the evaluation, how could you quantify AROM, particularly ankle dorsiflexion? (c) How much active dorsiflexion is considered normal during a walking gait?*

a. The most probable explanation for a lack of quantitative ROM findings as part of the physical examination is a lack of goniometer.

b. Goniometry is typically used to assess PROM, but it can be used to asses AROM as well. To assess ankle dorsiflexion, the patient is placed in short-sitting or long-sitting with the knee flexed 20° to 30° to reduce gastrocnemius tension. The axis of the goniometer is placed inferior to the lateral malleolus while the stationary arm is parallel to the long axis of the fibula and the movable arm is parallel to the sole of the foot.

c. During a normal walking gait, a patient should be able to produce 10° of ankle dorsiflexion from mid-stance to terminal stance.

# CASE 11.2 Deltoid Sprain with Fibula Fracture

11.2 / **1.** *Based on the information presented in the case, determine (a) the differential diagnoses and (b) the clinical diagnosis.*

a. Differential diagnoses: fibula fracture, medial malleolus fracture, talus fracture, calcaneus fracture, syndesmosis sprain, lateral ankle sprain, peroneal strain

b. Clinical diagnosis: deltoid sprain concomitant fibula fracture

11.2 / **2.** *Mary presented with tenderness over and inferior to the distal medial malleolus. Identify the structures responsible for providing medial ankle joint stability.*

The medial "deltoid" ligament is a fan-shaped (delta), broad complex with an apical attachment above to the medial malleolus and to the talus, calcaneus, and navicular bone, and spring ligament.[123] Although clinicians commonly refer to the ligament as a single unit, it is composed of superficial and deep fibers and is divisible into separate anatomical parts.[118,123] The superficial fibers are comprised of the tibiocalcaneal (TC) (apex of the medial malleolus to the calcaneus directly below the medial malleolus) and tibionavicular (TN) (runs beneath and slightly posterior to the anterior tibiotalar ligament, inserting onto the medial navicular surface) ligaments.[87,118] The deep fibers are composed of the anterior tibiotalar (ATT) (anteromedial medial malleolus to the superior medial talus) and posterior tibiotalar (PTT) (posterior medial malleolus to the posterior talus) ligaments. During maximum ankle dorsiflexion (10°–20°), the TC and PTT are taut; the ATT and TN are taut during 30°–40° of ankle plantarflexion.[118,131]

11.2 / **3.** *Based on the clinical presentation and the MOI, what is one pertinent history question Nichole could have asked to guide the physical examination?*

In this case, based on the MOI (forced ankle eversion) and the injury pattern (especially the medial popping sensation), Nichole would have been wise to ask about any other unusual sounds or sensations, such as cracking or snapping. A cracking or snapping sensation would correspond with trauma (fracture) to the distal fibula. The lower position of the lateral malleolus (distal fibula) limits eversion ankle injuries. However, in situations in which excessive eversion forces have been applied and there is direct trauma to the distal fibula, concomitant injury such as fibula fracture, or a bimalleolar fracture should be suspected with a medial ankle sprain.

11.2 / **4.** *As the evaluating clinician, in addition to the obvious anatomical landmarks (e.g., malleoli), what other bony anatomical landmarks would you have assessed to guide the physical examination?*

The answers to this question will vary among students. However, emphasis should be placed on structures such as the tibia, fibula (particularly the distal end), talus, calcaneus, navicular, cuienforms, cuboid, and metatarsals.

11.2 / **5.** *Overall, do you believe Nichole made the correct decision by removing Mary from the ice after completing her on-ice evaluation? If not, why? What would you have done differently?*

The answers to this question will vary among students. However, a review of the vital signs (blood pressure 126/90; radial pulse 124 bpm, rapid, weak; and respiration 21, shallow, labored) may suggest shock. Even though the pulse and respiration rate appear normal, given the case's clinical presentation (participating in athletics), the rhythm and quality are abnormal. The vital signs in this case mandate immediate medical intervention, including supplemental oxygen and activation of EMS.

11.2 / **6.** *As a new certified athletic trainer, how would you respond to the assistant coach's request for playing status? If a difference of opinion occurred, how and when should the situation be handled?*

This answer to this question will vary among students and should be discussed with the classroom instructor. In fact, this question is best answered as a group discussion, because there is not necessarily only one correct answer. Certainly, the actions of the coach were at best inappropriate and could have been handled much differently.

## CASE 11.3 Syndesmosis Sprain

11.3 / **1.** *Based on the information presented in the case, determine (a) the differential diagnoses and (b) the likely clinical diagnosis?*

a. Differential diagnoses: lateral ankle sprain, distal fibula fracture, fibula dislocation, peroneal tendon dislocation[112]

b. Clinical diagnosis: distal tibiofibular syndesmosis sprain, often referred to as a "high ankle sprain"

11.3 / **2.** *What is the typical MOI for this injury?*

A variety of mechanisms individually or in combination can result in a syndesmotic injury. The most common mechanisms, individually and particularly in combination, are external rotation of the leg and hyperdorsiflexion of the ankle.[96,152]

Syndesmotic sprains are an uncommon injury that has a reported incidence of between 1 and 11 percent of all ankle injuries.[27,56] It is a significant injury in athletes because of the extended lost time from participation[152] and if misdiagnosed or managed incorrectly, it may lead to unfavorable consequences later on.[152] There is no one specific MOI of a syndesmotic ankle sprain.[16] Besides occurring in combination with external rotation of the leg and hyperdorsiflexion of the ankle, other reported causes include eversion, plantarflexion, and pronation.[96] A syndesmotic sprain may occur in isolation or associated with other trauma such as a fibula fracture.[96,154] For a comprehensive review of the anatomy, biomechanics, and mechanisms of tibiofibular syndesmosis ankle sprains, please review *The Anatomy and Mechanisms of Syndesmotic Ankle Sprains* by Norkus and Floyd.

11.3 / **3.** *Obviously, the ICD-9 CM code provided by the PA was incorrect. (a) What is an ICD-9 CM code, and based on the clinical diagnosis, (b) what is the correct ICD-9 code for this injury?*

a. ICD-9-CM stands for International Classification of Disease, Ninth Revision, Clinical Modification and is used for medical billing purposes. The ICD-9 CM consists of three volumes. Volume 1 contains the diagnosis codes all providers need for billing and Volume 2 is an alphabetical index of Volume 1. Volume 3 contains inpatient hospital procedures. Because computerized searches do the same thing as a printed index, the second volume is not a useful data file. Outpatient diagnostic or treatment centers, like physician offices, need only Volume 1. The final volume contains procedure codes. These are used for billing inpatient hospital stays. The ICD-9 is used more by clinicians working in the outpatient rehabilitation or in billing situations. The code selected should most accurately describe the condition being treating based on the objective physical findings. When a clinician is treating more than one condition, a code is required for each condition.

b. According to the clinical diagnosis, a syndesmosis sprain would be coded as 845.03. The first three numbers (845) describe the condition (sprains and strains of ankle and foot). The number after the decimal (0) describes the joint (ankle). The final number (3) describes the special location; therefore, 845.03 means: sprain/strain of ankle, distal tibiofibular ligament.

11.3 / **4.** *During the physical examination, Dr. Angus performed a neurological assessment including dermatomes, myotomes, peripheral nerves, and deep tendon reflexes. What are the two main deep tendon reflexes in the lower extremity?*

The two main deep tendon reflexes in the lower extremity include the patellar tendon (L2, L3, L4) and the Achilles tendon (S1, S2). Please refer to your current assessment textbook for the correct procedures when assessing deep tendon reflexes.

11.3 / **5.** *Dr. Angus performed several provocative tests to determine the stability of the ankle. If the patient asked you to explain these tests and the purpose behind them, what would be your response?*

The external rotation test[20] and squeeze test[56] are two provocative tests used in the clinical diagnosis of syndesmotic ankle instability (anterior and posterior inferior tibiofibular, transverse tibiofibular, and interosseous ligaments).[16,154] To perform an external rotation test, the patient sits with the knee at 90° of flexion and the ankle held in neutral. The clinician sits in front of the patient, stabilizing the lower leg with one hand and grasping the medial aspect of the foot with the other while using the forearm for support. An external rotation stress is then applied to the involved forefoot in an attempt to reproduce external rotation of the talus, which increases pressure on the fibula, causing the injured ankle mortise to spread. A positive test produces pain over the anterior or posterior inferior tibiofibular ligaments and over the interosseous membrane.[20] The squeeze test is performed by manually compressing the fibula to the tibia above the midpoint of the calf.[56] The test is considered positive when proximal compression produces distal pain in the area over the distal tibiofibular and interosseous ligament. This test is also used to identify fibula fractures when pain is described along the fibular shaft, rather than at the distal tibiofibular joint.

Of these two tests, the external rotation test has demonstrated good interrater reliability (K = 0.75); the squeeze test was found to have moderate reliability (K = 0.50).[3] However, pain rather than displacement of the anterior and posterior inferior tibiofibular ligaments should be considered the outcome measure of these tests.[16,17] When making return-to-play decisions, patients with a positive external rotation test result took significantly longer to return to playing sports.[3]

11.3 / **6.** *If this dancer had been a football player and you were attempting to stabilize the ankle for further medical referral, describe how you could properly stabilize the joint.*

The answers will vary among students; however, there are several methods to stabilize an ankle injury, these include the following:

- Ankle stirrup: SAM SPLINT®, best used to immobilize injuries to the distal tibia and fibula and ankle
  (1) Stabilize and support the extremity.
  (2) Assess the distal neurovascular status.
  (3) Pad the splint and/or bony areas to prevent local pressure.
  (4) Fold a 36-inch SAM® SPLINT in half, creating a C-curve two thirds of the distance down each half. A reverse C-curve may be added for additional support.
  (5) Using the athletic trainer's leg as a model, mold the splint around the extremity so that the medial and lateral malleoli are located in the middle of the splint. The ankle should be held in a neutral position if possible.

(6) The splint is applied to the athlete from the heel and gently molded around the distal tibia and fibula. Padding may be applied to the malleoli for comfort.
(7) Secure the splint using the wrap of choice (e.g., elastic wrap, cravat).
(8) Beware of excessive pressure on the peroneal nerve when securing the splint.
(9) Re-assess the distal neurovascular status, and document findings.

- Cadillac Splint: SAM SPLINT®, used to immobilize injuries to the distal tibia, fibula ankle, and foot and may work well when a neutral ankle position cannot be maintained
  (1) Stabilize and support the extremity.
  (2) Assess the distal neurovascular status.
  (3) Pad splint and/or bony areas to prevent local pressure.
  (4) Fold a 36-inch SAM SPLINT® in half creating a "U". Form a C-curve two thirds of the distance down each half of the splint.
  (5) Cut an 18- to 24-inch splint.
  (6) A reverse C-curve may be added for additional support.
  (7) Using the athletic trainer's leg as a model, mold the shorter splint to form a posterior "L" splint from the toes to the popliteal fossa.
  (8) Mold the 36-inch "U" splint around the extremity so that the medial and lateral malleoli are located in the middle of the splint.
  (9) Apply the posterior splint "L" first from the toes to just distal to the popliteal fossa, followed by the "U" splint.
  (10) Padding may be applied to the malleoli for comfort.
  (11) Secure using the wrap of choice (e.g., elastic wrap, cravat, roller bandage).
  (12) Beware of excessive pressure on the peroneal nerve when securing the splint.
  (13) Re-assess the distal neurovascular status, and document findings.

- A soft splint can also be used to immobilize general injuries to the foot and ankle
  (1) Stabilize and support the extremity.
  (2) Assess the distal neurovascular status.
  (3) Prepare three cravats and slide under the Achilles tendon.
  (4) Mold a pillow or rolled-up blanket around the injured ankle.
  (5) Secure two cravats superior to the malleoli, and secure a third cravat around the foot.
  (6) Use additional cravats, if warranted, for greater support.
  (7) Re-assess the distal neurovascular status, and document findings.

## CASE 11.4 First MTP Joint Sprain (Turf Toe)

11.4 / **1.** *Based on the information presented in the case, determine (a) the differential diagnoses and (b) the clinical diagnosis and the common term used to describe the clinical diagnosis.*

a. Differential diagnoses: sesamoiditis, phalange fracture, flexor hallucis longus tenosynovitis, bursitis, nerve compression, contusion[5,119]

b. Clinical diagnosis: a possible grade II first metatarsophalangeal joint sprain. It is often referred to as "turf toe."[2,7,19] The term "turf toe" was first coined by Bowers and Martin when they described sprains of the plantar capsule ligament of the first metatarsophalangeal joint in football players and examined two predisposing factors: (1) playing surface hardness and (2) shoe stiffness.[19]

11.4 / **2.** *(a) In your opinion, was the MOI in this case typical for the injury? (b) What other mechanism, if any, may cause the injury?*

a. Turf toe is most commonly seen in football players, but it can occur in other sports when athletes wear lightweight, flexible shoes and play on artificial turf.[2,63,64,150] The combination of shoe flexibility and hard, unyielding surface causes the athlete's shoe to grasp the playing surface and the foot to slide forward, increasing the forward momentum of the body on the planted forefoot. As the down pressure on the forefoot increases, the MTPJ is forced into hyperextension and pushed beyond the biomechanical limits of the plantar-capsule ligament.[2,19,29,135]

b. Other plausible MOIs include excessive valgus stress from a strenuous push-off,[29] direct contact to the protruding heel by another player (which drives the distal aspect of the opposing player's planted and dorsiflexed foot and toes beyond the limits of the joint),[2] leaps by ballet dancers upon landing, and the kicking of a non-yielding surface.[49,124]

11.4 / **3.** *If you were the evaluating clinician in this case, based on the clinical presentation, what one other item would you expect to observe during the inspection phase of the physical examination?*

Based on the clinical diagnosis and clinical presentation in this case, including the diminished pain and AROM and PROM, an athletic trainer should expect to observe changes in the athlete's gait pattern[2] as he attempts to avoid dorsiflexing the MTPJ during the toe-off phase of the gait cycle.

11.4 / **4.** *(a) Identify the bony and soft tissue structures Al should have palpated as part of his evaluation specific to the foot. Then (b) identify the anatomical landmarks in textbook Figure 11.4.2.*

a. The exact anatomical structures palpated will depend on the extent of the athlete's pain and apprehension. Given the information presented in the case, Al would have been wise to palpate the structures listed below. Additionally, close attention should be given to the medial and lateral collateral ligaments and sesamoid bones to rule out concomitant injury.[64]

- Bony: forefoot—5 metatarsals and 14 phalanges, paying particular attention to the first MTP and 2 sesamoids; midfoot—navicular, cuboid, cuneiforms (medial, intermediate, lateral)
- Soft: tarsometatarsal joint, intermetatarsal joint, deep transverse ligament, collateral and plantar ligaments of the first MTP, intrinsic foot muscles (adductor

and abductor hallucis, plantar interosseous), flexor hallucis longus and brevis, flexor digitorum longus and brevis, plantar aponeurosis

b. Answers appear in Figure A11.4.1.

11.4 / **5.** *What is the purpose of the first MTPJ valgus stress test, and how is it performed? If you were the evaluating athletic trainer, would you have performed this test? If so, why? If not, what other test might you have performed?*

a. A first MTPJ valgus stress test is a provocative test used to diagnose damage to the medial collateral ligament and joint capsule of the first MTPJ. The test is performed with the athlete in long or short sitting and/or supine position, with the clinician stabilizing the distal metatarsal. With the first MTPJ in neutral, a clinician grasps the proximal distal phalange and attempts to move the phalange laterally. The clinician assesses for increased pain and/or laxity as compared with the uninvolved side.

b. Two other possible provocative tests are the intermetatarsal glide test (Figure A11.4.2), to assess for trauma to the deep transverse ligament, and the interosseous ligament. Assessment of the dorsal and plantar joint capsule can be accomplished using dorsal and plantar glides (Figure A11.4.3).

FIGURE A11.4.1 View of an adult ankle and foot with structures identified.

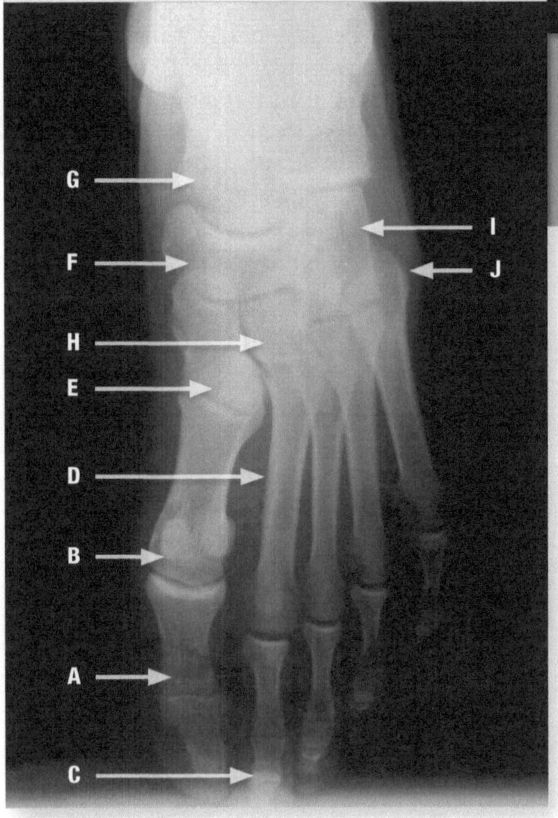


A = Proximal phalange
B = Sesamoids
C= Middle phalange
D = 2nd metatarsal
E = First cuneiform
F = Navicular
G = Talus
H = Second cuneiform
I = Cuboid
J = 5th metatarsal or styloid process

FIGURE A11.4.2 Intermetatarsal glide test.

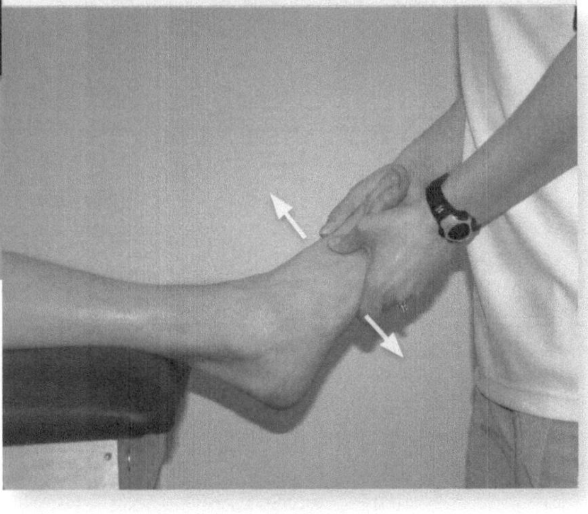

Arrows indicate direction of alternating forces.

FIGURE A11.4.3 Dorsal and plantar glides.

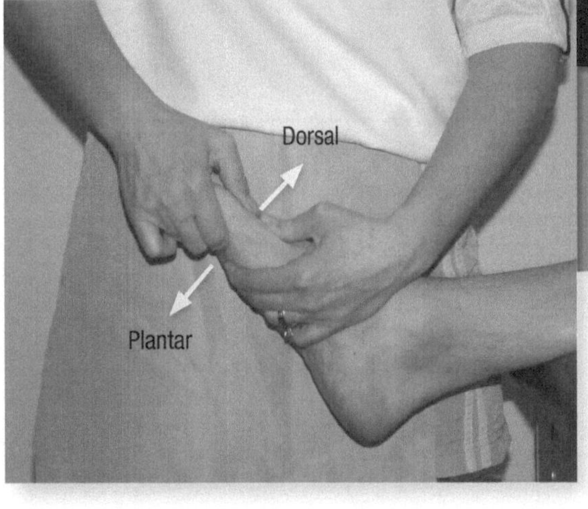

11.4 / **6.** *Clearly Ika'aka was extremely upset and annoyed by Al's decision to place him on the injured reserve list. If this were your athlete and he did not return for treatment or a follow-up evaluation, how would you handle this situation?*

The answers to this question will vary among students. Student-athletes should be made aware before the beginning of the season (in writing) that this type of behavior will not be tolerated. Failing to report to the athletic training room for medical care when an athlete has been told to do so jeopardizes his ability to return to full function, affects the team, and places the athletic trainer in a difficult situation with the coaching staff. An athlete's failure to comply with recommendations from the athletic trainer needs to be documented in the athlete's medical file. For further information, please discuss this case with your staff athletic trainer to determine how she would handle this situation.

## CASE 11.5 Posterior Tibialis Tendonitis with Spring Ligament Instability/Sprain

11.5 / **1.** *Based on the information presented in the case, determine (a) the differential diagnoses and (b) the clinical diagnosis.*

a. Differential diagnoses: tarsal tunnel syndrome, flexor digitorum longus tenosynovitis, posterior tibialis strain

b. Clinical diagnosis: posterior tibialis tendonitis with possible plantar calcaneonavicular ligament (spring ligament) trauma

11.5 / **2.** *During the observation component of the physical examination, Emma apparently performed a posterior evaluation of Carrie's posture and noted pes planus. If you were the evaluating clinician, what other lower extremity postural deviations, if any, would you want to note?*

Postural assessments should be viewed from all directions—anterior, lateral, and posterior—using a plumb line to detect any deviations from the ideal posture. In this case, when performing a posterior assessment of ideal posture of the lower extremity, a clinician should observe the following:

- Are the feet evenly spaced from the plumb line?
- What is the degree of rearfoot varus or valgus?
- What is the position of subtalar joint (i.e., what is the position of the navicular relative to the floor)?
- What is the degree of lower leg lateral (external) rotation, how many toes are visible bilaterally?
- Are the knees evenly spaced from the plumb line?
- Do the popliteal creases line up bilaterally?
- What is the degree of knee lateral (external) rotation?
- What is the symmetry of the soft tissue?

11.5 / **3.** *Emma noted palpable tenderness directly behind the medial malleolus up to the distal calf and from the sustentaculum tali to the navicular. (a) What structure is located between the sustentaculum tali and the navicular? (b) What is the clinical significance of this structure?*

a. The structure is the plantar calcaneonavicular ligament, often referred to as the spring ligament. It spans from the navicular beak to the sustentaculum tali (a horizontal eminence arising from the medial surface of the calcaneus that serves as a point of soft tissue attachment and support for the talus). The spring ligament, in combination with the deltoid ligament, forms a socket for the head of the talus and provides support to the medial longitudinal arch.[123,131,136]

b. Both the term "spring ligament" and the structure's functional role are in question.[136] According to Davis,[37] the consensus among researchers is that the spring ligament is composed of the superomedial calcaneonavicular and inferior calcaneonavicular.[136] However, Taniguchi believes that the spring ligament fibrocartilage complex consists of three components: superomedial calcaneonavicular ligament, inferior calcaneonavicular ligament, and a structure they termed the third ligament, which comprises fibers running from the notch between the calcaneal facets to the navicular tuberosity. When there is trauma to the spring ligament, fibrocartilage complex dysfunction of the posterior tibialis tendon can occur, resulting in a flat foot position as the support for the head of the talus collapses. Conversely, loss of function of the posterior tibialis tendon results in stretching of the calcaneonavicular ligament, failure of the medial longitudinal arch, and decreased push-off during ambulation.[136]

11.5 / **4.** *Do you believe that textbook Figure 11.5.2, the positive manual muscle testing, demonstrates the proper procedure for evaluating manual muscle strength of the ankle plantar flexors and foot invertors against gravity? If not, what if anything would you do differently?*

Figure 11.5.2 demonstrates the correct procedure in assessing muscle strength of the tibialis posterior muscle, which is a primary foot invertor and secondary ankle plantar flexor. In situations requiring that gravity be eliminated, place the patient in a supine position with the heel off the table and the foot and ankle in a neutral position.

11.5 / **5.** *Why did Emma apply a LowDye taping procedure? If you were the treating clinician, how would you perform the taping procedure?*

A LowDye taping procedure is used in treating pathologies such as an arch strain and plantar fasciitis. It provides support and corrects foot and lower leg structural abnormalities.[11] Materials needed include one-inch and two-inch non-elastic tape, two-inch elastic tape, and adherent spray. The application process is as follows:

- The patient assumes a long-sitting position with her foot over the edge of the table in a neutral position.
- Apply the adherent spray to the medial and lateral surface of the foot.
- Place an anchor (1-in non-elastic tape) directly to the skin from the lateral surface of the fifth MPTJ around the heel to the first MTPJ. Repeat this two or three times while overlapping half of the tape width.
- Apply an anchor strip using the two-inch elastic tape on the lateral dorsum of the proximal foot, across the plantar surface to the medial dorsum of the foot. Repeat two more times overlapping half of the tape width, ensuring that the one-inch tape is covered.
- Repeat the anchor strip (the 1-in non-elastic tape) from the lateral surface of the fifth MPTJ around the heel to the first MTPJ.
- Close the procedure using the two-inch elastic tape on the lateral dorsum, across the plantar surface, finishing back where the tape started (this encircles the foot).[11]
- Finally, determine patient comfort and effectiveness of the taping procedure.

Refer to your preferred taping text for alternative LowDye taping procedures.

## CASE 11.6 Achilles Tendon Rupture (Third Degree)

**11.6 / 1.** *Based on the information presented in the case, determine (a) the differential diagnoses and (b) the clinical diagnosis.*

a. Differential diagnoses: Achilles tendonitis, gastrocnemius, soleus and/or plantaris musculoskeletal pathology, ankle sprain, tarsal fracture, and tibia or fibula fracture[60]

b. Clinical diagnosis: Achilles tendon third-degree strain

**11.6 / 2.** *James asked several history questions to guide his physical examination. Identify three or four other history questions you, as the evaluating clinician, would have asked.*

To arrive at this clinical diagnosis, there are several other history questions a clinician could ask to assist in making the determination. These questions could include the following:

- What is your age? Males between the ages of 30 and 40 are at greatest risk.[65]
- Do you have a sedentary lifestyle? Do you feel like you overexert yourself when you do engage in physical activity? Do you tend to be much more active on the weekends?[65]
- What is your current level of training, technique, and footwear?[60]
- Do you have a history of previous injury[82] such as Achilles tendinopathies or contralateral tendon rupture? Did the patient hear and audible "snap"? Patients with a contralateral tendon injury are at an increased risk for Achilles tendon ruptures.[6]
- Do you have a history of prolonged corticosteroid therapy[108] or overuse of performance-enhancing drugs (anabolic steroids)?[95,100]
- Do you have a history of fluoroquinolone use? Fluoroquinolones are broad-spectrum antimicrobial medicines used to treat bacterial infections in many parts of the body, including skin infections, urinary tract infections, serious ear infections, bronchitis, pneumonia, tuberculosis, some sexually transmitted diseases (STDs). Studies have shown that the risk of Achilles tendon ruptures while using fluoroquinolone is greater in individuals over the age of 60 and is greater with simultaneous usage of corticosteroids.[145–147]

**11.6 / 3.** *(a) If you were the evaluating clinician, how would you assess plantarflexion strength based on the muscle strength grade found in the physical examination? (b) How do you explain Hancock's muscle strength, given the clinical diagnosis?*

a. Plantarflexion strength could be assessed two ways: in prone and standing positions. In a prone position, the gastrocnemius is assessed with the knee extended. Flexion of the knee to 45° places the gastrocnemius on slack and allows the clinician to assess the soleus.[31] In either position, resistance can be applied to the plantar surface of the foot (Figures A11.6.1 and A11.6.2) or to the posterior aspect of the calcaneus. However, because the gastrocnemius and soleus are very powerful muscles, assessment of the muscle in a weight-bearing position is often indicted. To assess strength in a weight-bearing position, a patient is asked to perform a single leg toe raise (i.e., heel raise) with the knee straight (isolates gastrocnemius) then with the knee flexed (isolates soleus).

b. In Hancock's case, a muscle grade of 3/5 would be obtained from testing the patient in a prone position. Even in the presence of a complete Achilles tendon rupture, a patient may continue to demonstrate active plantar flexion against resistance, because of the influence of the plantaris, peroneus longus, tibialis posterior, and great toe flexors, all which assist in ankle plantarflexion.[98,108,131,141] However, despite the activation of the secondary plantar flexors against gravity in a prone position, functional testing while bearing weight will be difficult to impossible with a complete Achilles tendon rupture.[65]

FIGURE A11.6.1

Isolating the gastrocnemius.

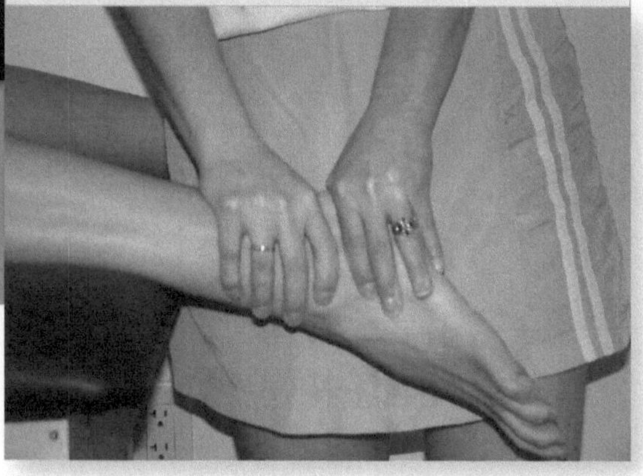

Knee should be extended over a table.

FIGURE A11.6.2

Isolating the soleus.

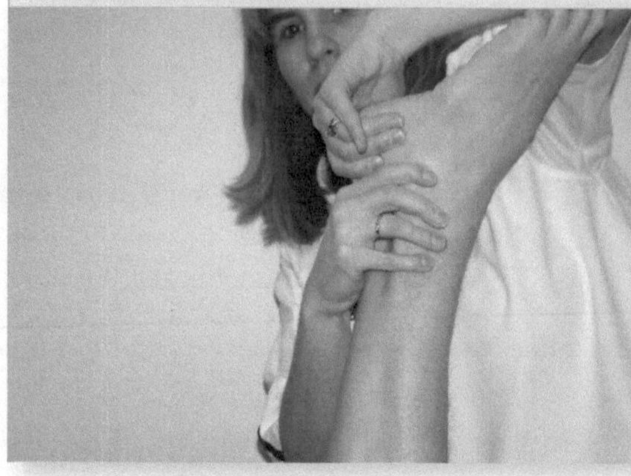

Knee should be flexed to 90°.

11.6 / **4.** *What is the name of the special test performed in textbook Figure 11.6.2? What is considered a positive finding?*

The special test performed in textbook Figure 11.6.2 is commonly referred to as the Thompson test,[128,138] Simmonds test[128], or the Simmonds–Thompson test.[40,125] Regardless of the name, the test is performed by placing the patient in a prone position with the feet hanging over the end of the plinth. In this position, a clinician squeezes the mid-calf, causing plantarflexion of the ankle. If no plantarflexion occurs, the test is positive for Achilles tendon rupture.[65,100] According to Scott and Chalabi, "The result of the Simmonds–Thompson test principally reflects the integrity of the soleus musculotendinous unit. Plantarflexion is caused by posterior bowing of the calf tendons and, to a lesser extent, by proximal displacement of the bellies of the gastrocnemius."[125] Thus, disruption of the soleus musculotendinous units seen in a complete Achilles tendon rupture will result in no movement of the foot into plantarflexion and is highly suggestive of a ruptured Achilles tendon.[62] However, Douglas[40] recently reported two cases in which patients with surgically treated Achilles tendon rupture and positive Simmonds–Thompson tests demonstrated rupture of only the gastrocnemius portion of the triceps surae complex and not the soleus. He suggests that when "treatment decisions are based on whether a rupture is partial or complete and whether the soleus is involved, the Simmonds–Thompson test alone is insufficient."[40,125]

11.6 / **5.** *During the physical examination, James assessed Hancock's dermatome patterns, which were unremarkable. (a) What are dermatomes? (b) If you were the evaluating clinician, what levels would you have assessed? Identify the location of these dermatome levels.*

a. Dermatomes are areas of skin supplied by cutaneous branches from a single spinal nerve and are used to determine the extent of spinal damage or neurological stenosis using a light stroking technique.

b. Based on the clinical diagnosis an assessment of L4–S2 would be warranted. Although dermatome patterns vary from author to author, the following are the dermatomes patterns as described in Schultz, Houglum, and Perrin.[124]

- L4: Level of L4, medial gluteals, lateral thigh and knee, anterior medial lower leg, dorsomedial aspect of foot and big toe
- L5: Level of L5, lateral knee and anterior leg, dorsum of foot (toes 2–4)
- S1: Level of S1, buttock, posterolateral thigh, plantar surface of lateral foot, fifth toe
- S2: buttock, posteromedial thigh, posterior, medial heel

# CASE 11.7 Plantar Heel Contusion

11.7 / **1.** *Based on the information presented in the case, determine (a) the differential diagnoses and (b) the clinical diagnosis.*

a. Differential diagnoses: plantar fasciitis, fat pad contusion, calcaneus stress fracture, Achilles tendon pathology, tarsal tunnel syndrome[101]

b. Clinical diagnosis: plantar heel contusion

11.7 / **2.** *(a) Was the MOI in this case typical for the injury? (b) What other mechanism, if any, may exist?*

a. In this case, compression on the heel upon landing from a jump was the primary mechanism, and marching 12 hours during his marching tour was most likely the event exacerbating the condition. This is a typical MOI.

b. A thick pad of fat covers the calcaneus. It is designed to compress under weight and absorb impact forces during activity. Injuries to the fat pad and the calcaneus (i.e., periosteum) normally occur in activities requiring sudden stop-and-go responses or sudden changes in horizontal or vertical positions (e.g., running and jumping),[49,106] which can overwhelm the fat pad's ability to dissipate force.

11.7 / **3.** *If you were the evaluating clinician in this case, what anatomical structures would you have palpated based on the clinical presentation?*

Based on the clinical presentation in this case, palpation of the rearfoot and midfoot would be warranted, particularly around the calcaneus. Tenderness at the origin of the plantar fascia on the medial tubercle may suggest plantar fasciitis; tenderness on the posterior calcaneus near the insertion of the Achilles may suggest retrocalcaneal bursitis. However, tenderness and increased pain beneath the heel and upon weight bearing (i.e., standing) and around the posterior plantar surface may suggest plantar fat pad syndrome.[94] The heel's fat pad, composed of an elastic fibrous tissue septa separating closely packed fat cells,[94] is optimized for load-bearing activities and acts as a shock absorber during a heel strike.[61]

11.7 / **4.** *(a) In your opinion, did Lt. Commander Logan make the correct decision in placing a single insert into Midshipman Brady's shoe? (b) What type of inserts would you consider using based on the clinical diagnosis?*

a. Based on the clinical findings of the physical examination, Lt. Commander Logan made an inappropriate decision by placing only one insert into the shoe.

b. The recommended inserts are heel pads or commercial heel cups, and they should be placed bilaterally to maintain a normal gait pattern. Two types exist, hard and soft, and both have been used with success.[13] Bedinghaus and Niedfeldt report that hard heel cups help to contain the heel pad under the calcaneus, assisting in restoration of fat-pad compressibility.[13] Soft cups aid in cushioning the fat pad while containing it at the same time.

11.7 / **5.** *Lt. Commander Logan requested that Midshipman Brady return to the athletic training facility so a staff athletic trainer can prepare him for practice. If you were the treating clinician, what would you do to prepare this athlete for athletic competition?*

The answers to this question will vary among students. One likely possibility is the application of either a donut pad or a taping procedure known as heel box technique.

Materials needed include half-inch or one-inch non-elastic tape and adherent spray. The application process is as follows:

- With the patient in a long-sitting position, with the foot over the edge of the table, spray the adherent spray on the heel.
- Place an anchor directly on the skin from the inferior medial malleolus, across the Achilles tendon, to the inferior lateral malleolus, using either half-inch or one-inch non-elastic tape.
- Apply another anchor strip from the inferior medial malleolus, across the plantar surface of the foot to the inferior lateral malleolus.
- Continue this pattern, overlapping the tape one-half width until the entire surface of the heel is covered.[11]

# CASE 11.8 Ankle Dislocation

**11.8 / 1.** *Based on the information presented in the case, determine (a) the differential diagnoses and (b) the clinical diagnosis.*

a. Differential diagnoses: tibia fracture, fibula fracture, tarsal dislocation, tarsal fracture

b. Clinical diagnosis: dislocation of the right talocrural joint

**11.8 / 2.** *Based on the clinical presentation and your clinical diagnosis, identify three to five additional history questions you may have asked as the evaluating clinician.*

The answers will vary among students, but may include the following:

- Do you have any previous history of ankle or foot injury or trauma? If so, are you currently wearing a brace?
- Do you feel any heaviness in the foot or ankle as a result of vascular trauma?
- Is your foot or ankle cold?
- Have you noticed any changes in sensitivity?
- Did you hear any sounds or feel any sensations other than the popping?

**11.8 / 3.** *Do you believe Jennifer and the EMTs adequately evaluated Georgia's condition? If not, what would you have done differently as the evaluating clinician?*

The answers to this question will vary among students. Given the patient's history and physical examination, Jennifer and the EMTs appear to have failed to assess Georgia's neurovascular status. Ankle dislocations typically present with concomitant trauma to the tibia, fibula, and/or neurovascular structures[53,67,126] and occur most often as a result of falls[66,134] and motor vehicle accidents.[113] The occurrence of ankle dislocations or fracture-dislocations in the athletic population is rare,[46,111,122,143] because a large amount of force is required to disrupt the inherent stability of the talocrural joint. Located adjacent to the tibia and fibula are neurovascular structures such as the common peroneal nerve and posterior tibial artery, all of which need to be carefully assessed during the physical examination to rule out neurovascular compromise (Table A11.8.1). Any change or compromise in the neurovascular status should be considered a medical emergency requiring immediate immobilization and transportation. Any change in the patient's neurovascular status, such as a dismissed pulse, cold feet, numbness, or loss of distal limb function, requires immediate medical attention to restore normal function.

**11.8 / 4.** *(a) If you were an athletic trainer at a high school or college/university and your athlete presented with signs and symptoms similar to those presented in the case, are there any equipment or clothing complications that may make the physical examination more challenging? (b) How would you handle this situation?*

a. The answers to this question will vary among students; however, shoe and athletic tape removal may complicate the situation.

b. "To remove or not remove the shoe, that is the question." Each actual situation will dictate the necessary care that must be provided by an athletic trainer. When a gross fracture-dislocation is suspected, the shoe may be loosened to the point where the dorsalis pedis and posterior tibial pulses are palpable.[131] In other situations, complete removal of the shoe may outweigh concerns over accessory foot movement, even when it is unknown if there is an associated fracture, in order to assess the athlete's neurovascular status.[67] Another factor making assessment of an ankle dislocation more complicated is the presence

**TABLE A11.8.1** Neurovascular assessment of the lower extremity.

| COMPARTMENT | LOCATION | ASSESSMENT |
|---|---|---|
| **Anterior compartment** | | |
| Anterior tibial artery | Originates opposite the inferior border of the popliteus muscle, terminating as the dorsalis pedis artery | Palpate the dorsalis pedis pulse on the dorsal surface of the foot lateral to the extensor hallucis longus tendon and distal to the dorsal most prominence of the navicular bone.[90] |
| Deep peroneal nerve | One of the two terminal branches of the common peroneal nerve; originates between the fibula and superior peroneus longus muscle, running inferomedial to the fibula deep to the extensor digitorum longus | Sensory: Assess sharp (pinwheel) and dull sensation (brush) located between dorsal web of the first and second digits.<br>Motor:* Assess muscle strength of extensor hallucis longus (i.e., great toe extension). |
| **Lateral compartment** | | |
| Superficial peroneal nerve | Second of the two terminal branches of the common peroneal nerve; begins between the fibula and superior peroneus longus muscle, running anterolateral to the fibula | Sensory: Assess sharp (pinwheel) and dull sensation (brush) located along the lateral aspect of leg and dorsum of foot.<br>Motor:* Assess muscle strength of ankle evertors (i.e., peroneus longus and brevis). |
| **Deep posterior compartment** | | |
| Tibial nerve | Terminal branch of the sciatic nerve, descending through the middle of the popliteal fossa, posterior to the popliteal artery and vein, descending the median plane of the calf, deep to the soleus and inferiorly on the tibialis posterior; terminates forming the medial and lateral plantar nerves | Sensory: Assess sharp (pinwheel) and dull sensation (brush) of the medial plantar nerve, which includes medial sole and medial three and one-half toes, and the lateral plantar nerve, which includes the lateral sole and lateral one and one-half toes.<br>Motor:* Assess muscle strength of ankle plantar flexors (i.e., soleus, gastrocnemius). |
| Posterior tibial artery | Terminal branch of the popliteal artery, passing deep to the origin of the soleus, passing inferomedially on the posterior surface of the tibialis posterior muscle until it runs posterior to the medial malleolus from which it is separated by the tendons of the tibialis posterior and flexor digitorum longus | Palpate for a pulse posterior and inferior to the medial malleolus. |

*More than one muscle or movement may be assessed to determine the integrity of the peripheral nerve. Please refer to your evaluation text for a complete list of peripheral nerves and their associated muscles.

of athletic tape, particularly when the tape is applied over the athlete's shoes. Given these two situations, a clinician should speak with the team physician and emergency medical personnel to determine the best course of action if a dislocated ankle ever does present itself and also should practice the removal of athletic tape applied over athletic shoes.

11.8 / **5.** *If you were the athletic trainer in this case, what type of immediate care would you have provided? Describe the steps you would have used.*

The answers to this question will vary among students. Immobilization of an ankle dislocation commonly requires the use of a vacuum splint to stabilize the joint in the position found. Remember to check for signs of circulation, sensation, and movement (CSM) before and after immobilization of the extremity. Cover all open wounds with sterile dressings, and apply cryotherapy in and around the area if necessary to decrease edema formation.

## CASE 11.9 Peroneal Tendon Subluxation

11.9 / **1.** *Based on the information presented in the case, determine (a) the differential diagnoses and (b) the clinical diagnosis.*

a. Differential diagnoses: peroneal tendon rupture, acute lateral ankle sprain, osteochondral lesion, lateral process fractures of the talus[105]

b. Clinical diagnosis: peroneal tendon subluxation

11.9 / **2.** *Jamie asked several specific history questions to guide the physical examination. However, there was one question that he did not appear to ask, which may have assisted in narrowing down the clinical diagnosis. Can you identify this question?*

"Did you hear or have any popping or snapping sensations when the injury occurred?" Jamie did a good job in taking an adequate history, but he failed to ask about any popping or snapping sensations related to either the acute injury or Tammy's current condition. Patients often report hearing a loud "pop" when the injury initially occurs and experience pain around the distal fibula.[79] In chronic cases, the patient reports a history of peroneal tendon instability and a "clicking" or snapping sensation behind the lateral malleolus.[79] He could also have questioned her further about the MOI in an attempt to determine if Tammy experienced sudden forced ankle dorsiflexion with a forceful reflex contraction of the peroneal muscles. This is the common MOI,[25,79,116] and it occurs when the resistance of the superior retinaculum is overcome and either tears or is subperiosteally stripped from its fibular insertion,[120] allowing the two peroneal tendons to dislocate or sublux from within the fibular groove.[25,43]

11.9 / **3.** *(a) If Tammy had presented immediately after her injury occurred, but with her current clinical features, a careful history and physical examination would be needed to rule out what similar condition? (b) What pieces of information from the physical exam or history could have led Jamie to differentiate and determine the clinical diagnosis?*

a. In an acute setting, the patient's diagnosis of peroneal tendon subluxation/dislocation is often determined based on the history and physical exam, but this can be mistaken for an acute lateral ankle sprain unless a careful history and physical examination are completed.[79]

b. Unlike lateral ankle sprains, which present with anterior fibula (lateral malleolus) pain and tenderness, peroneal tendon subluxation/dislocation presents with posterior fibula tenderness and pain, particularly over the peroneal retinaculum.[116] Patients with peroneal tendon trauma all demonstrate pain with eversion of the ankle, rather than inversion, which is commonly seen with lateral ankle sprains.

11.9 / **4.** *During the physical examination, Jamie was able to reproduce Tammy's feeling that the tendon was sliding by using RROM testing. If you were the evaluating clinician, what specific motion would you muscle test, and how would you perform it?*

Talocrural dorsiflexion and subtalar eversion resisted muscle testing have been recommended to reproduce the symptoms or show obvious dislocations of the peroneal tendons, with emphasis on subtalar eversion. To isolate the peroneus longus and brevis, the patient should be side-lying with the involved leg on top, hanging over the edge of the examination table. The clinician stabilizes the lower leg distal fibula and applies resistance to both the lateral border of the foot and the plantar surface of the first metatarsal

FIGURE A11.9.1 Manual muscle testing of peroneal muscles.

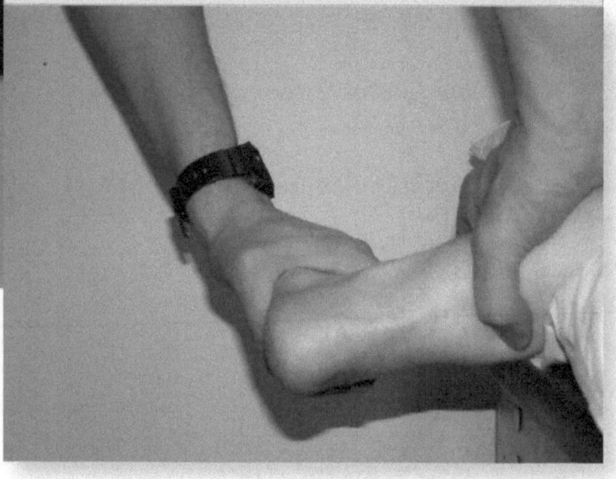

while the patient attempts to resist the foot from moving from eversion into inversion and elevating the first metatarsal[31] (Figure A11.9.1).

Safran, O'Malley, and Fu[120] suggest an alternative provocative test to determine dynamic instability of the peroneal tendon. In their method, a patient is instructed to lie prone on the examination table with the knee flexed to 90°. After visually inspecting the posterior lateral malleolar region for a subluxated or dislocated peroneal tendon, and for swelling, the ankle is then actively dorsiflexed and plantar flexed, then everted against resistance, which allows for visualization of peroneal tendon instability as the tendon dislocates or subluxes from the groove behind the lateral malleolus.

11.9 / **5.** *Given the MOI, clinical presentation, and date of initial injury, Tammy's condition appears to have progressed from an acute injury to a more recurrent chronic injury. (a) If Tammy had been treated within the first 24 hours, what type of conservative care approach would you have taken? (b) What are her options if this condition continues?*

a. The answers to this question will vary among students. However, acute dislocations of the peroneal tendon can be treated conservatively with immobilization, cryotherapy, and compression. Initial immobilization may include the use of a short-leg, non-weight-bearing splint. This is followed by placing a felt[79] or a U-shaped pad[105,126] against the peroneal tendon to allow the tendon to remain in place and adhere to the fibula when swelling has begun to subside. Heavy taping and wrapping can be used to allow the athlete to return to play in some situations.[105]

b. If conservative treatment fails to resolve the "popping" or "snapping," and the patient is diagnosed with a chronic subluxing peroneal tendon, surgical repair individualized to the patient's specific pathology is warranted.[120] Safran, O'Malley, and Fu report that there are more than 18 different surgical procedures, all with good to excellent results, and that the surgical approach employed depends on where the surgeon intends to deepen the peroneal groove, re-route the tendons (under the calcaneofibular ligament), repair the tendon, or perform reconstruction and reinforcement of the tissue.[25,79,120] Refer to your team's orthopedic surgeon for more information about the preferred method.

## CASE 11.10 Calcaneus Fracture

11.10 / **1.** *(a) Based on the information presented in the case, determine the clinical diagnosis. (b) What is the typical MOI?*

a. Clinical diagnosis: fracture of the calcaneus

b. Calcaneus fractures typically occur when an axial load is applied to the heel. This injury may result from jumping or falling from a height or from a motor vehicle accident when the foot is pressed firmly against the floor.[109,110]

11.10 / **2.** *Do you believe the EMT adequately evaluated the condition in this case? If not, what would you have done differently as the evaluating clinician?*

The answers to this question will vary among students. It would appear that the medical team provided adequate medical care given the information presented in the case. Any discussion addressing the need for spinal stabilization and helmet removal would be appropriate in this case scenario.

11.10 / **3.** *If you were an athletic trainer at a high school or college/university and your athlete presented with signs and symptoms similar to those in the case, what other type of functional testing could you perform to assist in making the clinical diagnosis?*

The calcaneus is the largest of all the tarsal bones and is the point of attachment for ankle ligaments, the Achilles tendon, plantar fascia, and intrinsic foot muscles. Together, the calcaneus, Achilles tendon, plantar fascia, and intrinsic foot muscles provide the foot with a mechanical advantage by acting as a long and strong lever arm during walking, standing, and crouching.[109,110] Thus, an athletic trainer, depending on the clinical presentation, may consider assessing the patient's ability to bear weight, because this will normally be compromised on the involved side.[109,110]

11.10 / **4.** *If you were an athletic trainer at a high school or college/university and your athlete presented with signs and symptoms similar to those presented in the case, how would you remove the athlete from the field?*

The answers to this question will vary among students; however, any removal from the field in this case should be accompanied with immobilization of the foot. Immobilization techniques may include the use of a soft splint, Cadillac splint, posterior splint, ankle stirrup, or vacuum splint. After the injury is immobilized, the athlete can safely be removed using a variety of techniques, including the simple two-person lift or backboard.

11.10 / **5.** *If you were the evaluating athletic trainer in this case, how would you have removed DJ's shoe when he was in the medical facility?*

To adequately assess an ankle or foot injury may require removal of the athlete's shoe. This is accomplished by removing or cutting the athlete's shoe laces, opening the shoe, and pulling the tongue down to the toes (Figure A11.10.1, (a) and (b)). The heel counter is then pulled away from the foot, and the shoe is slid up and off the foot as gently as possible, with assistance when possible.[131] In some instances, the athlete may elect to remove his own shoe. Ankle braces using Velcro or straps should be removed following

FIGURE A11.10.1 **Shoe removal for a suspected calcaneus fracture.**

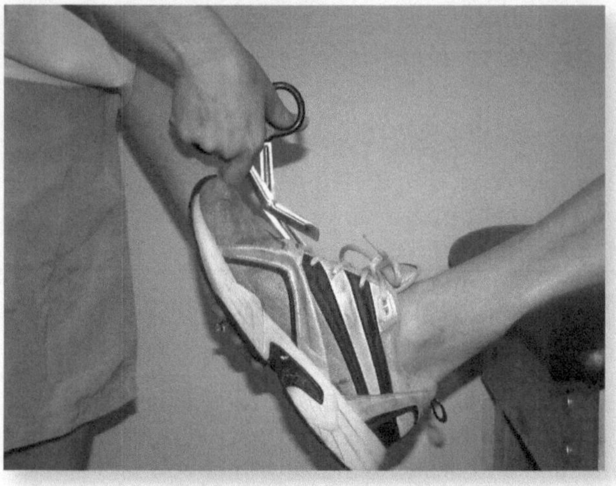

(a) Note: Using scissor or EMT shears, cut down along the laces.

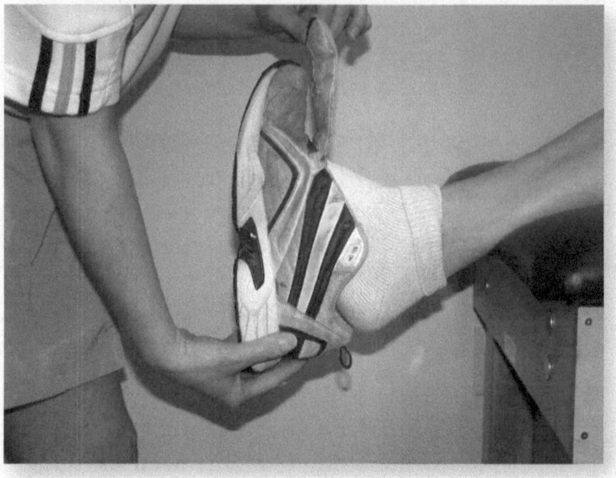

(b) Note: After pulling out the tongue, slide heel counter down and away from the heel.

the manufacturer's directions. Ankle tape can be removed using a tape cutter on the side opposite of pain beginning proximally and working distally along the plantar surface of the foot.[131] In the presence of a possible severe ankle fracture-dislocation, an athletic trainer should loosen the shoe or brace only enough to assess the neurovascular status of the athlete and then use the shoe as part of the splinting device.

## CASE 11.11 Metatarsal (Jones Fracture)

**11.11 / 1.** *Based on the information presented in the case, determine (a) the differential diagnoses and (b) the clinical diagnosis.*

a. Differential diagnoses: lateral ankle sprain, tibia, fibula and tarsal fracture, stress fracture[107]

b. Clinical diagnosis: Jones fracture

**11.11 / 2.** *What are the Ottawa Ankle Rules, and what information in the case led Mike to suspect the need for radiographs?*

The Ottawa Ankle Rules are a set of clinical parameters developed in 1990s to evaluate the need for ankle and midfoot radiographs based on simple, well-defined historical and physical findings.[132] If a patient does not exhibit any of the specific criteria outlined below, radiographs of the foot or ankle are not warranted after trauma.[97,132] The following are indications for ankle and midfoot radiographs[97]:

- Ankle: tenderness over the inferior or posterior pole of either malleolus, including the distal 6 cm; inability to bear weight (take 4 steps independently, even if limping) at the time of injury and at the time of evaluation
- Midfoot: tenderness along the base of the fifth metatarsal or navicular bone; inability to bear weight (4 steps) at the time of injury and at the time of examination

The establishment of the Ottawa Ankle Rules is believed to have reduced unneeded ankle films by 28 percent,[132] thereby saving millions of dollars annually in healthcare costs.[97,102] The Ottawa Rules have also been applied to the knee, cervical spine, and head. For a comprehensive review of the effects of the Ottawa Rules please review *Impact of Clinical Decision Rules on Clinical Care of Traumatic Injuries to the Foot and Ankle, Knee, Cervical Spine, and Head* by Perry and Stiell.[102]

**11.11 / 3.** *Mike asked several history questions to guide the physical examination. (a) Based on the information presented in the case, do you believe Mike took an adequate history? (b) If not, what additional questions would you ask as the evaluating clinician?*

a. The answers to this question will vary among students. Students should recognize the need to perform a more thorough history.

b. Some of the items a student may focus on based on the case include: (1) further examination of Lance's pain using OPQRTS, (2) questioning about previous injury or trauma to the foot, and (3) ability to bear weight and whether Mike was able to walk without assistance.

**11.11 / 4.** *Based on the clinical diagnosis above, why did Lance present with decreased ankle eversion and plantarflexion strength?*

Resisted ROM testing suggests trauma to the peroneus longus and brevis, most likely a strain. It is likely that as Lance stepped into the pothole the peroneal muscles (longus and brevis) eccentrically contracted to control inversion of the ankle. However, the force of the trauma overpowered the muscles, resulting in excessive lengthening of the tissue.

11.11 / **5.** *What injury should Mike suspect if Lance reported an MOI of forced inversion of the foot while the foot was plantar flexed. When does this commonly occur?*

Mike should suspect a pseudo-Jones fracture or what is commonly referred to as an avulsion fracture. This injury typically occurs when stepping off a curb or falling when climbing stairs.[107]

11.11 / **6.** *Overall, do you believe Mike adequately evaluated Lance's condition, given the information provided in the case? If not, what would you have done differently as the evaluating clinician?*

The answers to this question will vary among students. Given the athlete's history and physical examination, Mike appeared to perform a relatively complete physical examination, except for possibly two items. First, strength testing could have been performed in a side-lying position (against gravity position) to isolate the peroneal muscles. Second, ligamentous stress testing for a lateral ankle sprain and/or testing for fractures, such as a compression test, could have also been performed, considering the MOI.

## CASE 11.12 Sesamoid Fracture

11.12 / **1.** *Based on the information presented in the case, determine (a) the likely differential diagnoses and (b) the clinical diagnosis?*

a. Differential diagnoses: phalange fracture, MTPJ sprain, sesamoiditis, bursitis, hallux flexor strain[42,147,153]

b. Clinical diagnosis: fracture of one or both of the sesamoids located under the great toe

11.12 / **2.** *Based on the clinical diagnosis, is this mechanism of injury typical?*

Although sesamoid fractures can and do occur with acute direct trauma, such as a fall from a height, sudden loading of the foot, or a crush injury, patients will oftentimes report an insidious onset with no clear event or trauma to the first metatarsophalangeal joint.[5,12,89,153] Repetitive overuse of the first metatarsophalangeal joint can lead to sesamoid stress fractures[85] or sesamoditis, which when left untreated may result in a sesamoid fracture.

11.12 / **3.** *(a) What, if anything, could a clinician add to Nancy's evaluation to assist in determining the clinical diagnosis? (b) How would you perform the evaluation?*

a. The sesamoids of the great toe are located within the tendons of the flexor hallucis brevis (FHB) and are intratendinous except where they articulate with the cartilaginous bodies dorsally.[5] They are also the point of insertion for the abductor hallucis tendon on the medial (tibial) sesamoid and the adductor hallucis tendon on the lateral (fibular) sesamoid. This being the case, PROM may produce pain, and therefore, passive dorsiflexion and plantar flexion of the great toe should be performed.[147]

b. To isolate the MTPJ, an athletic trainer should stand to the side of the patient, stabilize the first metatarsal being assessed, then move the MTPJ to the limits of dorsiflexion and plantarflexion.

11.12 / **4.** *In your opinion, did Nancy make the correct decision in allowing Tiffany to return to play in the game? What, if anything, would you have done differently?*

The answers to this question will vary among students. However, based on the MOI, clinical findings of the physical examination, and the importance of the sesamoid of the hallux in absorbing body weight applied to the first ray and in aiding locomotion,[5] the conservative approach to the management of this case would be to withhold Tiffany from the match for referral to a physician for further diagnostic evaluation.

Trauma such as fracture, subluxation, dislocation, and medial plantar nerve compression[5,85] are possible and should be ruled out before returning to play in order not to affect normal gait patterns. Radiographs, including anteroposterior, lateral, and non–weight-bearing oblique views, are usually recommended.[5,12,85] If radiographs demonstrate a displaced sesamoid, or when conservative care fails, a repair or partial sesamoidectomy may be recommended.[5,12,85]

11.12 / **5.** *What type of initial care should Nancy provide Tiffany before she leaves for home after the match?*

The initial care for a sesamoid fracture would consist of RICE, anti-inflammatory medication (steroids in rare cases), and unloading of the involved foot. Nancy should consider the need for immobilization of the foot if a dislocated or fractured sesamoid is possible and place Tiffany in a walking boot or in a stiff-soled shoe until the symptoms subside.[12,85] If these are not readily available, Nancy may consider placing Tiffany on crutches to assist in unloading the involved joint until the proper device can be located or purchased.

## CASE 11.13 Metatarsal (March Fracture)

11.13 / **1.** *(a) Based on the information presented in the case, what is the clinical diagnosis? (b) What is the common term used to describe the clinical diagnosis?*

a. The most likely clinical diagnosis would be a stress fracture of the third metatarsal[26,38,39,55]

b. Stress fractures of the metatarsals were first described in the medical literature in 1855 by the Prussian military physician Breithaupt, who described what is now known as a "march fracture."[21]

11.13 / **2.** *Steve asked several history questions to guide the physical examination. (a) Based on the information presented in the case, do you believe Steve took an adequate history? If not, (b) what kinds of questions would you have asked as the evaluating clinician?*

a. According to the clinical diagnosis, there are several other questions Steve may have directed toward Pvt. Cross. He should have inquired about changes in Pvt. Cross's diet, eating behaviors (e.g., energy intake, eating disorders), and menstruation, because these are two of the three components of the female athlete triad which have been found to increase a women's risk of developing stress fractures.[114,133]

b. Inquiring about intrinsic risk factors such as anatomical, physiological, muscular, and bone characteristics may prove useful.[15,73,114,121] Other questions could be related to changes in running regime, type, age, and especially the cushioning properties (insoles) of her running shoes and boots.[15,44,54,114]

11.13 / **3.** *What are Pvt. Cook's PFT deficiency areas according to textbook Table 11.13.1?*

According to the United States Marine Corp Physical Fitness Testing formula, Pvt. Cook acquired enough points overall to meet the second class fitness rating (flexed-arm hang time, plus number of abdominal crunches in 2 minutes, plus 3-mile run score out of 100) in order to pass the semi-annual fitness test.[142] However, for her age group, she should be able to perform a minimum of 50 abdominal crunches in 2 minutes. Her three-mile score also places her in the lower half of the scoring scale, suggesting that, in addition to her mediocre abdominal strength, her lower leg strength is deficient.

11.13 / **4.** *(a) Why did Steve assess the wear pattern of Pvt. Cook's shoes? (b) If you were the evaluating clinician, what would you hope to observe? (c) Why didn't Steve see anything?*

a. Assessment of the shoes' wear patterns allows Steve to identify any possible structural deficits in the lower extremity and foot posture/biomechanics, because wear patterns are records of the usual long-term activity of the functioning foot. Generally the shoes should be observed for overall wear, uneven wear patterns (i.e., examining the last, outer sole, and shank), the type of last[23] (i.e., the form on which the shoe is built, whether it is straight, semi-curved, or curved), and the type of insoles that are being used.

b. Based on the clinical presentation in this case, excessive wear under the metatarsal head is a possibility. In fact, in one study examining metatarsal head loading in combat boots of the German armed forces, results suggest that the peak pressures under the metatarsal heads (MT) were as follows: MT-II > MT-III > MT-I > MT-IV > MT-V.[54] Furthermore, the researcher found that the neoprene insole resulted in the lowest peak pressures, with significant load reductions under MT-III when compared with synthetic mesh and EVA foam, suggesting that modified insoles might be able to reduce the incidence of march fractures.[54] A similar study of military infantry recruits found no significant difference in the incidence of stress fractures, ankle sprains, or foot problems among recruits using the different types of orthoses (soft custom, soft prefabricated, semi-rigid biomechanical, and semi-rigid prefabricated orthoses).[45] However, of the recruits completing training in their assigned orthoses, the soft custom (3.54) and soft prefabricated (3.43) orthoses had significantly higher comfort scores than the semi-rigid biomechanical (3.23) and prefabricated (3.17) orthoses, ($p = .0001$).[45]

c. The logical explanation for lack of an identifiable shoe/boot wear pattern would be that Pvt. Cook is wearing new sneakers and boots.

11.13 / **5.** *Given the information presented in the case, what diagnostic test would Dr. Weston most likely order first?*

Plain film radiography would be the first diagnostic test ordered in this case. Although they are unreliable during the early stages of a stress reaction (sensitivity of 15%–35% upon initial examination, increasing to 30%–70% at follow-up), they are mandatory to rule out differential diagnoses such as tumors, infection, or gross bone fractures.[14,73] If they are negative, more advanced imaging techniques may be considered. The technetium-99m biphosphate bone scintigraphy, once considered the gold standard, appears to have been replaced by the MRI, which has been shown to be as sensitive as scintigraphy while having significantly higher specificity.[73] Consult your team physician to determine which imaging technique she prefers and why.

11.13 / **6.** *As the case mentions, Steve documented his findings and sent a copy of the report to Maj. Weston. Please document your findings as if you were in Steve's position. If the case did not provide information you believe is pertinent to the clinical diagnosis, please feel free to add this information to your documentation.*

Answers will vary. Students should consider writing a SOAP note (see textbook Appendix B) using the ABCD format when writing the short- and long-term goals.

## CASE 11.14 Medial Tibial Stress Syndrome (MTSS) with Posterior Tibialis Tendonitis

**11.14 / 1.** *Based on the information presented in the case, determine the clinical diagnosis and the possible etiology.*

The clinical diagnosis, based on the history and physical exam, would suggest medial tibial stress syndrome (MTSS), particularly posterior tibialis tendonitis. Medial tibial stress syndrome describes an overuse injury producing inflammation of the periosteum and pain along the posteromedial aspect of the distal two thirds of the tibia.[34–36,70]

The term "shin splints" is commonly used interchangeably with MTSS. However, researchers advocate the use of MTSS "since it more aptly describes the location and presumptive etiology of this disorder."[70] There are a variety of possible causative and predisposing factors—excessive pronation, inflexibility of lower leg musculature (particularly the soleus), pes cavus, and pes planus foot—regarding the development of MTSS, and there is still confusion and controversy regarding the most appropriate terminology for the pathological mechanism.[34,70] For a further review of possible etiology, please consider consulting your team physician or the reviews by Craig,[34,35] Thacker,[137] and Kortebein.[70]

**11.14 / 2.** *Based on the physical examination, Valerie believed she identified a pes planus foot. Identify the common name for pes planus and describe it.*

Pes planus is known as flat foot. It is characterized by the lowering of the medial longitudinal arch as a result of increased ligament laxity (plantar calcaneonavicular or "spring" ligament), muscle weakness of the plantar surface of the foot, and rupture of the tibialis posterior or tibialis anterior tendon.[124,131] Increased talar beaking occurs as the lowered medial arch causes the talus to tilt medially, displacing the navicular inferiorly, and thereby causing the talus to become more prominent. Rearfoot valgus, which may be associated with pes planus, is characterized by eversion of the calcaneus and results in subtalar joint pronation and a possible hypermobile foot.

**11.14 / 3.** *Based on the case report, Valerie performed a non-weight-bearing assessment of Joan's foot and calcaneal alignment. If you were the evaluating clinician, describe how you would perform this exam. What does the result of Valerie's exam indicate?*

The answers to these questions may vary among students. However, an examination of forefoot position and rearfoot position (and their associated abnormalities) in a non-weight-bearing position often begins with an identification of the subtalar joint's neutral position (STJN). The "subtalar joint neutral position is regarded as being the most efficient position around which the foot functions during gait"[84] and is used as an important piece of information for orthotic fabrication.[58] The STJN, as defined by Root,[84] is "the position in which the joint is neither pronated nor supinated." Athletic training texts[124,131] typically describe using the prone figure-4 position, based on the work of Elveru,[41] when indentifying STJN in the non-weight-bearing position. The steps are as follows:

- Begin by placing the patient in a prone position on the table, with the involved leg straight and the foot extending over the table's edge.
- The opposite leg is placed in a figure-4 position (flexed knee with the ankle crossed over the knee of the leg under investigation). This position helps align the pelvis and hips, keeping the calcaneus parallel to the floor, and prevents unwanted movement of the lower leg.[58,124]
- Position yourself behind the patient, palpating the calcaneus, and draw a line from the medial to the lateral calcaneus (calcaneal line). The center of the calcaneus is identified near the insertion of the Achilles tendon, and a perpendicular line is drawn from the

center point of the calcaneus near the insertion of the Achilles tendon to the medial to lateral calcaneal line.

- Palpate and identify the midpoint of the lower leg, drawing a straight line to connect this point with the midcalcaneal point.[58,124]
- The STJN is found by palpating the talus (using your medial hand) by placing the thumb on the medial talar head and the index finger on the lateral aspect of the talar head. The lateral hand grasps the fourth and fifth metatarsal heads with the thumb on the plantar surface. Maximally invert and evert the foot, using lateral hand until you are able to equally palpate both medial and lateral aspects of the talus. Maintain a relaxed position, compare the line bisecting the lower leg (tibia) and the calcaneus; this should be straight (0°) or in slight varus (5°–8°).[58,124] A varus angle greater than 8° suggests rearfoot varus, while a heel angled in eversion is considered rearfoot valgus.

To determine forefoot-rearfoot alignment, follow the directions above, but this time, when STJN is found, visually inspect the relationship between the two by looking downward through the rearfoot to the forefoot. Normally the plantar surface of the calcaneus and metatarsal heads lie in the same plane. Forefoot varus occurs when the first metatarsal is elevated relative to the fifth metatarsal; forefoot valgus occurs when the fifth metatarsal is elevated relative to the first metatarsal.

In this case, Joan's forefoot varus in a non–weight-bearing position means increased periods of pronation during gait as the body attempts to compensate the extra time necessary to allow the first metatarsal to contact the ground.

11.14 / **4.** *(a) What is the name of the special test performed in textbook Figure 11.14.1? (b) What is considered a positive clinical finding? (c) If you were the evaluating clinician, would you have performed any other special tests?*

a. Figure 11.14.1 is a navicular drop test. The navicular drop test is a clinical measurement used to estimate the amount of pronation a patient has at the ankle-foot complex.[10,22,81] The test assesses the distance between the heights of the navicular tuberosity and the floor during the STJN position (quiet stance with no load on the foot) and during a relaxed tandem stance with a full load on the foot.[10,22,81] The most common technique used to assess navicular drop is described by Brody.[22] In this technique, the clinician identifies the STJN in a standing position, recording the height of the navicular on the index card. The patient then allows the foot to relax while bearing weight, and the clinician again records the height of the navicular on the index card. The difference between the two measurements is the patient's navicular drop.

b. Values between 0 mm and 10 mm are considered normal[69,131]; abnormal values are reportedly between 10 mm and 15.1 mm,[22,130,131] suggesting a lack of consensus about what is considered abnormal. Reliability studies have demonstrated an intra-rater reliability range between .61 and .95.[18,76,88,104] A recent study demonstrated that subjects with MTSS demonstrated a significantly larger navicular drop during quiet standing than controls.[10]

c. Two other tests that could be performed are the test for supple pes planus and a Feiss' line. The test for supple pes planus distinguishes between either rigid (structural) or flexible (supple) pes planus. A Feiss' line, similar to a navicular drop, measures the displacement of the navicular tuberosity and, in turn, determines rearfoot-forefoot alignment.[124]

11.14 / **5.** *Describe the anatomical landmarks you would use as the evaluating clinician in order to measure talocrural dorsiflexion.*

According to Clarkson,[30] the goniometric axis or fulcrum should be placed inferior to the lateral malleolus. The stationary arm is placed parallel to the long axis of the fibula, and the movable arm is parallel to the sole of the foot along the fifth metatarsal.

# CASE 11.15 Retrocalcaneal Bursitis

11.15 / **1.** *Based on the information presented in the case, determine (a) the differential diagnoses and (b) the clinical diagnosis.*

a. Differential diagnoses: Achilles tendon rupture, Achilles tendonitis, plantar fasciitis, calcaneus stress fracture[82,91]

b. Clinical diagnosis: retrocalcaneal bursitis, resulting in Haglund's deformity

11.15 / **2.** *Clay presented with end-range pain with PROM. (a) In what direction would you suspect the end-range pain? (b) Is there anything else that would also be palpable during AROM?*

a. Clay would present with pain during passive dorsiflexion of the foot,[74] as the inflamed bursa is compressed between the calcaneus and the insertion of the Achilles tendon. Pain could be accentuated if the Achilles tendon has thickened in response to increased activity.[82]

b. During AROM, a palpable bogginess may be noted along the medial and lateral aspects of the Achilles tendon at its insertion.[74]

11.15 / **3.** *Kevin asked several specific history questions to guide the physical examination. However, he did not appear to ask a certain question that could have assisted in determining the MOI and narrowing down the possibilities for the clinical diagnosis. Can you identify this question?*

Overall, Kevin gathered a decent history, but an important line of questioning he missed was, "How new are your boots, and did you break them in before wearing them to practice?" Haglund's deformity or "pump bump," sometimes known as "boot bump," was first identified by Haglund in 1927 when he observed a correlation between a combination of a prominent posterior-superior-lateral border of the calcaneus and wearing rigid low-back footwear while playing golf and hockey.[52] Because ice hockey players' boots are typically smaller than the foot, the extra pressure placed on the heel from the new boot's restrictive heel counter causes additional friction between the boot and the calcaneus (i.e., excessively prominent posterosuperior calcaneus). This results in hindfoot pain, inflammation, and secretion of additional fluid from the retrocalcaneal bursa.

11.15 / **4.** *Overall, do you believe Kevin adequately evaluated Clay's condition given the provided information? If not, what would you have done differently as the evaluating clinician?*

The answers to this question will vary among students, but it must be noted that Kevin performed an incorrect special test. Rather than performing a Thomas test, which assesses for hip flexor contractures, Kevin should have performed a Thompson test. A Thompson test assesses for trauma to the Achilles tendon (i.e., Achilles tendon rupture).[69,82]

11.15 / **5.** *What "trick," or form of conservative treatment, do you think Kevin utilized on Clay during the follow-up examination?*

In some situations it may be necessary to place the athlete in an open-back shoe to reduce pain[74,82] and to require night splinting. When this fails to resolve the condition, it is often necessary to debride the inflammatory tissue and eliminate the stimulus for repetitive mechanical trauma.

## CASE 11.16 Tarsal Tunnel Syndrome

**11.16 / 1.** *(a) Based on the information presented in the case, determine the clinical diagnosis. (b) What led you to this conclusion?*

a. The clinical diagnosis, based on the history and physical examination, would suggest tarsal tunnel syndrome. The tarsal tunnel is comprised of the tibia (anterior border), posterior process of the talus, calcaneus, and sustentaculum tali (lateral border) and is covered by the fibrous roof formed by the flexor retinaculum. Passing through the tunnel is the posterior tibial nerve (and its branches, calcaneal nerve and the medial and lateral plantar nerve), posterior tibial artery and vein, flexor digitorum longus, flexor hallucis longus, and tibialis posterior. Compression of the tunnel from trauma[115,140] (i.e., eversion ankle sprain, tarsal fracture), biomechanical deficiencies (i.e., pes planus, unstable medial longitudinal arch),[1,148] and space-occupying lesions[57,68,86] predisposes patients to the development of tarsal tunnel syndrome.

b. The answers to this question will vary among students. However, the apparent numbness along the plantar and medial aspect of the foot that increases with activity and decreases with rest should provide enough clinical features to lead to a diagnosis of tarsal tunnel syndrome.

**11.16 / 2.** *Jennifer presented with pain upon PROM. In which direction would you expect to find the end-range pain and why?*

Jennifer would present with pain during passive ankle dorsiflexion and heel eversion with maximal extension of the toes,[68,103] because the posterior tibial nerve or one of its medial or lateral branches passing behind the medial malleolus is within the tarsal tunnel and would be compressed from pressure by the flexor retinaculum.

Kinoshita,[68] was able to reproduce the symptoms of tarsal tunnel syndrome with a Tinel's sign by placing the patient's ankle in maximal dorsiflexion and eversion followed by dorsiflexion of the metatarsophalangeal joint even for a second (dorsiflexion-eversion test). Forty-four feet (belonging to 37 patients) were categorized into three groups based on symptoms and were evaluated using the dorsiflexion-eversion maneuver both before and after decompression of the tarsal tunnel (Table A11.16.1). During the surgical decompression, he observed changes in the anatomical relationship of the structures within the tarsal tunnel. In particular, when the "ankle joint was dorsiflexed and the foot was everted, the tibial nerve was stretched and bulged medially. When all of the toes were then forcibly dorsiflexed, the flexor hallucis longus muscle belly entered farther into the tarsal tunnel

**TABLE A11.16.1** Pre-Surgery dorsiflexion-eversion maneuver results from assessing tarsal tunnel syndrome.

| Numbness Group (n = 20) | | Pain Group (n = 17) | | Numbness and Pain (n = 7) | |
|---|---|---|---|---|---|
| **Number** | **Pre-Surgery Maneuver Results** | **Number** | **Pre-Surgery Maneuver Results** | **Number** | **Pre-Surgery Maneuver Results** |
| 9 | Increase in numbness | 15 | Increase in pain | 4 | Increase in pain |
| 6 | Increase in pain | 2 | No change | 2 | Increase in numbness |
| 5 | No change | | | 1 | No change |

A Tinel's sign was more pronounced in 41 (93%) of the 44 feet tested.

and pressed upon the stretched tibial nerve from behind. The tibial nerve became markedly constricted by the superior edge of the laciniate ligament (i.e., flexor retinaculum). This constriction of the nerve disappeared after the laciniate ligament was released." Post-surgical follow-up revealed no reproduction of symptoms in 91 percent (n=40) of the feet tested.

11.16 / **3.** *Based on the clinical diagnosis, where would you expect numbness and/or loss of function to occur?*

Because the tibial nerve (including its associated branches), the posterior tibial artery, and the posterior tibial vein pass through the tarsal tunnel, any and all of these structures could become entrapped within the tunnel. However, tarsal tunnel syndrome specifically describes the entrapment of the posterior tibial nerve at the level of the medial malleolus, resulting in numbness or a loss of tactile sensation along the medial position of the ankle and/or plantar surface of the foot,[68,140,148] depending on the nerve affected. More specifically, compression of the plantar nerves, which are purely sensory, results in a loss of tactile sensation about the heel. The medial plantar nerve provides cutaneous innervation to the medial aspect of the sole and medial three and one half toes and supplies the abductor hallucis, flexor digitorum brevis, flexor hallucis brevis, and first lumbrical. Finally, the lateral plantar nerve provides cutaneous innervation to the lateral sole and the lateral one-and-one-half toes and supplies the adductor hallucis, abductor digiti minimi, flexor digiti minimi brevis, dorsal and plantar interossei, and the second through fifth lumbricals.

11.16 / **4.** *Overall, do you believe Gena adequately evaluated Jennifer's condition, given the provided information? If not, what would you have done differently as the evaluating clinician?*

The answers to this question will vary among students. Overall, the history and physical examination should have provided enough information for the appropriate clinical diagnosis. However, Gena should have considered assessing for weakness of the intrinsic foot muscles and toe flexors because these are innervated by branches of the tibial nerve. She could also have considered the use of two-point discrimination to further assess the extent of sensory loss in the medial and plantar aspect of the foot.

11.16 / **5.** *What is dictation? As an experienced clinician, what pointers would you provide to Gena to improve this skill?*

Dictation is the form of medical documentation whereby a clinician speaks into a type of recorder and describes the results of her physical examination and treatment. The recording will be transcribed at a later date and placed into the patient's medical record. The transcription is most often done by a different person.

Probably one of the most important things to remember when dictating is to "think before you speak." The success of the transcription of the dictated note(s) depends on the transcriptionist's ability to hear and understand the note. There are several factors that will determine the success of any dictated note, including good sound quality, the clinician's delivery, the equipment, and background noise.[77] Therefore, if this is something done on a regular basis, spend the money to buy a quality recorder and tapes and extra batteries. Find a quiet, stress-free environment and organize your thoughts by referring to the notes you have taken using some type of standard medical documentation, most likely in a SOAP note format.[77] While recording, remember to slow down and enunciate. Do not talk with food in your mouth or carry on another conversation. When identifying the patient, consider spelling the patient's first and last name. Identify the patient's date of birth, date of the visit or service, medical record number, and spelling of the name of the referring or consulting physician or other health care provider, including first and last name. For further information, refer to the Internet and professional literature for pointers.

# CASE 11.17 Plantar Fasciitis

*by William Holcomb, Ph.D., ATC, CSCS-D, University of Nevada, Las Vegas*

11.17 / **1.** *Based on the information provided in the case, determine (a) the differential diagnoses and (b) the clinical diagnosis.*

a. Differential diagnoses: abductor hallucis strain, flexor digitorum brevis strain, abductor digiti minimi strain, plantar ligament sprain, subcutaneous plantar calcaneal bursitis, tendinous lesions (tendinitis, tenosynovitis), tibial nerve compression neuropathy and calcaneal stress fracture[33,94]

b. Clinical diagnosis: plantar fasciitis

11.17 / **2.** *What do the muscles involved in the differential diagnoses and the clinical diagnosis have in common?*

Each of the structures originates from the medial calcaneal tubercle.

11.17 / **3.** *Based on the results of the case, what led you to the clinical diagnosis?*

Two items in particular should have lead to the clinical diagnosis of plantar fasciitis. The first is the report of pain and point tenderness over the anteromedial portion of the plantar surface of the calcaneus.[94] The second is pain on the undersurface of the heel which worsens when moving from a non-weight-bearing to weight-bearing position, especially upon rising in the morning.[83,94]

11.17 / **4.** *Palpation is an important part of the assessment in making the clinical diagnosis. A good understanding of the anatomy is important for successful palpation. Describe the anatomy of the structures involved in the condition and the specific location that will be point tender.*

There is some variation in the anatomy of the plantar fascia. Typically, there are three distinct bands that have a common proximal insertion on the medial calcaneal tubercle. For the distal insertions, the central slip inserts on the distal heads of the five metatarsals; the medial slip inserts on the medial cuneiform; and the lateral slip inserts on the base of the fifth metatarsal.[87,149] Palpation of the proximal insertion typically reveals point tenderness, and the presence of an exostosis should be determined.

11.17 / **5.** *Emma was observed to have excessive pronation during tandem weight bearing, which is implicated in roughly 80 percent of those with this condition. What other foot abnormality has been implicated and why?*

Foot abnormalities such as rearfoot valgus, pes cavus, pes planus, Achilles tendon or triceps surae tightness are possible predisposing factors of plantar fasciitis.[33,131] In particular, athletes with pes cavus lack the ability to effectively dissipate tensile forces during weight bearing, which places added stress on the plantar fascia.[33]

11.17 / **6.** *Several authors have recommended a three-step approach for the management of this condition: (1) reduce pain and inflammation, (2) reduce tissue stress, and (3) restore muscle strength and flexibility. For each, list specific management techniques that have proven effective.*

Cryotherapy, hydrotherapy, iontophoresis, phonophoresis and NSAIDs have all proved to be effective in managing inflammation.[33,80] Corticosteroid injections can be effective but should be used with great caution because they have been associated with plantar fascia ruptures.[33]

Tape and/or hoses (e.g., rubber tubing) can be used to correct foot abnormalities such as excessive pronation and pes cavus, which will reduce stress.[11,33,80,117] Heel cups can pad the point tender area and put the ankle in a position of plantar flexion, which will also reduce stress.[80] Night splints that place the ankle in 90° of dorsiflexion, placing the heel cord under mild tension, help lengthen the fascia, which will decrease stress and pain experienced during weight bearing.[33,80,83]

The intrinsic and extrinsic muscles that act in plantar flexion and toe flexion should be stretched via passive dorsiflexion and toe extension.[33] The muscles on the plantar surface of the foot can be strengthened by gathering a towel with the toes.

11.17 / **7.** *Overall, do you believe Adrian adequately evaluated Emma's condition, according to the provided information? If not, what would you have done differently as the evaluating clinician?*

The answers to this question will vary among students. Given the athlete's history and physical examination, Adrian should have completed a neurovascular examination and performed a Tinel's sign, because entrapment of the posterior tibial nerve and/or medial calcaneal nerve (tarsal tunnel syndrome) can mimic or complicate plantar fasciitis.[83]

# CASE 11.18 Plantar Neuroma (Morton's Neuroma)

*by Kyle Blecha, MS, ATC, Western Michigan University, Kalamazoo*

11.18 / **1.** *Based on the information presented in the case, determine (a) the differential diagnoses and (b) the clinical diagnosis.*

a. Differential diagnoses: metatarsal stress fracture, metatarsalgia, ganglion cysts, intermetatarsal bursal fluid collections, rheumatoid arthritis and other systemic arthritis conditions, neoplasms, MTP synovitis, lumbar radiculopathy[8,28,51,72]

b. Clinical diagnosis: interdigital plantar neuroma, commonly referred to as Morton's neuroma

11.18 / **2.** *Vin asked several different history questions to guide the physical examination. However, do you believe that his method for obtaining all of the information gathered in this case was appropriate? What would you have done differently, if anything, as the evaluating clinician?*

Overall, Vin gathered a decent history. However, Vin asked a closed-ended question that made the assumption that numbness was present, rather than asking an open-ended question to allow Cameron to describe the nature of his condition. For example, a clinician may rephrase the question as, "Can you describe the type of pain you are having?" or "Does the pain cause any other abnormal sensations besides what you have already described?"

11.18 / **3.** *There is no report of the presence of any motor deficits in Cameron's right foot (i.e., intrinsic or extrinsic) or ankle. Given the clinical diagnosis, why are motor deficits not present?*

Morton's neuroma affects the third common digital nerve located in the region of the third webspace[8,51] and supplies cutaneous information on the adjacent sides of the third and fourth toes. This is also the area where the nerve is the thickest as it receives branches from the medial and lateral plantar nerves. The wider nerve is easily irritated from stretching and shearing stresses between the metatarsal heads and transverse intermetatarsal ligament.[28] Because the third common digital nerve provides only sensory information, motor deficits to the intrinsic or extrinsic muscles should not be noted, and any noted weakness should raise concerns that a different diagnosis may be in order.[50]

11.18 / **4.** *During the physical examination, Vin performed a couple of different special tests, including textbook Figure 11.18.2. (a) What is the name of this test, and how is it performed? (b) Do you believe this test is reliable?*

a. Figure 11.18.2 demonstrates how to perform a Mulder's sign, which was first described in 1951 by Mulder himself.[92] A clinician begins by placing the patient in a supine position. Standing lateral to the patient, he grasps the heads of the first and fifth metatarsals squeezing the two metatarsal heads together, while simultaneously putting pressure on the interdigital space with the other hand, using a thumb or object such as a pencil eraser on the plantar surface of the foot. A positive finding includes pain at the site of the neuroma, as well as a click. The click occurs because of the presence of a mass known as a fibrotic intermetatarsal neuroma, which is displaced as the strength of the compression between the metatarsal heads increases.[139]

b. In one study, a Mulder's sign or click was positive in 20 of 21 cases[32] at the time of surgery. Sixteen patients presented with a neuroma; four had an abnormally thickened, inflamed nerve, one had evidence of neuritis and underwent neurolysis (i.e., freeing of a nerve from inflammatory adhesions), and one patient had an epidermal cyst. Cloke and Greiss report 95 percent and 100 percent sensitivity and specificity, respectively.[32]

11.18 / **5.** *If you were in Vin's position, what type of changes in footwear would you recommend and why?*

Cameron reported wearing wing-tipped shoes while waiting tables. Shoes like these, that are narrow, pointed, and heeled have been reported to be a primary contributing factor to the development of Morton's neuroma.[8,28,32,50,72,99] Finally, figure skates are often laced very tightly to help support the ankle. So together, the pointed shoes and tight skates may work in combination to cause the metatarsal heads to be squeezed together, thereby exacerbating the condition. Given the clinical diagnosis, Cameron would be wise to wear a shoe with a wide toe box and flat heel to reduce the compressive force on the metatarsals.

# REFERENCES


1. Aldridge T. Diagnosing heel pain in adults. *Am Fam Physician.* 2004;70(2):332–338.
2. Allen L, Flemming D, Sanders T. Turf toe: Ligamentous injury of the first metatarsophalangeal joint. *Mil Med.* 2004;169(11):xix–xxiv.
3. Alonso A, Khoury L, Adams R. Clinical tests for ankle syndesmosis injury: reliability and prediction of return to function. *J Orthop Sports Phys Ther.* 1998;27(4):276–284.
4. Anderson SJ, Harmon KG, Rubin A. Acute ankle sprains. *Physician Sportsmed.* 2002;30(12):29.
5. Anwar R, Anjum S, Nicholl J. Sesamoids of the foot. *Curr Orthop.* 2005;19:40–48.
6. Aroen A, Helgo D, Granlund OG, Bahr R. Contralateral tendon rupture risk is increased in individuals with a previous Achilles tendon rupture. *Scand J Med Sci Sports.* 2004;14(1):30–33.
7. Ashman C, Klecker R, Yu J. Forefoot pain involving the metatarsal region: differential diagnosis with MR imaging. *Radiographics.* 2001;21:1425–1440.
8. Ayub A, Yale SH, Bibbo C. Common foot disorders. *Clin Med Res.* 2005;3(2):116–119.
9. Bahr R, Pena F, Shine J, Lew W, Conrad L, Tyrdal S, et al. Mechanics of the anterior drawer and talar tilt tests: a cadaveric study of lateral ligament injuries of the ankle. *Acta Orthop.* 1997;68(5):425–441.
10. Bandholm T, Boysen L, Haugaard S, Kreutzfeldt M, Bencke J. Foot medial longitudinal-arch deformation during quiet standing and gait in subjects with Medial Tibial Stress Syndrome. *J Foot Ankle Surg.* 2008;47(2):89–85.
11. Beam J. Foot and toes. In *Orthopedic Taping, Wrapping, Bracing, and Padding.* Philadelphia PA: F. A. Davis; 2006; 35–89.
12. Beaman D, Nigo L. Hallucal sesamoid injury. *Oper Tech Sports Med.* 1999;7(1):7–13.
13. Bedinghaus JM, Niedfeldt MW. Over-the-Counter foot remedies. *Am Fam Physician.* 2001;64(5):791.
14. Berger FH, de Jonge MC, Maas M. Stress fractures in the lower extremity: the importance of increasing awareness amongst radiologists. *Eur J Radiol.* 2007;62(1):16–26.
15. Berry DC. Diagnosis of a medial tibial stress fracture by ultrasound. *Athl Ther Today.* 2007;12(2):16–20.
16. Beumer A, Swierstra BA, Mulder PGH. Clinical diagnosis of syndesmotic ankle instability: evaluation of stress tests behind the curtains. *Acta Orthop Scand.* 2002;73(6): 667–669.
17. Beumer A, van Hemert WL, Swierstra BA, Jasper LE, Belkoff. A biomechanical evaluation of clinical stress tests for syndesmotic ankle instability. *Foot Ankle Int.* 2003;24(4):358–363.
18. Billis E, Katsakiori E, Kapodistrias C, Kapreli E. Assessment of foot posture: correlation between different clinical techniques. *Foot.* 2007;17(2):65–72.
19. Bowers K, Martin R. Turf-toe: a shoe-surface related football injury. *Med Sci Sports Exerc.* 1976;8(2):81–83.
20. Boytim MJ, Fischer DA, Neumann L. Syndesmotic ankle sprains. *Am J Sports Med.* 1991;19:294–298.
21. Briethaupt M. Zur Pathologie des Mensch lichen Fusses. *Med Zeitung.* 1855;24:169–171, 175–177.
22. Brody D. Techniques in the evaluation and treatment of the injured runner. *Orthop Clin N Am.* 1982;13(3): 541–558.
23. Browning KH. Hip and pelvis injuries in runners: careful evaluation and tailored management. *Physician Sportsmed.* 2001;29(1):23–28, 31–34.
24. Burks R, Morgan J. Anatomy of the lateral ankle ligaments. *Am J Sports Med.* 1994;22;72–7.
25. Burns B, Tansey C, Sproule J, Borton D. Recurrent peroneal tendons dislocation: a novel anatomic repair. *Foot.* 2004;14(2):80–85.
26. Carmont MR, Patrick JH, Cassar-Pullicino VN, Postans NJ, Hay SM. Sequential metatarsal fatigue fractures secondary to abnormal foot biomechanics. *Mil Med.* 2006;171(4):292–297.
27. Cedell C. Ankle lesions. *Acta Orthop Scand.* 1975;46: 425–445.
28. Childs S. Diagnosis and treatment of interdigital Perineural Fibroma (a.k.a. Morton's Neuroma). *Orthop Nurs.* 2002;21(6):35.
29. Childs S. Pathophysiology: the pathogenesis and biomechanics of turf toe. *Orthop Nurs.* 2006;25(4):276–282.
30. Clarkson H. *Musculoskeletal Assessment: Joint Range of Motion and Manual Muscle Strength.* Philadelphia PA: Lippincott Williams & Wilkins; 2000.
31. Clarkson H. *Joint Range of Motion and Function Assessment: A Research-Based Practical Guide.* 3rd ed. Baltimore MD: Lippincott Williams & Wilkins; 2006.
32. Cloke DJ, Greiss ME. The digital nerve stretch test: a sensitive indicator of Morton's neuroma and neuritis. *Foot Ankle Surg.* 2006;12(4):201–203.
33. Cornwall M, McPoil T. Plantar fasciitis: etiology and treatment. *J Orthop Sports Phys Ther.* 1999;29:756–760.
34. Craig D. Medial tibial stress syndrome: current etiological theories part 1—background. *Athl Ther Today.* 2008a;13(1):17–20.
35. Craig D. Medial tibial stress syndrome: etiological theories, part 2. *Athl Ther Today.* 2008b;13(2):34–36.
36. Craig D. Medial tibial stress syndrome: evidence-based prevention. *J Athl Train.* 2008c;43(3):316–318.
37. Davis WH, Sobel M, DiCarlo EF, Torzilli PA, Deng X., Geppert MJ, Patel MB, Deland J. Gross, histological, and microvascular anatomy and biomechanical testing of the spring ligament complex. *Foot Ankle Int.* 1996;17(2): 95–102.
38. Dhami S, Sheikh A. Metatarsal stress fracture. *GP: Gen Pract.* 2002;76.
39. Dixon S, Creaby M, Allsopp A. Comparison of static and dynamic biomechanical measures in military recruits with and without a history of third metatarsal stress fracture. *Clin Biomech.* 2006;21(4):412–419.
40. Douglas J, Kelly M, Blachut P. Clarification of the Simmonds–Thompson test for rupture of an Achilles tendon. *Can J Surg.* 2009;52(3):E40–E41.

41. Elveru, RA, Rothstein JM, Lamb RL, Riddle DC. Methods for taking subtalar joint measurement: A clinical report. *Phys Ther.* 1988;68(5):678-682.

42. Farber DC. Foot injuries in the sports population. *Curr Opin Orthop.* 2007;18:97–101.

43. Ferran N, Oliva F, Maffullo N. Recurrent subluxations of the peroneal tendons. *Sports Med.* 2006;36(10):839–846.

44. Finestone A, Giladi M, Elad H, Salmon A, Mendelson S, Eldad A, et al. Prevention of stress fractures using custom biomechanical shoe orthoses. *Clin Orthop Relat Res.* 1999;369:182–90.

45. Finestone A, Novack V, Farfel A, Berg A, Amir H, Milgrom C. A prospective study of the effect of foot orthoses composition and fabrication on comfort and the incidence of overuse injuries. *Foot Ankle Int.* 2004;25(7):462–466.

46. Frankel M, Tucker D. Ankle dislocation without fracture in a young athlete. *Foot Ankle Surg.* 1998;37(4):334–338.

47. Fujii T, Luo ZP, Kitaoka HB, An KN. The manual stress test may not be sufficient to differentiate ankle ligament injuries. *Clin Biomech.* 2000;15(8):619–623.

48. Gaebler C, Kukla C, Breitenseher M, Nellas Z, Mittlboeck M, Trattnig S, et al. Diagnosis of lateral ankle ligament injuries: comparison between talar tilt, MRI and operative findings in 112 athletes. *Acta Orthop Scand.* 1997;68(3):286–290.

49. Gallaspy JB, May JD. *Signs and Symptoms of Athletic Injuries.* St. Louis MO: Mosby; 1996.

50. Gonzalez P, Berry K, Bowman R. *Morton neuroma* [electronic version]. 2010. Available from: http://emedicine.medscape.com/article/308284-overview. Accessed May 20, 2010.

51. Gulick DT, Charles TK. Differential diagnosis of Morton's Neuroma. *Athl Ther Today.* 2002;7(1):39–42.

52. Haglund P. Beitrag zur Klinik der Achillesseh. *Z Orthop Chir.* 1927;49:49–58.

53. Hammouda A, Rayes ME, Kordy SE. Posteromedial dislocation of the ankle without fracture. *Foot Ankle Surg.* 2006;12(3):169–171.

54. Hinz P, Henningsen A, Matthes G, Jäger B, Ekkernkamp A, Rosenbaum D. Analysis of pressure distribution below the metatarsals with different insoles in combat boots of the German army for prevention of march fractures. *Gait Posture.* 2008;27(3):535–538.

55. Hod N, Ashkenazi I, Levi Y, Fire G, Drori M, Cohen I, et al. Characteristics of skeletal stress fractures in female military recruits of the Israel defense forces on bone scintigraphy. *Clin Nucl Med.* 2006;31(12):742–749.

56. Hopkinson W, St. Pierre P, Ryan J, Wheeler J. Syndesmosis sprains of the ankle. *Foot Ankle.* 1990;10:325–330.

57. Hu Liang L, Stephenson G. These boots weren't made for walking: tarsal tunnel syndrome. *CMAJ Suppl.* 2007;176(10):1415–1416.

58. Hunter S, Burnett G. Subtalar joint neutral and orthotic fitting. *Athl Ther Today.* 2000;5(1):6–9.

59. Ivins D. Acute ankle sprain: an update. *Am Fam Physician.* 2006;74:1714–1720.

60. Jacobs BA, Lin D, Schwartz E. Achilles tendon rupture. *eMedicine* [electronic version]. 2009. Available from: http://emedicine.medscape.com/article/85024-overview. Accessed December 30, 2009.

61. Jahss M, Kummer F, Michelson J. Investigations into the fat pads of the sole of the foot: heel pressure studies. *Foot Ankle.* 1992;13(5):227–232.

62. Johnson D, Morelii M. Clinical case challenge: Achilles tendon rupture *Medscape Orthop Sports Med eJournal* [electronic version]. 2001. Available from: www.medscape.com/viewarticle/404350. Accessed June 30, 2008.

63. Kennedy J, Hodgkins CW, Colombier J, Guyette S, Hamilton WG. Foot and ankle injuries in dancers. *Int SportMed J.* 2007;8(3):141–165.

64. Kennedy J, Knowles B, Dolan M, Bohne W. Foot and ankle injuries in the adolescent runner. *Curr Opin Pediatr.* 2005;17(1):34–42.

65. Kerr J. Achilles tendon injury: assessment and management in the emergency department. *Emerg Nurse.* 2005;13(2):32–38.

66. Khan R, MacDowell A, Lloyd C, Bayliss S. An uncommon case of fracture-dislocation of the ankle: traction revisited. *Injury.* 2000;31(8):644–647.

67. Kiefer E, Wikstrom E, Douglas McDonald J. Ankle dislocation without fracture: an on-field perspective. *Clin J Sport Med.* 2006;16(3):269–270.

68. Kinoshita M, Okuda R, Morikawa J, Jotoku T, Abe M. The dorsiflexion-eversion test for diagnosis of tarsal tunnel syndrome. *J Bone Joint Surg Am.* 2001;83-A(12):1835.

69. Konin JG, Wiksten D, Isear JA, Brader H. *Special Tests for Orthopedic Examination.* 3rd ed. Thorofare NJ: Slack; 2006.

70. Kortebein P, Kaufman K, Basford J, Stuart M. Medial tibial stress syndrome. *Med Sci Sports Exerc.* 2000;32(3 Supple):S27–S33.

71. Kovaleski J, Norrell P, Heitman RJ, Hollis JM, Pearsall IV, Albert W. Knee and ankle position, anterior drawer laxity, and stiffness of the ankle complex. *J Athl Train.* 2008;43(3):242–248.

72. Lackey E, Sutton R. Morton's neuroma. *GP: Gen Pract.* 2008;25–25.

73. Lassus J, Tulikoura I, Konttinen Y, Salo J, Santavirta S. Bone stress injuries of the lower extremity: a review. *Acta Orthop Scand.* 2002;73:359–68.

74. Leitze Z, Sella E, Aversa J. Endoscopic decompression of the retrocalcaneal space. *J Bone Joint Surg Am.* 2003;85-A(8):1488–1496.

75. Liu W, Maitland M, Nigg B. The effect of axial load on the in vivo anterior drawer test of the ankle joint complex. *Foot Ankle Int.* 2000;21(5):420–426.

76. Loudon J, Jenkins W, Loudon K. The relationship between static posture and ACL injury in female athletes. *J Orthop Sports Phys Ther.* 1996;24(2):91–97.

77. Lowes R. Practice pointers: how to be a supreme dictator. *Med Econ.* 2002;79(17):69–72, 75.

78. Lynch S. Assessment of the injured ankle in the athlete. *J Athl Train.* 2002;37(4):406–412.

79. Mann R. Subluxation and dislocation of the peroneal tendons. *Oper Tech Sports Med.* 1999;7(1):2–6.

80. Martin R, Irrgang J, Conti S. Outcome study of subjects with insertional plantar fasciitis. *Foot Ankle Int.* 1998;19:803–811.

81. Mattacola CG, Kelly JJ. Using navicular-drop measurements to determine subtalar pronation. *Athl Ther Today.* 2003;8(6):60–61.
82. Mazzone M, McCue T. Common conditions of the Achilles tendon. *Am Fam Physician.* 2002;65(9):1805–1810.
83. McBryde Jr AM, Hoffman JL. Injuries to the foot and ankle in athletes. *South Med J.* 2004;97(8):738–741.
84. Menz HB. Clinical hindfoot measurement: a critical review of the literature. *Foot.* 1995;5(2):57–64.
85. Mittlmeier T, Haar P. Sesamoid and toe fractures. *Injury.* 2004;35(2):87–97.
86. Mizel MS, Hecht PJ, Marymont JV, Temple HT. Evaluation and treatment of chronic ankle pain. *J Bone Joint Surg Am.* 2004;86-A(3):622–632.
87. Moore K, Dalley A. *Clinically Oriented Anatomy.* (5th ed.) Baltimore MD: Lippincott Williams & Wilkins; 2005.
88. Morrison SC, Durward BR, Watt GF, Donaldson MDC. The intra-rater reliability of anthropometric data collection conducted on the peripubescent foot: A pilot study. *Foot.* 2005;15(4):180–184.
89. Mouhsine E, Leyvraz PF, Borens O, Ribordy M, Arlettaz Y, Garofalo R. Acute fractures of medial and lateral great toe sesamoids in an athlete. *Knee Surg Sports Traumatol Arthroscop.* 2004;12(5):463–464.
90. Mowlavi A, Whiteman J, Wilhelmi B, Neumeister M, McLafferty R. Dorsalis pedis arterial pulse: Palpation using a bony landmark. *Postgrad Med J.* 2002;78(926):746–747.
91. Moye P, Stitik T, Nadler S. Retrocalcaneal bursitis. *eMedicine* [electronic version]. 2009. Available from: http://emedicine.medscape.com/article/86297-overview. Accessed May 20, 2010.
92. Mulder J. The causative mechanisms in Morton's metatarsalgia. *J Bone Joint Surg Br.* 1951;33-B:94 –95.
93. Muresanu M, Quinn A. Ankle injury, soft tissue. *eMedicine* [electronic version]. 2009. Available from: http://emedicine.medscape.com/article/822378-overview. Accessed May 20, 2010.
94. Narvaez JA, Narvaez J, Ortega R, Aguilera C, Sanchez A, Andia E. Painful heel: MR imaging findings. *Radiographics.* 2000;20(2):333–352.
95. Newham D, Douglas J, Legge J, Friend J. Achilles tendon rupture: an underrated complication of corticosteroid treatment. *Thorax.* 1991;46(11):843–854.
96. Norkus S, Floyd R. The anatomy and mechanisms of syndesmotic ankle sprains. *J Athl Train.* 2001;36(1):68–73.
97. Nugent PJ. Ottawa Ankle Rules accurately assess injuries and reduce reliance on radiographs. *J Fam Pract* 53 [electronic version]. 2004. Available from: http://www.jfponline.com/Pages.asp?AID=1789.
98. O'Kane JW, Sallis RE. Beyond the Thompson Test. *Physician Sportsmed.* 2003;31(6):45.
99. Oh SJ. Neuropathies of the foot. *Clin Neurophysiol.* 2007;118(5):954–980.
100. Paige NM, Nouvong A. The top 10 things foot and ankle specialists wish every primary care physician knew. *Mayo Clin Proc.* 2006;81(6):818–822.
101. Panchbhavi VK. Plantar heel pain. *eMedicine* [electronic version]. 2008. Available from: http://emedicine.medscape.com/article/1233178-overview. Accessed May 20, 2010.
102. Perry JJ, Stiell IG. Impact of clinical decision rules on clinical care of traumatic injuries to the foot and ankle, knee, cervical spine, and head. *Injury.* 2006;37(12):1157–1165.
103. Persich G, Touliopolous S. Tarsal tunnel syndrome. *eMedicine* [electronic version]. 2009. Available from: http://emedicine.medscape.com/article/1236852-overview. Accessed May 20, 2010.
104. Picciano A, Rowlands M, Worrell T. Reliability of open and closed kinetic chain subtalar joint neutral positions and navicular drop test. *J Orthop Sports Phys Ther.* 1983;18(4):553–558.
105. Porter D, Barill E. Acute peroneal tendon dislocation in a collegiate baseball player. In: DeCarlo M, Oneacre, K, eds. *Current Topics in Musculoskeletal Medicine: A Case Study Approach.* Thorofare NJ: Slack; 2001:227–233.
106. Prentice WE. *Arnheim's Principles of Athletic Training: A Competency-Based Approach.* 13th ed. Boston MA: McGraw Hill Publishing; 2009.
107. Rajiah P, Karthikeyan S. Metatarsals, fracture. *eMedicine* [electronic version]. 2009. Available from: http://emedicine.medscape.com/article/399372-overview. Accessed May 20, 2010.
108. Ramelli F. Diagnosis, management and post-surgical rehabilitation of an Achilles tendon rupture: a case report. *J Can Chiropract Assoc.* 2003;47(4):261–268.
109. Rammelt S, Zwipp H. Calcaneus fractures: facts, controversies and recent developments. *Injury.* 2004;35(5): 443–461.
110. Rammelt S, Zwipp H. Calcaneus fractures. *Trauma.* 2006;8(3):197–212.
111. Ricci RD, Cerullo J, Blanc RO, et al. Talocrural dislocation with associated Weber Type C fibular fracture in a collegiate football player: a case report. *J Athl Train.* 2008;43(3):319–325.
112. Rimando MP. Ankle sprain. *eMedicine* [electronic version]. 2008. Available from: http://emedicine.medscape.com/article/307466-overview. Accessed May 10, 2010.
113. Rivera F, Bertone C, De Martino M, Pietrobono D, Ghisellini F. Pure dislocation of the ankle: three case reports and literature review. *Clin Orthop Relat Res.* 2001;382:179–184.
114. Romani W, Gieck J, Perrin D, Saliba E, Kahler D. Mechanisms and management of stress fractures in physically active persons. *J Athl Train.* 2002;37(3):306–314.
115. Romani W, Perrin D. Tarsal tunnel syndrome: case study of a male collegiate athlete. *J Sport Rehabil.* 1997;6(4):364.
116. Rosenfeld P. Acute and chronic peroneal tendon dislocations. *Foot Ankle Clin N Am.* 2007;12(4):643–657.
117. Ross M. Use of the tissue stress model as a paradigm for developing an examination and management plan for a patient with plantar fasciitis. *J Am Podiatr Med Assoc.* 2002;92:499–506.
118. Rubin A, Sallis R. Evaluation and diagnosis of ankle injuries. *Am Fam Physician.* 1996;54(5):1609–1618.
119. Rupp TJ, Karageanes S. Athletic foot injuries. *eMedicine* [electronic version]. 2008. Available from: http://emedicine.medscape.com/article/84613-overview. Accessed May 10, 2010.

120. Safran M, O'Malley D, Fu F. Peroneal tendon subluxation in athletes: new exam technique, case reports, and review. *Med Sci Sports Exerc.* 1999;31(7 Suppl):S487–S492.

121. Sanderlin B, Raspa R. Common stress fractures. *Am Fam Physician.* 2003;68(6):1527–1532.

122. Savoie F, Wilkinson M, Bryan A, Barrett G, Shelton W, Manning J. Maisonneuve fracture dislocation of the ankle. *J Athl Train.* 1992;27(3):268–269.

123. Schneck CD, Mesgarzadeh M, Bonakdarpour A, Ross GJ. MR imaging of the most commonly injured ankle ligaments. Part I. Normal anatomy. *Radiology.* 1992;184(2):499–506.

124. Schultz SJ, Houglum PA, Perrin DH. *Examination of Musculoskeletal Injuries.* 2nd ed. Champaign IL: Human Kinetics; 2005.

125. Scott B, Chalabi A. How the Simmonds-Thompson test works. *J Bone Joint Surg Br.* 1992;74-B(2):314–315.

126. Segal LS, Lynch CJ, Stauffer ES. Anterior ankle dislocation with associated trigonal process fracture. *Clin Orthop Relat Res.* 1992;278:171–176.

127. Sharma D, Harris A. Clinical: management of ankle sprains. *GP: Gen Pract.* 2005;53–55.

128. Simmonds F. The diagnosis of the ruptured Achilles tendon. *Practitioner.* 1957;179:56–58.

129. Smith AH, Bach BR, Jr. High ankle sprains: minimizing the frustration of a prolonged recovery. *Physician Sportsmed.* 2004;32(12):39–43.

130. Snock A. The relationship between excessive pronation as measured by navicular drop and isokinetic strength of the ankle musculature. *Foot Ankle Int.* 2001;22(3):234–240.

131. Starkey C, Ryan J. *Evaluation of Orthopedic and Athletic Injuries.* 2nd ed. Philadelphia PA: F. A. Davis; 2002.

132. Stiell IG, McKnight RD, Greenberg GH, McDowell I, Nair RC, Wells GA, et al. Implementation of the Ottawa Ankle Rules. *JAMA.* 1994;271:827–832.

133. Subcommittee on Body Composition Nutrition, Health of Military Women. Reducing stress fracture in physically active military women. 1998. Available from: http://books.nap.edu/catalog/6295.html. Accessed July 12, 2008.

134. Syed A, Agarwal M, Dosani A, Giannoudis P, Matthews S. Medial subtalar dislocation: importance of clinical diagnosis in distinguishing from other dislocations. *Eur J Emerg Med.* 2003;10(3):232–235.

135. Tallia A, Cardone D. Diagnostic and therapeutic injection of the ankle and foot. *Am Fam Physician.* 2003;68: 1356–1362.

136. Taniguchi A, Tanaka Y, Takakura Y, Kadono K, Maeda M, Yamamoto H. Anatomy of the spring ligament. *J Bone Joint Surg Am.* 2003;85-A(11):2174–2178.

137. Thacker S, Gilchrist J, Stroup D, Kimsey, C. The prevention of shin splints in sports: a systematic review of literature. *Med Sci Sports Exerc.* 2002;34(1):32–40.

138. Thompson T. A test for rupture of the tendo Achillis. *Acta Orthop Scand.* 1962;32:461–465.

139. Torriani M, Kattapuram SV. Dynamic sonography of the forefoot: the sonographic Mulder Sign. *Am J Roentgenol.* 2003;180(4):1121–1123.

140. Toth C, McNeil S, Feasby T. Peripheral nervous system injuries in sport and recreation: a systematic review. *Sports Med.* 2005;35(8):717–738.

141. Ufberg J, Harrigan RA, Cruz T, Perron AD. Orthopedic pitfalls in the ED: Achilles tendon rupture. *Am J Emerg Med.* 2004;22(7):596–600.

142. U.S. Marine Corps. Marine Corps Physical Fitness Charts: Females. 2008. Available from: http://usmilitary.about.com/od/marines/l/blfitfemale.htm. Accessed May 24, 2009.

143. Uyar M, Tan A, Isler M, Cetinus E. Closed posteromedial dislocation of the tibiotalar joint without fracture in a basketball player. *Br J Sports Med.* 2004;38(3):342–343.

144. van der Linden PD, Sturkenboom MC, Herings RM, Leufkens HM, Rowlands S, Stricker BH. Increased risk of Achilles tendon rupture with quinolone antibacterial use, especially in elderly patients taking oral corticosteroids. *Arch Intern Med.* 2003;163:1801–1807.

145. van der Linden PD, Sturkenboom MC, Herings RC, Leufkens HM, Stricker BH. Fluoroquinolones and risk of Achilles tendon disorders: case-control study. *BMJ.* 2002;324(7349):1306–1307.

146. van der Linden PD, van de Lei J, Nab HW, Knol A, Stricker BH. Achilles tendinitis associated with fluoroquinolones. *Br J Clin Pharmacol.* 1999;48(3):433–437.

147. Vanore J, Christensen J, Kravitz S, et al. Clinical practice guideline first metatarsophalangeal joint disorders panel of the American College of Foot and Ankle Surgeons. *Foot Ankle Surg.* 2003;42(3):112–154.

148. Ward PJ, Porter ML. Tarsal tunnel syndrome: a study of the clinical and neurophysiological results of decompression. *J R Coll Surg Edinb.* 1998;43(1):35–36.

149. Wearing S, Smeathers J, Urry S, Henning E, Hills A. The pathomechanics of plantar fasciitis. *Sports Med.* 2006;36, 585–611.

150. Wilson L, Dimeff R, Miniaci A, Sundaram M. Radiologic case study: first metarsophalangeal plantar plate injury (turf toe). *Orthopedics.* 2005;28(4):417–419.

151. Wolfe MW. Management of ankle sprains. *Am Fam Physician.* 2001;63(1):93.

152. Wright R, Barile R, Surprenant D, Matava M. Ankle syndesmosis sprains in National Hockey League players. *Am J Sports Med.* 2004;32(8):1941–1945.

153. Wuelker N, Wirth CJ. The great toe sesamoids. *J Foot Ankle Surg.* 1996;2:167–174.

154. Zalavras C, Thordarson D. Ankle syndesmotic injury. *J Am Acad Orthop Surg.* 2007;15(6):330–339.

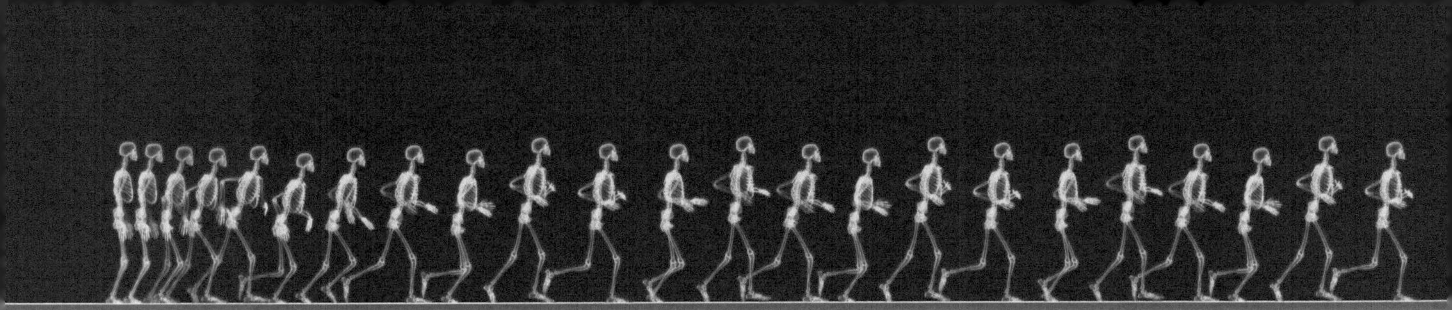

# Appendix

BOARD OF CERTIFICATION

***Role Delineation Study/Practice Analysis, Sixth Edition***

Content Outline

Domain Descriptions and Task Statements

| DOMAIN | TITLE | DESCRIPTION |
|---|---|---|
| 1 | **Injury/Illness Prevention and Wellness Protection** | Educating participants and managing risk for safe performance and function. |

A key aspect of the athletic trainer's (AT) education and training is in the area of prevention and risk management. The AT is the front-line professional charged with this duty. Many individuals come to activity in less than ideal condition. They may suffer from disorders such as sickle-cell trait, diabetes or have other conditions predisposing them to injury or illness. Pre-participation screenings are critical to identifying risks and putting prevention plans into action. Additional prevention and risk management strategies undertaken by the AT range from on-site reviews for hazards, monitoring environmental conditions and educating participants on nutrition and performance enhancing drugs to monitoring for overtraining, maintenance of clinical and treatment areas, and development of emergency action plans.

| Task | Description |
|---|---|
| 0101 | Minimize risk of injury and illness of individuals and groups impacted by or involved in a specific activity through awareness, education, and intervention. |
| 0102 | Interpret individual and group pre participation and other relevant screening information (e.g., verbal, observed, written) in accordance with accepted and applicable guidelines to minimize the risk of injury and illness. |
| 0103 | Identify and educate individual(s) and groups through appropriate communication methods (e.g., verbal, written) about the appropriate use of personal equipment (e.g., clothing, shoes, protective gear, and braces) by following accepted procedures and guidelines. |
| 0104 | Maintain physical activity, clinical treatment, and rehabilitation areas by complying with regulatory standards to minimize the risk of injury and illness. |
| 0105 | Monitor environmental conditions (e.g., weather, surfaces, client work setting) using appropriate methods and guidelines to facilitate individual and group safety. |
| 0106 | Maintain or improve physical conditioning for the individual or group by designing and implementing programs (e.g., strength, flexibility, CV fitness) to minimize the risk of injury and illness. |
| 0107 | Promote healthy lifestyle behaviors using appropriate education and communication strategies to enhance wellness and minimize the risk of injury and illness. |

*(continued)*

| DOMAIN | TITLE | DESCRIPTION |
|---|---|---|
| 2 | **Clinical Evaluation and Diagnosis** | Implementing standard evaluation techniques and formulating a clinical impression for the determination of a course of action. |

The profession of athletic training is unique in that the athletic trainer may be present at the time of an injury or emergency. This requires the clinician be prepared and proficient in all aspects of emergency care. Preparation includes writing, rehearsing and executing emergency action plans for every venue for which the AT is responsible. The AT must demonstrate excellent communication skills, both verbal and/or written, in order to transfer vital assessment information to the healthcare provider, parent, supervisors and others that are involved in the healthcare of the individual.

The recognition of signs and symptoms of life-threatening conditions is the cornerstone of effective management of emergencies. ATs have a vast knowledge of medical conditions that can quickly become emergencies and because the AT is often on-site, they are the primary healthcare professional able to intervene. There are times that injuries require care that warrant referrals. It is the AT who recognizes these conditions and selects the most effective and safest method to transport the individual to the appropriate healthcare professional.

| Task | Description |
|---|---|
| 0201 | Obtain an individual's history through observation, interview, and/or review of relevant records to assess current or potential injury, illness, or health-related condition. |
| 0202 | Examine by appropriate visual and palpation techniques the involved area(s) of an individual's body to determine the type and extent of the injury, illness, or health related condition. |
| 0203 | Examine by appropriate and specific tests (e.g., ROM, special tests, neurological tests) the involved area(s) of an individual's body to determine the type and extent of the injury, illness, or health-related condition. |
| 0204 | Formulate a clinical diagnosis by interpreting the signs, symptoms, and predisposing factors of the injury, illness, or health related condition to determine the appropriate course of action. |
| 0205 | Educate the appropriate individual(s) about the clinical evaluation by communicating information about the current or potential injury, illness, or health-related condition to encourage compliance with recommended care. |

| DOMAIN | TITLE | DESCRIPTION |
|---|---|---|
| 3 | **Immediate and Emergency Care** | Employing standard care procedures and communicating outcomes for efficient and appropriate care of the injured. |

Following injury, the AT serves as the clinician who designs, administers and executes a plan of care. Included within this plan of care is the implementation of appropriate techniques, procedures, practices and methods that are designed to provide the patient with optimal outcomes. Acting under the direction of a physician and within the scope of practice acts and/or BOC Standards of Professional Practice, the athletic trainer provides a plan of care that is realized through the evaluation of the patient.

Protection from additional insult and appropriate steps toward optimal recovery are included in the AT's plan and execution of care. Effective and clear communication to the patient and appropriate individuals concerned with the patient's care is critical to achieving full return to activity. Treatment objectives are outlined using short and long-term goals. These goals are achieved using appropriate treatment/rehabilitation methods available to the AT. Selection of various treatment/rehabilitation modes is based on sound rationale, appropriate standards of health care, reliable clinical judgment and when available, evidence based medicine.

| Task | Description |
|---|---|
| 0301 | Coordinate care of individual(s) through appropriate communication (e.g., verbal, written, demonstrative) of assessment findings to pertinent individual(s). |
| 0302 | Apply the appropriate immediate and emergency care procedures to prevent the exacerbation of non-life-threatening and life-threatening health conditions to reduce the risk factors for morbidity and mortality. |
| 0303 | Implement appropriate referral strategies, which stabilize and/or prevent exacerbation of the condition(s), to facilitate the timely transfer of care for conditions beyond the scope of practice of the Athletic Trainer. |
| 0304 | Demonstrate how to implement and direct immediate care strategies (e.g., first aid, Emergency Action Plan) using established communication and administrative practices to provide effective care. |

*(continued)*

| DOMAIN | TITLE | DESCRIPTION |
|---|---|---|
| 4 | **Treatment and Rehabilitation** | Reconditioning participants for optimal performance and function. |

An AT may be asked to perform in one or more distinct evaluation areas: (1) the pre-participation examination which assists in determining the readiness of an individual to participate in physical activities, (2) an on-field evaluation for acute conditions that had occurred during activity using the primary and secondary survey models, (3) a clinical evaluation, often occurring in a clinical or athletic training facility and 4) the ongoing evaluation of progress of an injury or illness assisting the AT in advancing or modifying current care and making return to play decisions.

Through the use of a sequential evaluation process and with the understanding of the injury pathology and any co-morbidities of the affected individual the AT provides a clinical diagnosis, determine appropriate immediate care, and establish short and long term goals for the affected individual.

| Task | Description |
|---|---|
| 0401 | Administer therapeutic and conditioning exercise(s) using appropriate techniques and procedures in order to aid recovery and restoration of function. |
| 0402 | Administer therapeutic modalities (e.g., electromagnetic, manual, mechanical) using appropriate techniques and procedures based on the individual's phase of recovery to restore functioning. |
| 0403 | Apply braces, splints, or other assistive devices according to appropriate practices in order to facilitate injury protection to achieve optimal functioning for the individual. |
| 0404 | Administer treatment for injury, illness, and/or health-related conditions using appropriate methods to facilitate injury protection, recovery, and/or optimal functioning for individual(s). |
| 0405 | Reassess the status of injuries, illnesses, and/or conditions using appropriate techniques and documentation strategies to determine appropriate treatment, rehabilitation, and/or reconditioning and to evaluate readiness to return to a desired level of activity. |
| 0406 | Provide guidance and/or referral to specialist for individual(s) and groups through appropriate communication strategies (e.g., oral and education materials) to restore an individual(s) optimal functioning. |

| DOMAIN | TITLE | DESCRIPTION |
|---|---|---|
| 5 | **Organizational and Professional Health and Well-being** | Understanding and adhering to approved organizational and professional practices and guidelines to ensure individual and organizational well-being. |

ATs are charged with many responsibilities including: (1) injury/illness prevention and wellness protection, (2) clinical evaluation and diagnosis, (3) immediate and emergency are, and (4) treatment and rehabilitation. However, in order to properly implement any type of comprehensive athletic training services, an organization must demonstrate and support an appropriate level of organizational and professional health and well-being. Together, organizational and professional health and well-being is defined as an organization's or professional association's ability to function effectively, to cope adequately, to change appropriately, and to grow from within. It is also the process by which the AT empowers patients and employees in the improvement of their health-related physical, mental and social well-being as well has physical and professional well-being of the institution and/or organization.

Whether covering a youth soccer tournament, working in one of several hospital satellite clinics, or running a collegiate athletic training program, the AT relies on these practices, standards, and guidelines. Maintenance of records and accurate documentation is mandatory for communication, reimbursement, risk management, and determining best practices. Emergency action plans with consideration for staffing, coordination of resources, liability, and equipment reduce the risk to the individual and organization. When organizing a health care team or making referrals related to injuries, illness and unhealthy lifestyle behaviors, the AT must be knowledgeable of their scope of practice and the state statutes that regulate their profession and the health professionals with whom they work. Additionally the AT engages in ongoing professional education to ensure the care provided by the organization and healthcare professionals adheres to best practices .For organizations and professions to maintain financial health, the AT must demonstrate the ability to utilize basic internal business skills including, strategic planning, human resource management, budgeting, and facility design. They must be able to apply external business skills, such as marketing and public relations to support organizational sustainability, growth, and development.

| Task | Description |
|---|---|
| 0501 | Apply basic internal business functions (e.g., business planning, financial operations, staffing) to support individual and organizational growth and development. |
| 0502 | Apply basic external business functions (e.g., marketing and public relations) to support organizational sustainability, growth, and development. |
| 0503 | Maintain records and documentation that comply with organizational, association, and regulatory standards to provide quality of care and to enable internal surveillance for program validation and evidence based interventions. |
| 0504 | Demonstrate appropriate planning for coordination of resources (e.g., personnel, equipment, liability, scope of service) in event medical management and emergency action plans. |
| 0505 | Demonstrate an understanding of statutory and regulatory provisions and professional standards of the practice of Athletic Training in order to provide for the safety and welfare of individual(s) and groups. |
| 0506 | Develop a support/referral process for interventions to address unhealthy lifestyle behaviors. |

Reprinted with permission from the Board of Certification. *Role Delineation/Practice Analysis.* 6th ed. Available at http://www.bocatc.org/index.php?option=com_content&view=article&id=109&Itemid=117.